Review for USMLE

United States Medical Licensing Examination *STEP 1*

7th EDITION

Review for USMLE

United States Medical Licensing Examination STEP 1

7th EDITION

John S. Lazo, PhD

Allegheny Foundation Professor
Department of Pharmacology
Director, Fiske Drug Discovery Laboratory
University of Pittsburgh School of Medicine
Co-Director, Molecular Therapeutics/Drug Discovery Program
University of Pittsburgh Cancer Institute
Pittsburgh, Pennsylvania

Bruce R. Pitt, PhD

Professor and Chairman
Department of Environmental and Occupational Health
University of Pittsburgh Graduate School of Public Health
Professor, Department of Pharmacology
University of Pittsburgh School of Medicine
Pittsburgh, Pennsylvania

Joseph C. Glorioso III, PhD

William S. McEllroy Professor of Biochemistry and Chairman
Department of Molecular Genetics and Biochemistry
Director, Molecular Medicine Institute
University of Pittsburgh School of Medicine
Pittsburgh, Pennsylvania

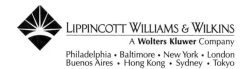

LIPPINCOTT WILLIAMS & WILKINS
A **Wolters Kluwer** Company
Philadelphia • Baltimore • New York • London
Buenos Aires • Hong Kong • Sydney • Tokyo

Editor: Donna Balado
Managing Editor: Cheryl W. Stringfellow
Marketing Manager: Emilie Linkins
Production Editor: Kevin Johnson
Designer: Holly McLaughlin
Compositor: Maryland Composition
Printer: Courier Kendallville

351 West Camden Street
Baltimore, MD 21201

530 Walnut St.
Philadelphia, PA 19106

The publisher is not responsible (as a matter of product liability, negligence, or otherwise) for any injury resulting from any material contained herein. This publication contains information relating to general principles of medical care that should not be construed as specific instructions for individual patients. Manufacturers' product information and package inserts should be reviewed for current information, including contraindications, dosages, and precautions.

Printed in the United States of America

First Edition, 2005

Library of Congress Cataloging-in-Publication Data

Lazo, John S.
   Review for USMLE : United States medical licensing examination, step
1 / John S. Lazo, Bruce R. Pitt, Joseph C. Glorioso III.– 7th ed.
      p. ; cm. – (The national medical series for independent study)
   Includes index.
   ISBN 0-7817-7921-9
  1. Medicine–Examinations, questions, etc. I. Pitt, Bruce R. II.
Glorioso, Joseph C. III. Title. IV. Series.
   [DNLM: 1. Medicine–Examination Questions. W 18.2 L431r 2006]
R834.5.L393 2006
610′.76–dc22

                                        2005021678

The publishers have made every effort to trace the copyright holders for borrowed material. If they have inadvertently overlooked any, they will be pleased to make the necessary arrangements at the first opportunity.

To purchase additional copies of this book, call our customer service department at **(800) 638-3030** or fax orders to **(301) 223-2320.** International customers should call **(301) 223-2300.**

Visit Lippincott Williams & Wilkins on the Internet: http://www.LWW.com. Lippincott Williams & Wilkins customer service representatives are available from 8:30 am to 6:00 pm, EST.

01 02 03 04 05
1 2 3 4 5 6 7 8 9 10

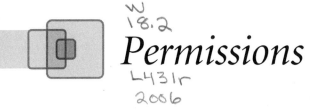

Permissions

Test 2

The figure in question 5 is reprinted from Berne RM, Levy MN (eds): *Physiology,* 3rd edition. St. Louis: CV Mosby, 1993, with permission from Elsevier.

The figure in question 11 is reprinted from Murray J: *The Normal Lung.* Philadelphia: WB Saunders, 1976, with permission from Elsevier.

The figure in question 16 is reprinted with permission from Gilman AG, Rall TW, Nies AS (eds): *Goodman and Gilman's The Pharmacological Basis of Therapeutics,* 8th edition. Elmsford, NY: Pergamon Press, 1990.

The figure in question 28 is reprinted with permission from Hoffman BF, Cranefield PF: *Electrophysiology of the Heart.* New York: McGraw-Hill, 1960.

Test 8

The figure in question 13 is reprinted from Robbins SL: *Pathologic Basis of Disease,* 3rd edition. Philadelphia: WB Saunders, 1989, with permission from Elsevier.

The figure in question 40 is reprinted from Bates DV, Macklem PT, Christie RV: *Respiratory Function in Disease,* 2nd edition. Philadelphia: WB Saunders, 1971, with permission from Elsevier.

Test 9

The figure in question 34 is reprinted with permission from Wilson JD, Braunwald E, Isselbacher KJ, et al (eds): *Harrison's Principles of Internal Medicine,* 12th edition. New York: McGraw-Hill, 1991.

Test 11

The figure in question 24 is reprinted from Guyton AC: *Textbook of Medical Physiology,* 8th edition. Philadelphia: WB Saunders, 1991, with permission from Elsevier.

Test 13

The figure in question 29 is reprinted from Guyton AC: *Textbook of Medical Physiology,* 8th edition. Philadelphia: WB Saunders, 1991, with permission from Elsevier.

Contents

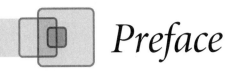

Preface

Because medical education and testing paradigms continue to evolve in the United States, we are especially pleased to present the seventh edition of the Lippincott Williams & Wilkins *Review for USMLE Step 1*. This edition incorporates a deep appreciation for the rapid advances in our understanding of the molecular basis of disease, stimulated in part by the completion of the Human Genome Project, the enormous increase in the data that can be presented to medical students, and a consensus that an integrated presentation of information during the first 2 years of medical school is desirable.

With the advent of the USMLE Step 1 that initially de-emphasized the traditional basic science disciplines and stressed the integrated approach, we believe it is especially important to provide students with a series of questions that accurately reflects this new format and prepares students for the test. Since the first edition, the *Review for USMLE Step 1* has undergone several iterations, reflecting the thoughtful comments of both students and faculty. In this new edition, we have expunged questions using the matching format and the "except" format, and we have continued to increase the patient-based questions that we hope will test your ability to integrate key basic science concepts with relevant clinical problems.

This book provides question types that are now used on the USMLE and will continue to be used for the new computer-based format. We appreciate all of the complimentary and thoughtful comments that readers have provided to help improve the book. We hope you will also find this book useful, and we and the publisher welcome any comments you may have.

Acknowledgments

The successful completion of this edition and the previous six could not have been accomplished without the generous assistance of many individuals in the Departments of Pharmacology, Molecular Genetics and Biochemistry, Pathology, and Environmental and Occupational Health at the University of Pittsburgh. We are particularly grateful to Alex Ducruet, PhD, who is a Postdoctoral Associate, and Christin Glorioso, who is a MD student at the University of Pittsburgh. We also thank David M. Krisky, MD, PhD, who helped formulate some of the questions; Sharon Webb for her secretarial assistance; and Donna Balado, Emilie Linkins, Cheryl Stringfellow, and Kelly Pavlovsky at Lippincott Williams & Wilkins.

test **1**

Questions

Directions: Single best answer questions consist of numbered items or incomplete statements followed by answers or by completions of the statement. Select the ONE lettered answer or completion that is BEST in each case.

1 Commensal microbes are commonly found within certain organs in the human body, yet they do not cause disease. However, such microbes can act as opportunistic pathogens if given access to other human tissue. Which of the following species of microbes is found only as an opportunistic pathogen?

(A) *Propionibacterium*
(B) *Bacteroides*
(C) *Pseudomonas*
(D) *Fusobacterium*
(E) *Clostridium*

2 Figure 1 from the color plate section depicts a soft hemorrhagic brain lesion that crosses the corpus callosum. Which of the following classifications best describes this lesion?

(A) Anaplastic astrocytoma
(B) Oligodendroglioma
(C) Meningioma
(D) Glioblastoma multiforme

3 A 60-year-old man has an abscess for which his physician prescribes a 7-day course of clindamycin. Before completion of the course, the patient returns to the office with cramps, diarrhea, and a fever of 39°C. The patient is admitted to the hospital, and a sigmoidoscopy is performed. Results demonstrate yellowish-white patchy areas on the wall of the colon. Which of the following is true of the causative agent?

(A) A Gram stain from the pseudomembrane would yield numerous red rods
(B) The pseudomembranes are classically caused by staphylococcal organisms
(C) The causative agent of the pseudomembranes produces toxins that act as monoglucosyltransferases that are specific for mammalian Rho protein
(D) The causative agent of the pseudomembranes is rarely found among the gut flora of the general population
(E) Clindamycin therapy should be discontinued, and an aminoglycoside should be used until the pseudomembranes resolve

4 A young child has a low-grade fever and malaise and is unwilling to eat. On physical examination, enlarged cervical lymph nodes and a gray membrane covering the tonsils and throat are found. A throat specimen shows gram-positive rods shaped like clubs that grew in "Chinese letter" forms. Which of the following statements concerning the illness is correct?

(A) The gene for the toxin that is present in this disease is carried on a bacteriophage
(B) This illness could have been prevented by vaccination with a killed suspension of organisms
(C) The causative organism expresses its toxin only in high-iron environments
(D) An adequate dose of penicillin will lead to the child's complete recovery
(E) The causative organism's most common reservoir is in the saliva of domesticated pets

5 A 55-year-old white man states that he has been having occasional episodes of chest pain for the past several months but that the discomfort usually goes away after a few minutes. Then, 3 days ago, the patient had an episode of chest pain that lasted more than 20 minutes. Which one of the following statements is most likely correct?

(A) The patient's creatine kinase (CK-MB) levels are normal; therefore, he could not have had a myocardial infarction

(B) The patient's electrocardiogram (ECG) shows ST-segment elevation in leads II, III, and aVF; therefore, he had a myocardial infarction in the anterior wall of the heart

(C) The patient's lactate dehydrogenase (LDH_1) levels are normal; however, if he had a myocardial infarction 3 days ago, they could have been elevated earlier but returned to normal by now

(D) Based on the history alone, it is clear that the patient did not have a myocardial infarction

(E) ECG changes seen in leads I, V_5, and V_6 indicate that the left circumflex coronary artery was likely involved

(F) A decrease in serum myoglobin was detected

6 A 21-year-old man dies suddenly during his track workout. The man had a history of occasional fainting, as does his brother. On autopsy, his heart showed a hypertrophic interventricular septum out of proportion with the rest of the heart. Which one of the following is the most likely diagnosis?

(A) Sarcoidosis
(B) Amyloidosis
(C) Idiopathic hypertrophic cardiomyopathy
(D) Hemochromatosis
(E) Hypertensive heart disease
(F) Acute respiratory distress syndrome

7 Which of the following statements about mitral valve prolapse is correct?

(A) Diagnosis of mitral valve prolapse rarely can be made before symptoms occur

(B) Mitral valve prolapse is seen in approximately 0.7% of the population

(C) Mitral valve prolapse usually causes a mid-diastolic click

(D) Ehlers–Danlos syndrome and other connective tissue diseases are associated with mitral valve prolapse

(E) Mitral valve prolapse is most common in men more than 40 years of age

8 Which of the following statements about rheumatic heart disease is correct?

(A) It has no known infectious disease etiology

(B) Only two layers of the heart—endocardium and myocardium—can be affected

(C) Rheumatic heart disease cannot be distinguished from other forms of carditis on the basis of microscopic analysis of biopsies alone

(D) The five major criteria for diagnosis of acute rheumatic fever are carditis, polyarthritis, chorea, erythema marginatum, and subcutaneous nodules

(E) The aortic valve is the most commonly affected valve in chronic rheumatic heart disease

9 A correct description of the individual curves depicted in the log–dose response relationship shown here includes which of the following?

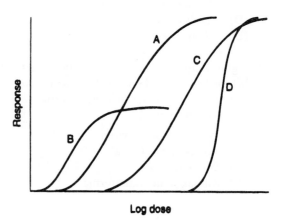

(A) Curves A and D: a full agonist (drug A) and a partial agonist (drug D)

(B) Curves B and C: an agonist in the absence of a noncompetitive inhibitor (curve B) and in the presence of one (curve C)

(C) Curves A, C, and D: three agonists with similar efficacy but different potency

(D) Curves A and C: an agonist in the absence of a competitive inhibitor (curve C) and in the presence of one (curve A)

(E) Curves A and C: drug A is less potent than drug C

10 The cerebellar tumor depicted in Figure 2 from the color plate section is frequently associated with which of the following conditions?

(A) Von Hippel–Lindau disease
(B) Pancreatic cysts
(C) Renal cell carcinoma
(D) Adenoma sebaceum

11 The most common type of Ehlers–Danlos syndrome (i.e., type VI) is inherited in an autosomal recessive fashion. Which one of the following extracellular matrix molecules is affected?

(A) Laminin, which is the most abundant glycoprotein in all basement membranes

(B) Type II collagen, which is an important component of cartilage and the vitreous humor

(C) Types I and III collagen, which together have wide distributions in the skin, blood vessels, tendons, and bone

(D) Proteoglycans, which regulate connective tissue structure and permeability

(E) Fibronectin, which is an essential macromolecule secreted by endothelial cells and fibroblasts

13 Which of the following pathophysiologic changes may be most useful in documenting, within less than 6 hours, that a patient had a myocardial infarction?

(A) Inverted or biphasic T wave on an ECG
(B) Elevated serum levels of CK-MB
(C) Elevated serum levels of myocardial LDH_1
(D) Maximal indices of coagulative necrosis
(E) Peak tissue infiltration of neutrophils

14 A patient has a throbbing right frontal headache. A cord-like subcutaneous abnormality in the right side of the head is sampled for biopsy, and the tissue is depicted in Figure 3 from the color plate section. The correct diagnosis is

(A) Wallerian degeneration of a nerve
(B) temporal arteritis
(C) helminthic infection (i.e., cutaneous larval migrans)
(D) ganglion cysts

12 A 34-year-old woman presented with pelvic pain, and ultrasound revealed a cystic ovarian mass. The multiloculated cyst pictured here was removed. The tumor can best be described as

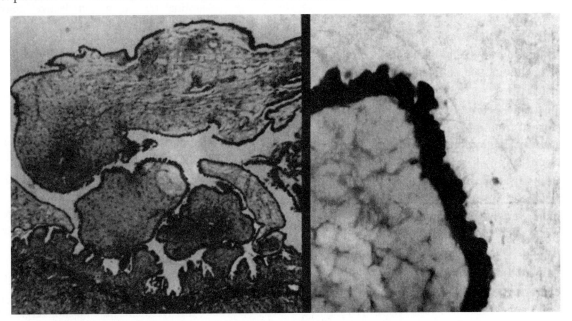

(A) associated with elevated production of the beta subunit of human chorionic gonadotropin (hCG)

(B) a germ cell tumor requiring interventional chemotherapy

(C) rare outside of the elderly female population

(D) an indolent low-grade neoplasm

15 On the basis of this schematic drawing of a cholinergic synapse, which of the following statements about neurons is correct?

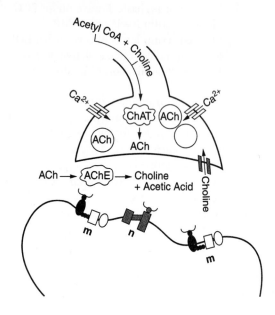

(A) Presynaptic neurons do not usually have receptors for the neurotransmitters that they release

(B) Neurons that release acetylcholine (ACh) are found only in the parasympathetic branch of the autonomic nervous system

(C) Cholinergic neurons in the substantia nigra selectively degenerate in the brains of patients with confirmed Alzheimer's dementia

(D) The toxin produced by the bacterium *Clostridium tetani* blocks excitatory signals to cholinergic motor neurons in the anterior horn

(E) Neurons releasing Ach make connections with cell types other than neurons, including cells found in glands, muscles, and blood vessels

16 Which of the following statements about muscarinic and nicotinic receptors are true?

(A) Muscarinic receptors have been found to carry signals via closely associated M proteins

(B) Nicotinic receptors activate the inositol triphosphate pathway, leading to the release of stored calcium

(C) Drugs that act at nicotinic sites are important in blocking the undesirable side effect of salivation during the administration of inhaled anesthetics

(D) Drugs that act at nicotinic sites are important for temporarily paralyzing patients before tracheal intubation

(E) Muscarinic receptors bind the endogenous ligand norepinephrine with high affinity

17 Inhibitors of cyclo-oxygenase II are used in the treatment of rheumatoid arthritis because they

(A) have less severe adverse effects on the gastrointestinal tract than nonselective inhibitors of cyclo-oxygenase

(B) inhibit the underlying cellular proliferation accompanying this disorder

(C) do not affect cardiovascular function

(D) are also efficacious in treating severe pain

(E) also inhibit 5′-lipoxygenase

18 Which of the following statements about ACh release and deactivation is true?

(A) ACh release is blocked by the toxin associated with *Clostridium tetani*

(B) Uptake of ACh into the presynaptic receptor is the most important mechanism in terminating the ACh signal

(C) Acetylcholinesterase (AChE) inhibitors, such as physostigmine, are not effective in the treatment of myasthenia gravis because patients with myasthenia have no cholinergic nerve terminals to release ACh

(D) The influx of Ca^{2+} into the depolarized axon terminal is a prerequisite for the release of stored ACh

(E) Inhibitors of the enzyme monoamine oxidase (MAO) are important in the treatment of depression because they inhibit the breakdown of ACh into its constituents, acetic acid, and choline

19 Glyceryl trinitrate (GTN or nitroglycerin) is a long-standing agent in the treatment of ischemic heart disease. Its mechanism of action is most likely due to

(A) elevation of cyclic guanasine monophosphate (cGMP) secondary to inhibition of phosphodi-esterase V

(B) relaxation of venous capacitance vessels and reduced myocardial oxygen consumption

(C) inhibition of baroreceptor reflex pathway

(D) direct relaxation of coronary vessels

(E) inhibition of NaK-ATPase in cardiac myocytes

20 The incubation period for hepatitis A is

(A) less than 15 days

(B) 15 to 40 days

(C) 40 to 60 days

(D) 60 to 160 days

(E) more than 160 days

21 A healthy person is flying in an airplane that has been pressurized to 10,000 feet (523 mm Hg). Which of the following statements concerning the effects of this barometric pressure is true?

(A) It will not affect alveolar P_{O_2} because inspired oxygen remains at 0.21

(B) It will be associated with significant desaturation of arterial hemoglobin

(C) It will shift the subject's oxyhemoglobin dissociation curve to the left

(D) It will decrease the vapor pressure of water in the airways

(E) It will cause a modest reduction in arterial P_{O_2}

22 The tuberculin test is used to determine if a patient has ever been exposed to *Mycobacterium tuberculosis*. If the patient has been exposed to the organism, the site where *M. tuberculosis* proteins were injected will trigger a type IV hypersensitivity response that causes the site to become red and swollen because of

(A) specific T cells recognizing the processed antigen and releasing inflammatory cytokines that increase blood vessel permeability to other immune effector cells and fluid

(B) antibodies binding the proteins and triggering neutrophils to release inflammatory cytokines that increase blood vessel permeability to other immune effector cells and fluid

(C) proteins binding to antibodies on mast cells and triggering mast cell degranulation

(D) unbound antibodies binding the proteins and the immune complex, then depositing protein in the tissue, which triggers a cell-mediated response

(E) cytotoxic CD8 + T cells recognizing the processed protein and releasing inflammatory cytokines as well as causing the antigen-presenting cells to undergo apoptosis

23 Cyclosporin A and FK-506 are often used in the treatment of transplant recipients. Both drugs interfere with the synthesis of the cytokine interleukin (IL) 2. These drugs are used to

(A) decrease plasma levels of IL-2 so that it will not bind to the foreign cells of the transplanted organ and cause rejection

(B) inhibit the IL-2 stimulus for proliferation of T cells and prevent organ rejection

(C) prevent the activation of macrophages by IL-2 and prevent organ rejection

(D) decrease the IL-2 stimulation of immunoglob-ulin-E (IgE) producing plasma cells and therefore hinder the recipient's allergic response to the foreign cells of the transplanted organ

(E) inhibit the suppression of T cells by IL-2 and prevent organ rejection

24 A 50-year-old man with a history of hemochromatosis presents to the emergency department coughing up bright red blood. He had his most recent phlebotomy yesterday. His blood pressure is 110/85, his pulse is 115; his face is flushed, and he is diaphoretic. During the physical examination, splenomegaly and a venous pattern on his chest and abdomen are noted. He seems somewhat drowsy and confused but has no focal neurologic signs. What is the most likely cause of this patient's bleeding?

(A) Portal hypertension
(B) Hemoglobin deficiency
(C) Eroded gastric ulcer
(D) Bronchogenic carcinoma
(E) Protein C deficiency

25 A premenopausal woman has a history of galactorrhea and amenorrhea with blurred vision. Clinical tests should be performed to pursue a likely diagnosis of

(A) prolactinoma
(B) hyperthyroidism
(C) Addison's disease
(D) iatrogenic disorder secondary to use of bromocryptine
(E) diabetes insipidus

26 Which of the following statements concerning the etiology and pathology of hemochromatosis is true?

(A) The excess iron accumulates primarily in cells of the mononuclear phagocyte system
(B) The most severe form of the disease is found in patients with thalassemia and sideroblastic anemia
(C) The iron accumulates due to a failure of renal excretion
(D) Approximately two-thirds of patients with hemochromatosis share a common human leukocyte antigen
(E) The organ damage resulting from hemochromatosis is characteristically confined to the liver

27 The multicystic tumor depicted in Figure 4 from the color plate section arose in the epiphysis of the femur and was associated with bone pain. The correct diagnosis is

(A) osteosarcoma
(B) chondroblastoma
(C) giant cell tumor
(D) chondromyxoid fibroma

28 Peripheral lymphoid tissues are the sites that antigen-specific lymphocytes migrate to after developing in central lymphoid tissues. Which one of the following statements concerning lymphoid tissue is correct?

(A) The gastrointestinal system contains peripheral lymphoid tissue called gut-associated lymphoid tissue that is the site of collection of food antigens
(B) T cells develop in the bone marrow and then migrate to the thyroid for maturation
(C) The spleen is the primary site plasma cells migrate to after being activated by antigen recognition; most antibodies are released into the blood from this peripheral lymphoid tissue
(D) B cells develop in the thymus and migrate to the bone marrow for maturation
(E) Lymph nodes contain germinal centers, which are sites of massive T cell proliferation during an infection

29 Carbon monoxide is an odorless and colorless combustion byproduct that accounts for a significant number of suicides and accidental poisonings. Carbon monoxide exerts its toxic effects by

(A) shifting the oxyhemoglobin dissociation curve to the right
(B) having an affinity for hemoglobin considerably less than oxygen
(C) reducing the ability of oxyhemoglobin to deliver oxygen in peripheral circulation
(D) stimulating the respiratory center
(E) activating cytochrome oxidase

30 The probability of hepatitis B $[P(D+)]$ in a certain patient population is known to be 0.20 [conversely, $P(D-) = 0.80$]. In a study of a new diagnostic test for hepatitis B, the probability of a positive test result among patients known to have hepatitis, $P(T+|D+)$, is shown to be 0.90, whereas the probability that a healthy patient will have a negative result, $P(T-|D-)$, is shown to be 0.95. What is the probability that a new patient with a negative test result is truly healthy?

(A) 0.95
(B) $(0.95)(0.80) [(0.95)(0.80) + (0.10)(0.20)]$
(C) $(0.90)(0.20) [(0.90)(0.20) + (0.05)(0.80)]$
(D) $(0.95)(0.80) [(0.95)(0.80) + (0.90)(0.20)]$

31 The well-circumscribed, 3-cm tumor of the breast depicted in Figure 5 from the color plate section bulged from the plane of cutting and had a gray, glistening appearance. The correct diagnosis is

(A) infiltrating ductal adenocarcinoma
(B) infiltrating lobular adenocarcinoma
(C) tubular adenoma
(D) fibroadenoma

32 Antibodies play multiple roles in the host's immune response. Which of the following statements concerning antibodies is correct?

(A) Mature antibodies are found only in serum
(B) Opsonization is mediated by binding the Fc portion of the antibody to the bacterial surface
(C) The Fc portions of cross-linked antibodies can trigger the complement cascade and lead to the destruction of bacteria that the antibodies have bound
(D) The process of antibody-dependent, cell-mediated cytotoxicity relies on neutrophil recognition of antibodies bound to a target cell's Fc receptor
(E) Antibodies are normally present in the urine of healthy individuals

33 The following data were obtained from an arterial blood sample drawn from a hospitalized patient: pH = 7.55, P_{CO_2} = 25 mm Hg, [HCO_3^-] = 22.5 mEq/L, and recall that CO_2 = 0.03 × P_{CO_2} (in mmol/L). This patient's arterial blood findings are consistent with a diagnosis of

(A) metabolic alkalosis
(B) respiratory alkalosis
(C) metabolic acidosis
(D) respiratory acidosis

34 Like single-unit smooth muscle, skeletal muscle fiber

(A) uses myosin as site of calcium regulation
(B) has similar thick and thin filaments
(C) reveals spontaneous production of action potentials
(D) maintains intrinsic tone
(E) contracts in response to stretch of fibers

35 A 63-year-old man has been having episodes of angina, syncope, and dyspnea on exertion for "quite some time." On auscultation, his physician notices a late-peaking systolic ejection murmur that increases in intensity with longer cardiac cycle lengths, a gallop in the fourth heart sound (S_4), and a soft aortic valve component in the second heart sound (A_2). An ECG shows abnormally high R waves in lead aVL. Which one of the following is the most likely diagnosis?

(A) Mitral stenosis caused by rheumatic fever
(B) Aortic stenosis caused by a congenital bicuspid aortic valve
(C) Mitral regurgitation caused by infective endocarditis
(D) Aortic regurgitation caused by aortic root dilation

36 Which of the following descriptions of cardiac conduction abnormalities is correct?

(A) Complete heart block—no detectable P waves and wide QRS complexes
(B) First-degree atrioventricular block (AV) block—prolonged PR interval with normal QRS complex
(C) High-grade AV block—prolonged PR interval when a beat occurs and a wide QRS complex
(D) Left bundle branch block—narrow QRS complexes with a short R wave in V_6 and a deep S wave in V_1
(E) Second-degree AV block, Mobitz type II—PR interval increasing with each successive beat until a P wave is blocked at the AV node; normal QRS complexes

37 A 75-year-old woman is admitted to the hospital after a cerebrovascular accident. Her CT shows a focal nonhemorrhagic infarction in the right hemisphere. During physical examination, no muscular weakness is noted; however, the patient is not responding to any visual, auditory, or tactile stimuli on the left side of her body. The woman also has a deficit involving only the inferior portion of her visual field in both eyes. Which lobe of the brain has been principally affected by this stroke?

(A) Parietal
(B) Frontal
(C) Occipital
(D) Temporal

38 The high metabolic needs of the heart and its relative exclusive reliance on aerobic metabolism require a high degree of regulation of coronary blood flow to maintain myocardial oxygen demands. As such, coronary perfusion

(A)   is greatest during systole

(B)   increases directly over a broad range of arterial pressures

(C)   is controlled mainly by local metabolic factors

(D)   is greatly decreased by direct sympathetic stimulation of resistance vessels

(E)   is achieved primarily via collateral vessels in healthy subjects

39 Rofecoxib (Vioxx) was recently voluntarily withdrawn from the market by its manufacturer. This unusual move was prompted by

(A)   a new study suggesting that it was equieffective in inhibiting COX-I and COX-II.

(B)   the results of a clinical trial for sporadic nonmalignant adenomas revealing increased incidence of adverse thromboembolic events compared to placebo

(C)   increased incidence of severe gastrointestinal side effects in users of rofecoxib compared to traditional nonsteroidal anti-inflammatory drugs

(D)   new founded concerns over prolonged bleeding times with rofecoxib

(E)   concerns that pregnant patients might have premature labor

40 Which of the following statements concerning the mechanism of clot formation is correct?

(A)   Activation of thrombin by factor VIII is the final common pathway in converting soluble fibrinogen to insoluble fibrin

(B)   The extrinsic pathway is activated by a lipoprotein called tissue factor, whereas the intrinsic pathway is activated by contact with foreign surfaces

(C)   Thrombin and several other cascade proteins are kinases that activate the next molecule in the pathway

(D)   Antithrombin III, an important regulator of the clotting cascade, acts by covalently crosslinking fibrin monomers into large meshworks in which platelets become lodged

(E)   Vitamin K is involved in the spleen's synthesis of factors that are calcium chelators

41 Which of the following statements correctly pairs a commonly used anticoagulant with its mechanism of action?

(A)   Heparin acts to cleave the covalent linkage between fibrin monomers

(B)   Tissue plasminogen activator acts by irreversibly inhibiting thrombin

(C)   Dicumarol (warfarin) is a natural product that competitively inhibits the vitamin K-dependent γ-carboxylation of several cascade proteins

(D)   Aspirin irreversibly binds fibrinogen, which decreases the pool of available fibrin monomers that can participate in clot formation

(E)   Streptokinase is a bacterial product that causes platelet lysis, therefore inhibiting platelet aggregation

42 A bone marrow transplant recipient developed progressive alveolar infiltrates visible on chest radiographs, and a lung biopsy was performed. The biopsy tissue, treated with silver stain, is depicted in Figure 6 from the color plate section. The agent responsible for this infection is most likely

(A)   *Pneumocystis carinii*

(B)   *Cryptococcus neoformans*

(C)   *Histoplasma capsulatum*

(D)   *Nocardia asteroids*

43 About 5% of individuals in a particular population are known to carry a recessive gene for poliodystrophy, an inherited disorder characterized by recurrent seizures and dementia with onset in early childhood. A 32-year-old healthy woman who had a brother with this disorder seeks genetic counseling. The patient's husband, an only child, does not know if his family has a history of the disorder. What is the probability that the patient is a carrier of poliodystrophy?

(A)   1/20

(B)   1/10

(C)   3/8

(D)   2/3

(E)   3/4

44 In contrast to aspirin, acetaminophen

(A)   has no anti-inflammatory effects

(B)   can lower normal body temperature

(C)   is equally effective at inhibiting COX-I and COX-II

(D)   is useful in the treatment of severe pain such as that from visceral organs

(E)   use in children with viral infections is associated with Reye's syndrome

45 A 68-year-old woman who is a volunteer at a church-sponsored kindergarten suddenly one evening develops a fever of 38.2°C and a severe headache. The following morning she also has a stiff neck and uncharacteristic drowsiness. At the emergency department, her temperature is 38.8°C, and pain and resistance manifest on flexion of her neck. The patient is noted to be mentally competent although lethargic. A cerebrospinal fluid (CSF) sample is obtained by lumbar puncture. On the basis of the history and physical examination of this patient, what is the most probable diagnosis?

(A) Viral meningitis
(B) Fungal meningitis
(C) Bacterial meningitis
(D) Viral encephalitis
(E) Brain abscess

46 Aspirin hypersensitivity is

(A) an unusual (<0.5% incidence) adverse effect of aspirin
(B) peculiar to acetylsalicylic acid
(C) also noted in some patients using acetaminophen
(D) an IgE-mediated anaphylactic-type reaction
(E) possibly due to shuttling of arachidonic acid via lipoxygenase pathway

47 Which of the following microscopic changes are indicative of reversible cellular injury?

(A) Swelling of mitochondria
(B) Cytoplasmic blebbing
(C) Cell shrinkage
(D) Chromatin condensation
(E) Cellular eosinophilia

48 Which of the following molecular errors is not a proven cause of the development of lysosomal storage diseases?

(A) Enzyme deficiency or enzyme inactivity
(B) Enzyme activator deficiency
(C) Mutant form of substrate
(D) Defective posttranslational processing of enzyme
(E) Lack of transport protein for egress of digested substrate

49 Of the following cell types, which would contain many mitochondria in the apical portion of the cell?

(A) Smooth muscle cells
(B) Ciliated epithelium cells
(C) Steroid-secreting cells
(D) Liver parenchymal cells
(E) Skeletal muscle cells

50 Which one of the following statements concerning infectious hepatitis is correct?

(A) Hepatitis C infection requires hepatitis B infection
(B) Diagnosis with hepatitis B carries a grave prognosis: many people die of fulminant hepatitis, and nearly 25% of infected patients progress to hepatocellular carcinoma
(C) Hepatitis B surface antigen (HBsAg) indicates active hepatitis infection
(D) The carrier state is common in patients infected with hepatitis A
(E) Hepatitis A infection accounts for approximately 25% of hepatitis cases in the United States

Answer Key

1-C	11-C	21-E	31-D	41-C
2-D	12-D	22-A	32-C	42-A
3-C	13-A	23-B	33-B	43-D
4-A	14-B	24-A	34-B	44-A
5-E	15-E	25-A	35-B	45-C
6-C	16-D	26-D	36-B	46-E
7-D	17-A	27-C	37-A	47-A
8-D	18-D	28-A	38-C	48-C
9-C	19-B	29-C	39-B	49-B
10-A	20-B	30-B	40-B	50-C

Answers and Explanations

1 **The answer is C** *General Principles / Microbiology / Anaerobic flora*

Pseudomonas are gram-negative aerobic motile rods that are not normally found within healthy tissue. *Propionibacterium* organisms are anaerobes found in the skin. *Bacteroides* are anaerobes that are found in the mouth, colon, and vagina. *Fusobacterium* organisms are anaerobes that live in the mouth. *Clostridium* organisms are anaerobes that are found in the colon.

2 **The answer is D** *Central and peripheral nervous system / Pathology / Gliomas of the brain*

Gliomas of the brain are divided into low-grade (e.g., benign astrocytoma), intermediate-grade (e.g., anaplastic astrocytoma), and high-grade variants. The most aggressive form is glioblastoma multiforme. Glioblastomas characteristically involve the cerebral hemispheres. They frequently cross the corpus callosum, and they cause progressive neurologic defects. Glioblastomas are characterized by a variegated gross appearance with zones of yellow necrosis, hemorrhage, and cystic change. Microscopically, the characteristic features of glioblastomas include cellular anaplasia, necrosis with pseudopalisading, and a dramatic endothelial proliferation in which small clusters of capillaries called glomeruli are formed. These tumors are extremely aggressive. Mortality within the first year after diagnosis is high.

3 **The answer is C** *Gastrointestinal system / Microbiology / Clostridium difficile*

The patient developed pseudomembranous colitis caused by *Clostridium difficile,* an anaerobic, gram-positive, spore-forming rod. The patient has been receiving clindamycin to treat the abscess. Treatment with clindamycin suppressed the normal colonic flora, thus permitting multiplication of *C. difficile.* The patient should stop taking clindamycin and should be given a prescription for vancomycin or metronidazole. Aminoglycosides are not appropriate because they are not effective against anaerobes. If untreated, *C. difficile* pseudomembranous colitis can be fatal. *C. difficile* produces at least two toxins (A and B). These toxins are monoglucosyltransferases specific for mammalian Rho protein, which is involved in cytoskeletal assembly (disassembly and signal transduction).

4 **The answer is A** *Hematopoietic and lymphoreticular system / Microbiology / Corynebacterium diphtheriae*

Corynebacterium diphtheriae is recognized by its unusual "Chinese letter" shape. Treatment for diphtheria involves disposal of the infecting organisms and administration of the appropriate antitoxin. The gene that encodes the diphtheria toxin is located on the β-corynephage, a bacteriophage, which lysogenizes into the *C. diphtheriae* chromosome. The only known host for *C. diphtheriae* is the human body. The diphtheria toxin is produced only in low-iron environments, like the human body, and is transmitted by aerosols. Prevention of diphtheria is possible with the diphtheria–pertussis–tetanus (DPT) vaccine. The tetanus and diphtheria components of DPT vaccine consist of inactive toxoid proteins, not preparations of the organism in question.

5 **The answer is E** *Cardiovascular system / Pathology / Myocardial infarction*

The patient's history, particularly chest pain for 20 minutes or longer, is consistent with a myocardial infarction. Both CK-MB and LDH_1 levels are typically elevated after a myocardial infarction; however, the timing of these changes is not the same for both markers. CK-MB levels increase several hours after an infarction, peak approximately 24 hours after the infarction, and may return to normal by 48 hours. Thus, CK-MB levels may be normal in a patient presenting a few days after having symptoms. Myoglobin is one of the first cardiac markers to increase after a myocardial infarction, but blood levels return to normal within 24 hours. LDH_1 levels do not peak until 48 to 72 hours after onset, but they remain elevated for 7 to 10 days. ST-segment elevation is also commonly seen after a myocardial infarction. Although changes in leads I, V_5, and V_6 are characteristic of involvement of the left circumflex coronary, changes in leads II, III, and aVF usually are associated with inferior infarcts with right coronary involvement.

6 **The answer is C** *Cardiovascular system / Pathology / Cardiomyopathies*

Idiopathic hypertrophic cardiomyopathy occurs as either autosomal dominant or sporadic disease, most often in young men. It commonly causes syncopal attacks, and it is recognized pathologically by the presence of a disproportionately enlarged interventricular septum, which differs from the concentric left ventricular hypertrophy of hypertensive heart disease. Sarcoidosis, amyloidosis, and hemochromatosis are not associated with hypertrophy but rather are restrictive cardiomyopathies that can be differentiated from each other on the basis of myocardial biopsies. Acute respiratory distress syndrome (ARDS) is a condition characterized by acute hypoxemic respiratory failure due to pulmonary edema caused by increased permeability of the alveolar capillary barrier. As the name implies, this is an acute, not chronic, syndrome.

7 **The answer is D** *Cardiovascular system / Pathology / Cardiac valvular diseases*

Diagnosis of mitral valve prolapse can be made on the basis of the presence of a midsystolic click with confirmation by echocardiography. This abnormality occurs in approximately 7% of the population and even more frequently in those with connective tissue diseases, including Ehlers–Danlos syndrome. The clinical importance of mitral valve prolapse is questionable, because it is often asymptomatic. Mitral regurgitation and infective endocarditis are rare complications. Mitral valve prolapse is more common in girls and women, especially those between ages 14 and 30.

8 **The answer is D** *Cardiovascular system / Pathology / Rheumatic heart disease*

Rheumatic heart disease is a complication of a group A β-hemolytic streptococcal pharyngitis characterized by carditis, polyarthritis, chorea, erythema marginatum, and subcutaneous nodules as major diagnostic criteria. This pancarditis affects all three layers of the heart. The mitral valve is most commonly affected, followed by the aortic valve. On microscopic examination, Aschoff bodies, which are areas of fibrinoid necrosis with histiocytes and Anitschkow's cells, are pathognomonic.

9 **The answer is C** *General principles / Pharmacology / Log–dose response relationships*

Curves A, C, and D all reach approximately the same maximal response and thus are similar in efficacy. However, curve A is more potent than C, which in turn is more potent than D. Potency is based on the relative positions of the curves along the x-axis. A competitive inhibitor would shift the curve to the right. For instance, curves A and C might be responses to an agonist in the absence (curve A) and presence (curve C) of a competitive inhibitor. Noncompetitive inhibitors decrease the efficacy (as a partial agonist might do). Thus, curves A and B may be the response to an agent in the absence (curve A) and the presence (curve B) of a noncompetitive inhibitor.

10 **The answer is A** *Central and peripheral nervous system / Pathology / Cerebellar tumors*

Hemangioblastomas are well-circumscribed, frequently cystic lesions that classically involve the cerebellar hemispheres. A tumor is characterized by an anastomosing network of capillary-sized vessels associated with a proliferation of stromal cells—large, polygonal cells with abundant, pale cytoplasm rich in fat. The nuclei of these cells are small but display significant pleomorphism. The histogenesis of these cells is uncertain. Many researchers believe they are related to endothelial cells and pericytes. Others believe they derive from precursors of macrophages and monocytes.

11 **The answer is C** *Skin and related connective tissue / Biochemistry / Ehlers–Danlos syndrome*

Ehlers–Danlos syndrome comprises a spectrum of disordered collagen biosynthesis. The clinical features of Ehlers–Danlos syndrome depend on the exact underlying abnormality but can include hyperextensible skin, hypermobile joints, large vessel fragility, and vulnerability to retinal detachment. The defect in type VI Ehlers–Danlos syndrome involves the collagens that predominate in the skin, bone, tendons, and vessels (i.e., types I and III). The syndrome results from decreased lysyl hydroxylase activity. Since hydroxylysine residues are critical to proper cross-linking, the structural stability of collagen in patients with Ehlers–Danlos syndrome is compromised. No common Ehlers–Danlos syndromes principally involve the cartilage and vitreous humor, which are structures that contain type II collagen. The characteristics describing laminin, proteoglycans, and fibronectin are all correct; however, none of these macromolecules is implicated in any of the Ehlers–Danlos syndromes.

12 **The answer is D** *Reproductive system / Pathology / Serous intermediate ovarian tumor*

The papillary tumor pictured is a serous intermediate (borderline) tumor of the ovary, which is commonly seen in young women. The tumor behaves in an indolent fashion, with repeated recurrences but rare metastases outside of the abdominal cavity, resulting in a high incidence of intestinal obstruction and long survival. The tumor is characterized by edematous papillae lined by stratified cuboidal to columnar cells, which have atypical cytology. Unlike serous adenocarcinomas, serous intermediate tumors do not invade ovarian stroma.

13 **The answer is A** *Cardiovascular system / Pathology / Myocardial infarction*

Immediately after a person has a myocardial infarction, changes are often evident on an ECG. Alterations in electrical events in the ventricles, including prolonged depolarization, are common and are manifested by abnormalities in the T wave. Although changes in circulating enzyme levels are helpful for diagnostic and prognostic purposes, they usually occur 6 hours or more after the attack and are more helpful 24 to 72 hours after the myocardial infarction.

14 **The answer is B** *Central and peripheral nervous system / Pathology / Vasculitis*

This slide shows the classic histologic features of temporal arteritis. The cylindrical structure is a large artery with focal areas of granulomatous inflammation in its wall. Giant cells are visible surrounding fragments of the mural elastic lamina. It is important to recognize temporal arteritis because it may be associated with coexistent involvement of the retinal artery and may lead to blindness if not treated appropriately.

15 **The answer is E** *Central and peripheral nervous system / Pharmacology / Synaptic neurotransmission*

ACh is among the first of the neurotransmitters to have its synthesis, localization, signal transduction, and pharmacology described. Presynaptic neurons frequently have receptors for the transmitter that they release, and these autoreceptors are often important for regulating the subsequent amount of transmitter release. Cholinergic neurons are found in the cerebral cortex and the anterior horn of the spinal cord. All preganglionic neurons in the autonomic nervous system (parasympathetic and sympathetic divisions) release ACh, and postganglionic neurons of the parsympathetic branch are also cholinergic. A small subset of postganglionic neurons in the cholinergic sympathetic branch release Ach onto eccrine sweat glands and blood vessels. Alzheimer's dementia is characterized by a relatively focal loss of cholinergic neurons in the basal nucleus of Meynert. Tetanus toxin is rapidly transported in a retrograde fashion from peripheral nerve terminals to the anterior horn cell bodies where it is released; inhibitory interneurons take up the toxin in the spinal cord, and the tetanus protein blocks inhibitory transmission of these neurons.

16 **The answer is D** *General principles / Pharmacology / Synaptic neurotransmission*

Release of inositol triphosphate and diacylglycerol is not a direct result of nicotinic receptor activation. Nicotinic receptors are found in the cerebral cortex and in the neuromuscular junction as well as postsynaptically in the autonomic ganglia. They are complex proteins with an ACh-binding site coupled to a cation-permeable channel. When activated, the receptors conduct sodium and potassium ions. Drugs such as succinylcholine produce paralysis during intubation by blocking the nicotinic receptors at neuromuscular junctions. Muscarinic receptors are universally coupled to either excitatory or inhibitory G proteins. They are important in mediating the effects of parasympathetic activation; thus, their blockade with drugs such as atropine results in decreased salivation (as well as other effects). Both receptor types are activated endogenously by ACh. Muscarinic receptors do not bind norepinephrine.

17 **The answer is A** *Musculoskeletal system / Pharmacology / Nonsteroidal anti-inflammatory drugs*

Drugs such as celecoxib (Celebrex) are selective inhibitors of cyclooxygenase II and at therapeutic doses neither inhibit cyclo-oxygenase I nor 5′-lipoxygenase. Their utility in the therapy of rheumatoid arthritis is in large part due to their well-documented reduced toxicity in the gastrointestinal tract compared to nonselective cyclo-oxygenase inhibitors (including aspirin). It is noteworthy that acetaminophen has minimal toxicity in the gastrointestinal tract but is devoid of anti-inflammatory effects and its use in rheumatoid arthritis is restricted to its analgesic action. Nonsteroidal anti-inflammatory drugs (whether selective for COX-II or not) are only useful in therapy of mild to moderate pain and none of these agents are known to affect the course of the rheumatoid arthritis, including underlying cellular proliferation. Some COX-II selective inhibitors, such as rofecoxib have been associated with enhanced risk of cardiovascular disease and have been withdrawn from the market. It remains to be determined if all COX-II drugs share this profile.

18 **The answer is D** *General principles / Pharmacology / Synaptic neurotransmission*

The influx of calcium is a prerequisite for the release of any neurotransmitter from the terminal of an axon. ACh release is blocked by toxin from *Clostridium botulinum*. Whereas high-affinity uptake of choline is important for the synthesis of new ACh, termination of the cholinergic transmission is mainly the function of fast-acting AChE. Cholinesterase inhibition is an important therapy for patients with myasthenia gravis. Myasthenic patients have an autoimmune disorder directed against the nicotinic receptors, not the nerve terminals. MAO inhibitors are important therapeutic agents used to treat depression because of their effects on the dopaminergic and adrenergic systems.

19 **The answer is B** *Cardiovascular system / Pharmacology of ischemic heart disease / Nitrovasodilators*

GTN is the prototype of nitrovasodilators that remain as important agents in the therapy of ischemic heart disease. These agents release either nitric oxide or nitrosothiols and activate soluble guanylyl cyclase in target tissues, including vascular smooth muscle. In therapeutic concentrations, they effectively relax capacitive veins thereby increasing their compliance and reducing venous return. Reduced venous return results in decreased preload and hence decreased myocardial work (or oxygen consumption) accounting for a significant component of mechanism of action of these agents. Unlike agents such as sildenafil, GTN does not affect phosphdiesterase V and indeed concomitant use of sildenafil with GTN is contraindicated to avoid potential excessive vasorelaxation that may be associated with reflex tachycardia and myocardial contractility. In this regard, it is apparent that GTN does not interfere with baroreceptor reflex pathways. Although the evidence is somewhat contradictory, it appears that GTN does not directly relax resistance coronary arteries but may favorably enhance perfusion of collateral vessels. Although GTN may have application in the treatment of congestive heart failure, it does not inhibit Na-K ATPase as is apparent in agents such as digitalis.

20 **The answer is B** *General principles / Microbiology / Hepatitis A*

Hepatitis A has a short incubation period: 15 to 40 days. The infection is transmitted by the fecal–oral route and takes hold very quickly. The virus replicates in the gastrointestinal tract and is shed in the feces during the incubation and acute phases of the disease.

21 **The answer is E** *General principles / Physiology / Gas exchange and partial pressure of oxygen*

The change in cabin air pressure will cause a modest reduction in arterial P_{O_2}. The partial pressure of a gas is proportional to the fractional concentration of the gas and total gas pressure. Predictably, P_{O_2} would decrease from the normal range of 97 to 100 mm Hg to approximately 67 mm Hg following decreases in alveolar P_{O_2}. This decrease is partially due to water vapor pressure, which remains constant at 47 mm Hg, and P_{CO_2}, which may decrease slightly due to stimulation from ventilation. This modest decline in P_{O_2} would not be associated with a decrease in oxygen saturation of arterial hemoglobin. A compensatory response would shift the oxyhemoglobin dissociation curve to the right because of the production of 2,3-diphosphoglycerate (2,3-DPG); however, this response usually takes more time than the average plane flight.

22 **The answer is A** *General principles / Immunology / Type IV hypersensitivity*

Type IV, or delayed, hypersensitivity reactions involve reactive lymphocytes recognizing an antigen and directing the immune response by the release of cytokines. Antibodies are not involved in this type of immune response. Neutrophils and mast cells are part of the nonspecific immune response, so they would not be major mediators of the specific response to the tuberculin test. Cytotoxic CD8+ T cells recognize antigen presented only by major histocompatability complex (MHC) I, which would not present proteins that the cell obtained from its environment but only proteins made within the cell. Therefore, these cells would not be part of the type IV response.

23 **The answer is B** *General principles / Immunology / Immune suppression*

IL-2, also known as T cell growth factor, is produced by T cells and leads to T cell activation by recognition of a combination of peptide and major MHC in the presence of costimulator molecules. IL-2 stimulates (not suppresses) the activated T cells to proliferate, as well as to differentiate to effector T cells. IL-2 has no effect on somatic cells of the body or on macrophages. Although other T cell cytokines can influence the type of antibody made by plasma cells (e.g., IL-4 directs IgE synthesis and IL-5 directs IgA synthesis), IL-2 does not have this role.

24 **The answer is A** *Cardiovascular system / Pathology / Hemochromatosis and clinical findings in cirrhosis*

Identification of hemochromatosis in its early stages facilitates effective treatment of this otherwise relentlessly progressive disease. Although he is being treated, this patient has already progressed to the late stages of the disease, and he is now displaying the classic signs of cirrhosis. The bleeding is most likely the result of ruptured esophageal varices. Portal hypertension causes the development of several collateral circulations; these other vessels offer less resistance to flow, and they enlarge over time to accommodate the increased volume. The rectal and esophageal veins dilate to become varices, which may allow significant blood loss if they tear. The caput medusae vascular pattern over the abdomen indicates enlargement of another collateral circulation. Portal hypertension also causes blood flow to back up in the spleen, which results in splenomegaly. Hemoglobin synthesis is limited by iron availability. A hemochromatosis patient has excess iron and will probably not be hemoglobin deficient. Protein C is an anticoagulant whose exact mechanism of action remains unknown. Deficiency of protein C has been demonstrated in some cases of disseminated intravascular coagulation. Although neither eroded gastric ulcer nor bronchogenic carcinoma is excluded by hemochromatosis, hemochromatosis does not predispose to either of those conditions. The patient's bleeding is more likely the result of portal hypertension.

25 **The answer is A** *Endocrine system / Physiology / Anterior pituitary*

The coexistence of galactorrhea and amenorrhea in a premenopausal woman is consistent with hyperprolactinemia. Additional symptoms of visual problems may be secondary to space-related lesions of tumor mass. Prolactinomas are the most frequent secretory tumors. Elevated plasma levels of prolactin (PRL) are directly correlated with tumor diameter and levels >200 ng/ml are strongly associated with a PRL-secretory tumor. Computed tomography (CT) or magnetic resonance imaging (MRI) examination can be used to reveal micro- or macroadenomas and distinguish hyperprolactenima that is idiopathic or secondary to other types of mass lesions compressing stalk and interfering with dopamine inhibition. Galactorrhea is a result of direct effect of PRL on breast tissue. Amenorrhea is usually secondary to PRL-suppression of GnRH. Medical therapy with dopamine agonist such as bromocryptine and/or transsphenoidal surgical approaches are useful after diagnosis. Radiation therapy may be an alternative. Although prolactin levels may increase in hypothyrodism (due to decreased clearance of prolactin, increased levels of estrogen, or enhanced TRH receptors in lactotrophs), hyperthyroidism is not associated with elevated levels of PRL or the physical symptoms described above. Addison's disease is a rare condition of primary hypoadrenalism and is not associated with galactorrhea. Galactorrhea can indeed be drug-induced but agents that interfere with dopamine effects (such as psychotropic agents that are dopamine antagonists) rather than dopamine agonists (like bromocryptine) may produce such symptoms. Diabetes insipidus is a disorder of posterior pituitary involving insufficiency in arginine vasopressin and does not cause symptoms in reproductive tissues.

26 **The answer is D** *Hematopoietic and lymphoreticular system / Pathology / Hemochromatosis and clinical findings in cirrhosis*

Hemochromatosis is an autosomal recessive disorder that is five times more common in men than in women, and it is related to the human leukocyte antigen A3 in 70% of cases. Renal excretion of iron is inherently limited to approximately 1 mg/day. Thus, in developed countries, the regulation of iron homeostasis requires absolute control of absorption. Unfortunately, the normal mechanisms of regulation are not well understood. The iron buildup seen as a physiologic response to anemia is almost entirely confined to phagocytic cells of the reticuloendothelial system. Yet, in hemochromatosis patients, parenchymal cells of the liver, pancreas, and heart accumulate large amounts of iron, whereas phagocytes remain normal. Thus, although there is clearly a regulatory problem at the absorptive stage, the reticuloendothelial system is also functioning improperly. Patients with various erythropoietic difficulties and a resultant physiologically normal iron accumulation almost never have the extensive pathology seen in patients with primary hemochromatosis. Involvement of the pancreas commonly leads to diabetes mellitus, and skin pigmentation is a routine finding.

27 The answer is C *Musculoskeletal system / Pathology / Bone neoplasms*

Giant cell tumors of bone classically involve the epiphysis of the long bones and are associated with a lytic expansile lesion occasionally associated with bone sclerosis. Grossly, these tumors are hemorrhagic. Microscopically, as shown in this photograph, they are characterized by two main cellular components: stromal cells and giant cells. The stromal cells probably are the neoplastic component. These tumors may be locally aggressive, and metastasis is rare. If completely excised or curetted, however, they usually have a benign clinical course.

28 The answer is A *Hematopoietic and lymphoreticular system / Immunology / Lymphoid tissues*

The central lymphoid tissues are the bone marrow and the thymus. Both T cells and B cells develop in the bone marrow. B cells also mature in the marrow, whereas T cells migrate to the thymus for maturation. Gut-associated lymphoid tissue, bronchial-associated lymphoid tissue, and other mucosal-associated lymphoid tissues are peripheral lymphoid tissues. The gut-associated lymphoid tissue collects any antigens entering the body through the gastrointestinal tract, and the proper immune response may begin. The spleen is the site of filtration of antigens in the blood and of red blood cell destruction. Most plasma cells migrate to the bone marrow, making it the site for most antibody production. Germinal centers are sites for B cell proliferation after they encounter antigen in the context of the proper cytokines.

29 The answer is C *Respiratory system / Toxicology / Carbon monoxide*

The toxicity of carbon monoxide is due to its significantly greater affinity for hemoglobin ($210\times$) than oxygen, shifting the oxyhemoglobin curve to the left and depression of respiratory drive. In addition to reducing hemoglobin saturation, carbon monoxide reduces the ability of oxyhemoglobin to deliver oxygen to the periperhy by shifting the dissociation curve to the left (not right). Carbon monoxide can also inhibit other heme-containing proteins such as cytochromce oxidase and cytochrome P450, but the significance of such inhibition in pathophysiological conditions is unclear.

30 The answer is B *General principles / Biostatistics / Probability of hepatitis B*

Given that $P(D+) = 0.20$, $P(D!) = 0.80$, $P(T+|D+) = 0.90$, and $P(T-|D-) = 0.95$, the probability that a patient with a negative test result does not have hepatitis B, $P(D-|T-)$, is

$$P(D-|T-) = [P(T-|D-)P(D-)]/[P(T-|D-)P(D-) + P(T-|D+)P(D+)]$$
$$= (0.95)(0.80)/[(0.95)(0.80) + (1-0.90)(0.20)]$$

31 The answer is D *Reproductive system / Pathology / Breast tumors*

Fibroadenoma of the breast is a common, benign lesion affecting the breast of young to middle-aged women. They are characterized by a proliferation of stromal cells associated with a similar proliferation of ductal cells. Visible at low magnification are slit-like spaces, some having a leaf-like configuration, that are lined by hyperplastic ductal epithelium with a surrounding cellular stroma. Malignant lesions that mimic fibroadenomas include phyllodes tumors.

32 The answer is C *General principles / Immunology / Functions of antibodies*

Antibodies have two active ends, Fab and Fc. The Fab (for antigen binding) portion binds specifically to one antigen. If the antibody is attached to the immature B cells that synthesized it, binding of the antigen to the Fab portion can lead to activation of the B cell. Free antibodies in the blood can bind to bacteria or their toxins. Then macrophages or other cells can ingest the antibody–antigen complexes using Fc receptors for recognition. The Fc (for constant) portion is responsible for the effector functions of antibodies. It binds to Fc receptors on neutrophils or macrophages to trigger phagocytosis of the antibody–antigen complex. Bound antibodies that cross-link their Fc portions can trigger the classical complement pathway. Antibody-dependent, cell-mediated cytotoxicity occurs when antibodies attach to specific antigens on tumor cells (or other cells recognized as foreign) and designate those cells to be killed by either natural killer (NK) cells or macrophages. The NK cells and macrophages have Fc receptors that allow them to identify the cells that are to be killed.

33 **The answer is B** *Respiratory system / Physiology / Acid–base disturbances*

The blood findings indicate that this patient has respiratory alkalosis, an acid–base disturbance characterized by increased arterial pH (or decreased $[H^+]$), decreased P_{CO_2} (hypocapnia), and decreased plasma $[HCO_3^-]$. Both $[H^+]$ and $[HCO_3^-]$ are decreased in this patient, which is consistent with the axiom that $[H^+]$ and $[HCO_3^-]$ change in the same direction in respiratory acid–base imbalances. The decline in $[HCO_3^-]$ indicates that renal compensation has begun.

34 **The answer is B** *Musculoskeletal system / Physiology / Muscle*

Smooth muscle and skeletal muscle cells use cross-bridge movements between actin (thin) and myosin (thick) filaments to generate force but differ in many other cellular features. Smooth muscle cells lack the sarcomeres of skeletal muscle and are innervated by the autonomic nervous system rather than the somatic nervous system. Skeletal muscle uses the calcium binding protein, troponin, rather than calmodulin/myosin light chain kinase complex to affect cross-bridge activation. In some smooth muscles, basal cytosolic calcium is sufficient to maintain a contractile state in the absence of external stimuli (e.g., intrinsic tone). In addition, some smooth muscle cells can generate action potentials without external stimuli and hence manifest pacemaker activity. Many types of smooth muscle have an intrinsic property in which mechanical stretch produces contraction.

35 **The answer is B** *Cardiovascular system / Pathology / Valvular heart disease*

Aortic stenosis commonly presents with symptoms of angina, syncope, and dyspnea on exertion. On physical examination, a delayed upstroke of the carotid pulse may be noted, as well as a late-peaking systolic ejection murmur and soft A_2 on auscultation. Over time, left ventricular hypertrophy may develop, leading to an S_4 gallop and ECG abnormalities. Aortic stenosis may be differentiated from mitral stenosis and aortic regurgitation by the systolic murmur rather than the diastolic murmurs caused by these two lesions. Similarly, the murmur heard in mitral regurgitation is holosystolic rather than ejection type, and it does not vary with changes in the cardiac cycle length. However, mitral regurgitation intensity does vary with the administration of amyl nitrite, a vasodilator that causes decreased intensity of the murmur.

36 **The answer is B** *Cardiovascular system / Pathology / Cardiac conduction abnormalities*

High-grade AV block is characterized by blockage of several P waves (skipped beats) but a normal PR interval and a normal QRS complex when a P wave is conducted to the ventricles. Second-degree AV block, Mobitz type II, is characterized by single skipped beats without a prolonged PR interval and frequently a wide QRS complex. Left bundle branch block is characterized by a long QRS complex with a tall R wave in V_6 and a deep S wave in V_1. First-degree AV block is associated with prolonged PR interval but a normal QRS complex. Complete heart block is associated with a narrow QRS.

37 **The answer is A** *Central and peripheral nervous system / Neuroanatomy / Stroke, lateral neglect syndrome*

The absence of motor defects rules out much of the frontal lobe, and the presence of partial visual field defects (as well as the striking cognitive disturbance) indicates temporal or parietal lesions. The patient is displaying signs of lateral neglect syndrome, in which lesions to the nondominant parietal lobe cause severe disturbances in a person's ability to respond to any stimuli contralaterally. Thus, sensory stimuli administered to the left side are attributed to the homologous region on the right side of the body; persons or objects in the left visual field are ignored. However, there is clearly no primary sensory loss; the deficit is purely perceptual (i.e., secondary and tertiary processing are dysfunctional). The visual deficit described is commonly called pie-on-the-floor because the two homologous lower quadrants are lost. This pattern of visual loss coupled with the features of lateral neglect strongly suggest a parietal lesion, because half of the optic radiations from the thalamus proceed upward through the parietal lobe before reaching the calcarine cortex.

38 **The answer is C** *Cardiovascular system / Physiology / Myocardial metabolism*

The high extraction ratio of oxygen across the heart (>50%), even at rest, suggests a limited reserve for further oxygen utilization and thus a close relationship between myocardial metabolism and underlying blood flow. Accordingly, it appears that local metabolic factors (such as adenosine) closely couple perfusion with myocardial demands. Compression of collapsible vessels within the myocardial wall result in perfusion being maximal during diastole. The heart exhibits extraordinary autoregulation and perfusion is thus constant over a broad range of arterial pressures. Although vessels are innervated by sympathetic fibers that can produce constriction in response to sympathetic activation, the concomitant increase in myocardial metabolism overrides this phenomenon and results in vasodilation in response to sympathetic stimulation. Healthy subjects have minimal collateral vessels and, even in patients with severe myocardial disease, perfusion via collateral vessels is only sufficient to maintain basal metabolism and cannot enable large increases in blood flow in response to exercise or other stimuli.

39 **The answer is B** *Cardiovascular system / Toxicology / Nonsteroidal anti-inflammatory drugs; thromboemboli*

Rofecoxib was withdrawn by the Merck Company late in 2004 as the results of a clinical trial (APPROVe) in patients with sporadic nonmalignant adenomas was revealed. Patients who took rofecoxib had a significant increase in incidence of severe thromboembolic events and also suffered a significant increase in incidence of heart attacks and strokes compared to those taking placebo. A previous large trial assessing the effect of rofecoxib (versus naproxen) on gastrointestinal side effects (VIGOR) also showed increased cardiovascular and heart disease but reservations on its conclusions related to the presumed cytoprotective effects of naproxen. Rofecoxib was a prototype of a group of agents that had significant selectivity towards inhibition of COX-II and were proven to have significantly less major adverse effects on the GI tract (as ascertained by endoscopy). These agents have been proven not to prolong bleeding times as is the case with COX-I inhibitors or traditional NSAIDs. COX-I and COX-II inhibitors are associated with prolonged labor.

40 **The answer is B** *Hematopoietic and lymphoreticular system / Hematology / Clot formation*

The liver synthesizes most of the substances in the clotting cascade as zymogen (inactive) proteins, which are either cofactors or enzymes. Many of the enzymes are members of a class known as serine proteases, because a serine residue forms the active site and cleaves the ester or amide linkage on the substrate. Tissue factor, which is derived from endothelial cells, is released after tissue damage to activate the extrinsic pathway. High-molecular-weight kininogen, prekallikrein, and Hageman factor interact to activate the intrinsic cascade. The final common pathway is activation of the serine protease thrombin by factor V; thrombin cleaves platelet-bound fibrinogen to create the fibrin monomer. Vitamin K is essential in the liver synthesis of γ-carboxyglutamate. The large negative charge afforded by the extra carboxylic acid is critical in the calcium-binding properties of several clotting factors. Antithrombin III is an important regulatory protein, but as its name implies, it antagonizes the clotting cascade by irreversibly binding to activated thrombin. Antithrombin III is similar to the protein α_1-antitrypsin, which inhibits elastase in the lung.

41 **The answer is C** *Hematopoietic and lymphoreticular system / Hematology / Anticoagulation*

Heparin, a large, negatively charged polysaccharide, acts by increasing the speed of binding of antithrombin III to thrombin, increasing the effectiveness of antithrombin III. Because it directly affects the clotting cascade, heparin's onset of action is relatively acute. Tissue plasminogen activator and urokinase both cleave plasminogen to plasmin, the active form. Plasmin cleaves the cross-linked fibrin clot in the connector rod regions, converting the clot to a multitude of fibrin monomers. Thus, tissue plasminogen activator and urokinase act in an extremely direct fashion to dissolve established clots (which may be growing); therefore, they are the mainstay in the treatment of acute myocardial infarction. Aspirin irreversibly inhibits cyclo-oxygenase in all cells of the body. For platelets, this irreversible enzyme inhibition means irreversible platelet inhibition because platelets have no protein synthesis machinery. Because platelet activation depends on enzymatic release of arachidonic acid metabolites, such as thromboxane, inhibition of the enzyme permanently inactivates the platelet. Streptokinase acts by aiding the enzymatic cleavage of inactive plasminogen to active plasmin. Its action is similar to that of urokinase and tissue plasminogen activator; however, it is much less specific, markedly antigenic, and no longer the drug of choice. Warfarin competitively inhibits vitamin K from binding to the liver enzymes that are responsible for carboxylation. Vitamin K antagonists like dicumarol have a slow onset of action, are easily overcome by vitamin K injections, and are important therapeutics in patients with a need for chronic anticoagulation.

42 **The answer is A** *Cardiovascular system / Microbiology / Pneumocystis pneumonia*

Silver stains are used in tissue sections to identify fungi and some protozoa. This silver stain demonstrates black cysts of *Pneumocystis carinii* with a green background counterstain. Infection by *P. carinii* is characterized by cup-shaped cysts 4 to 7 mm in diameter, frequently with a dot-like black accentuation of the cyst wall visible upon silver staining. These cysts resemble schistocytes in red blood cell smears. Pneumocystis pneumonia is characterized by alveolar filling by a frothy, honeycomb exudate, and silver staining highlights the cysts within this proteinaceous matrix.

43 **The answer is D** *Central and peripheral nervous system / Biostatistics / Genetic disorders*

The patient had a brother with poliodystrophy; therefore, the patient's mother and father must be carriers. The patient herself may be heterozygous or homozygous for the dominant allele of the poliodystrophy gene. The probability that a child born to two known carriers will be healthy is 3/4; the probability that such a child is also a carrier is 1/2. Thus,

$$P(\text{patient carrier} - \text{patient healthy}) = P(\text{patient carrier and patient healthy})/P(\text{patient healthy})$$
$$= (1/2) \div (3/4)$$
$$= 2/3$$

44 **The answer is A** *Musculoskeletal system / Pharmacology / Nonsteroidal anti-inflammatory drugs; inflammation; cyclo-oxygenase*

Although acetaminophen is traditionally grouped with nonsteroidal anti-inflammatory drugs (NSAIDs), it has no anti-inflammatory effects. Its use in clinical forms of arthritis presumably is secondary to its analgesic effects. Acetaminophen in pharmacological concentrations does not inhibit either COX-I or COX-II but, rather, has activity against a variant of the former gene (COX-III). This form is expressed in the central nervous system and accounts for the antipyretic effects of acetaminophen. Like aspirin, however, acetaminophen does not lower a normal body temperature nor is it useful for severe pain from visceral organs (that is often times treated with narcotic analgesics). Unlike aspirin, there is no association of acetaminophen with Reyes syndrome.

45 The answer is C *General principles / Microbiology / Bacterial meningitis*

The findings of fever, headache, nuchal rigidity, and lethargy with an acute onset and the lack of dramatic neurologic manifestations suggest acute bacterial meningitis. Viral meningitis causes much the same symptoms, but the onset is more insidious and the patient usually is less acutely ill. Patients with viral encephalitis display the same general symptoms as those with viral meningitis, but encephalitis is differentiated by dramatic neurologic manifestations and a much poorer prognosis. Fungal meningitis is more chronic and is frequently seen with other systemic signs of mycotic disease. Brain abscess usually is seen with other foci of infection, and the patient typically has deficits that reflect the location of the lesion.

46 The answer is E *General principles / Toxicology / Nonsteroidal anti-inflammatory drugs*

Aspirin hypersensitivity is a common adverse effect of the use of aspirin. It results in a cross-tolerance to most other NSAIDs except acetaminophen. The hypersensitivity involves urticaria, bronchial hyperreactivity, pruritis, and other symptoms of a non-IgE-mediated anaphylactoid-like phenomenon. Although the basis of it is unclear, it is noteworthy that it can be prevented in many patients by administration of leukotriene receptor antagonist supporting the notion that arachidonic acid is shuttled via lipoxygenase pathway when COX-I (or -II) is inhibited.

47 The answer is A *General principles / Pathology / Cellular injury*

Microscopic indicators of reversible cellular injury include plasma membrane alterations including blebbing and loosening of intercellular attachments, swelling of mitochondria, and dilation of the endoplasmic reticulum. Microscopic indicators of irreversible cell injury and apoptotic demise include cell shrinkage, chromatin condensation, and severe blebbing of cytoplasmic membrane and formation of apoptotic bodies. Cellular eosinophilia is seen in necrotic tissue and is caused by reduction in cellular RNA content.

48 The answer is C *General principles / Pathology / Lysosomal storage diseases*

Mechanisms for the development of lysosomal storage diseases include enzyme deficiency or inactivity, enzyme activator deficiency, defective posttranslational processing of enzyme (mannose 6-phosphate marker for routing to lysosomes), or lack of the proper transport proteins for the egress of digested materials from the lysosome.

49 The answer is B *General principles / Histology / Mitochondrial intracellular localization*

Mitochondria typically exist in cell areas that use substantial amounts of adenosine triphosphate (ATP). They are abundant in the apices of ciliated cells because the beating action of cilia consumes ATP. Mitochondria are distributed evenly throughout the cytoplasm of smooth muscle cells, steroid-secreting cells, skeletal muscle cells, and liver parenchymal cells rather than existing in apical concentrations.

50 The answer is C *Gastrointestinal system / Microbiology / Infectious hepatitis*

HBsAg is the earliest serologic marker of the hepatitis B virus infection. It indicates active infection (acute or chronic) and usually appears before the onset of symptoms. By the end of 6 months, HBsAg has declined to undetectable levels in most patients. Hepatitis C, also called non-A, non-B, or transfusion-associated hepatitis, progresses to chronic hepatitis in as many as 60% of infected individuals; 2% to 3% of the general population may be HCV carriers. Hepatitis D infection requires coexisting hepatitis B infection because it needs the hepatitis B virus encapsulation (i.e., surface antigen). Hepatitis B causes subclinical disease in two-thirds of infected individuals; fulminant hepatitis occurs in fewer than 1% of affected individuals, and progression to hepatocellular carcinoma occurs in fewer than 5%. Hepatitis A is not common in the United States but is very common in developing countries because it is spread by the fecal–oral route. The carrier state does not exist for hepatitis A infections.

test **2**

Questions

Directions: Single best answer questions consist of numbered items or incomplete statements followed by answers or by completions of the statement. Select the ONE lettered answer or completion that is BEST in each case.

1 The figure depicts log concentration time curves for three drugs (X, Y, and Z) after identical amounts of each drug were administered as a bolus at time zero. Which of the following statements regarding these drugs is correct?

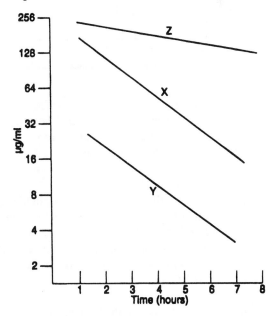

(A)   Volume of distribution (V_d) of X = Z < Y
(B)   Half-time of elimination ($t_{1/2}$) of X = Y > Z
(C)   Clearance of X (CL_X) = CL_Y
(D) CL_Z > CL_X
(E)   Elimination rate constant (k) of X < (k) of Y

2 The swollen-belly appearance of patients suffering from some forms of malnutrition may be ascribed to

(A)   lowered hydrostatic capillary pressure
(B)   decreased plasma oncotic pressure
(C)   elevated interstitial hydrostatic pressure
(D)   increased interstitial oncotic pressure
(E)   increased contraction of lymphatic smooth muscle

3 A 29-year-old man whose father died of Huntington's chorea when he was an infant is obsessively worried about developing the disease, symptoms of which appear in one's 30s or 40s. Although he knows little about the genetic disorder, he is aware that there is a 50% likelihood that he has the dominant Huntington's gene. One day, he impulsively rushes to a testing center and demands to initiate presymptomatic testing, making no attempt to hide his intention to commit suicide if he receives positive results. It would be ethically defensible for the testing center staff to

(A)   refuse to initiate testing
(B)   educate him about the disease and initiate testing
(C)   initiate counseling to alleviate his anxieties, educate him about the disease, and defer testing until he is more stable
(D)   test him and report negative results regardless of the actual results
(E)   test him for other diseases

4 A 57-year-old man complains of having episodes of chest pain. His blood pressure is 160/100 mm Hg, he has been smoking one pack of cigarettes every day for the past 40 years, and both his legs are amputated at the knee. Which one of the following actions is most appropriate?

(A) Because of the patient's amputations, a coronary angiogram should be performed in lieu of an exercise test

(B) The patient does not need an exercise test because his possible coronary artery disease can easily be assessed at rest

(C) The patient should immediately be rushed to the operating room for emergency bypass surgery

(D) Administration of dipyridamole should be used as a substitute for exercise in assessing the extent of the patient's potential coronary artery disease

(E) The patient is advised to quit smoking and to take one aspirin per day; he can safely return to work

5 Which one of the following statements accurately describes pressure–volume relationships, as shown in the accompanying figure, in the lungs of a healthy individual?

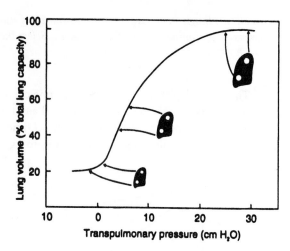

(A) At lung volumes close to functional residual capacity (FRC), alveoli at the base of the lung are smaller than alveoli at the top

(B) At lung volumes close to vital capacity (VC), alveoli at the top of the lung are smaller than alveoli at the base

(C) Alveoli in the base of the lung begin filling first during inspiration from residual volume

(D) Alveoli in the apex receive greater ventilation during inspiration from volumes near FRC

(E) Alveoli in the base of the lung close at volumes near VC

6 In the general format of the Henderson–Hasselbalch equation,

$$\log([\text{protonated form}]/[\text{unprotonated form}]) + pK'_a = pH.$$

Phenobarbital is a weak acid. In an emergency, a useful maneuver to hasten its elimination in an intoxicated person might be

(A) inhalation of CO_2

(B) infusion of $NaHCO_3$

(C) infusion of NH_4Cl

(D) induction of P_{450} enzymes with a separate barbiturate

(E) infusion of dextrose

7 The stain demonstrating the mycobacterial organisms depicted in Figure 7 from the color plate section is best classified as a

(A) Gram stain
(B) acid-fast stain
(C) silver stain
(D) mucicarmine stain

8 Which of the following statements most accurately describes specific features of neuromuscular transmission?

(A) Each muscle fiber contains multiple axon terminals
(B) The end plate is highly enriched in electrically excitable gates
(C) Enzymatic degradation of the transmitter can terminate transmission
(D) Acetylcholine (ACh) causes chloride channels to open as a result of membrane depolarization

9 A man acquires a cold sore from his girlfriend through ordinary kissing. Assuming that this man will exhibit recurrent infections, which nerve axon might this disease traverse during reinfection?

(A) Cranial nerve (CN) VII (upper and lower buccal branches)
(B) CN V and the marginal mandibular branch of CN VII
(C) CN V_2 and CN V_3
(D) CN V_1 only

10 DNA replication can be best described by which of the following statements? It

(A) initiates at random sites on the chromosome
(B) begins at multiple origins on the *Escherichia coli* chromosome
(C) is unidirectional for all DNAs
(D) is not dependent on the synthesis of RNA primers
(E) occurs during the S phase of the cell cycle

11 The accompanying figure shows volume–pressure curves from three subjects of the same age, sex, and body size. If subject B is normal, which one of the following statements is most accurate?

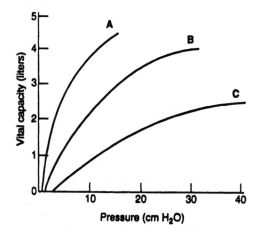

(A) Subject A has a stiff lung (fibrosis)
(B) Subject A has a flabby lung (emphysema)
(C) Subject A has a higher elastic recoil pressure than the other subjects
(D) Subject C is likely to have a higher functional residual capacity than the others
(E) Subject C has the lowest elastic recoil pressure of the three

12 A 20-year-old man has a penile lesion that is crateriform, moist, and indurated. The patient revealed that this lesion has been present for about 20 days and is not painful. Which one of the following groups of tests is most appropriate?

(A) Gram stain, Venereal Disease Research Laboratory (VDRL) test, and culture of the lesion for *Treponema pallidum*
(B) Gram stain and culture of the lesion for *T. pallidum*
(C) VDRL and dark-field examination
(D) Fluorescent treponemal antibody absorption (FTA-ABS) test

13 Which one of the following techniques would be the best way to study a new kind of growth factor that induces proliferation of certain cell types?

(A) Measure uptake of radiolabeled methionine into cells after addition of the growth factor
(B) Measure uptake of radiolabeled thymidine into cells after addition of the growth factor
(C) Measure uptake of radiolabeled uracil into cells after addition of the growth factor
(D) Trypan blue exclusion

14 Which one of the following statements concerning expiration is correct?

(A) At lung volumes close to VC, expiratory air flow is independent of expiratory effort

(B) At lung volumes close to VC, airway resistance is at its peak

(C) At lung volumes close to VC, expiratory air flow increases with increasing pleural pressures

(D) At 50% of VC, increased expiratory effort results in decreased airway resistance

(E) At lung volumes close to residual volume, the elastic recoil of the chest wall is directed inward

15 A 70-year-old woman is brought to the emergency department by her daughter, who noticed that her mother is not as energetic as she was previously. In the emergency department, the patient relates a history of increasing fatigability and shortness of breath over the past several months. On examination, the patient has elevated neck veins, rales in the back, and a third heart sound (S_3 gallop rhythm). Chest radiography reveals an enlarged cardiac silhouette and increased vascular markings. The patient has a heart rate of 90 and a blood pressure of 150/100. Based on this history and physical examination, the patient is most like to have

(A) atrial fibrillation

(B) ventricular paroxysmal tachycardia

(C) congestive heart failure

(D) adult respiratory distress syndrome

(E) rebound hypertensive crisis

16 The accompanying figure shows a hypothetical series of pressure–volume loops of the left ventricle of a control subject and a patient with congestive heart failure before and after digitalis. Based on these data, which of the following is correct?

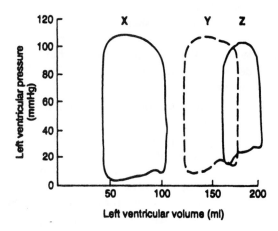

(A) X: control; Y: before digitalis; Z: after digitalis

(B) X: control; Z: before digitalis; Y: after digitalis

(C) Z: control; X: before digitalis; Y: after digitalis

(D) Z: control; Y: before digitalis; X: after digitalis

17 Figure 8 from the color plate section depicts tissue taken from a skin lesion of a 35-year-old homosexual man. Grossly, the lesion had a purple appearance. The correct diagnosis is

(A) Kaposi's sarcoma

(B) hemangiopericytoma

(C) bacillary angiomatosis

(D) arteriovenous malformation

18 Which of the following areas of the central nervous system (CNS) contain structures that are considered to be phylogenically the oldest parts of the brain?

(A) Frontal lobe

(B) Limbic system

(C) Cerebellum

(D) Visual cortex

19 RNA processing can be best described by which of the following statements? It

(A) occurs in the cytoplasm

(B) results in the addition of nucleotides to the primary transcript of ribosomal RNA (rRNA)

(C) results in the formation of new covalent bonds between RNA and DNA

(D) includes the addition of a tail of polyadenylic acid at the 5′ end

(E) includes the methylation of nucleotides in RNA

20 A 10-year-old girl is seen by her pediatrician for flu-like symptoms that were followed weeks later by a peculiar expanding skin rash (erythema chronicum migrans) and months later by monoauricular arthritis. Clinical laboratory findings include a positive titer against *Borrelia burgdorferi*. A likely diagnosis for this child includes which one of the following diseases?

(A) Leptospirosis
(B) Lyme disease
(C) Rocky Mountain spotted fever
(D) Relapsing fever
(E) Yaws

21 Histamine increases the vascular permeability of which of the following?

(A) Arterioles
(B) Large arteries
(C) Venules
(D) Capillaries
(E) Lymphatics

22 The following sequence is a part of a globular protein. Which of the following statements best describes this peptide? SER-VAL-ASP-ASP-VAL-PHE-SER-GLU-VAL-CYS-HIS-MET-ARG.

(A) At pH 7.4, the peptide has a net negative charge
(B) It has only one sulfur-containing amino acid
(C) The hydrophobic amino acid content exceeds the hydrophilic content
(D) Treatment with chymotrypsin would generate four smaller fragments
(E) Only three of the side chains are capable of forming hydrogen bonds

23 A rational approach to the treatment of ventricular tachycardia associated with myocardial ischemia in a hospitalized patient includes

(A) digitalis
(B) diltiazem
(C) lidocaine
(D) propranolol
(E) verapamil

24 What color would the kidney tumor in the accompanying figure be?

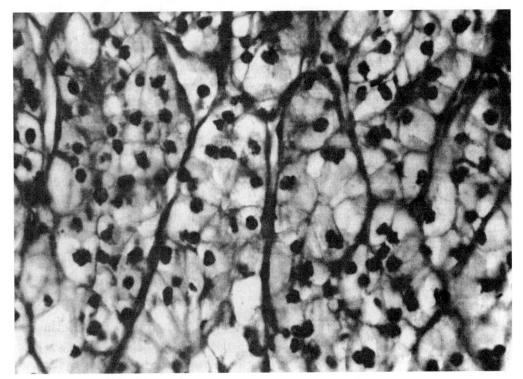

(A) Gray
(B) Translucent with a pink hue
(C) White
(D) Yellow

25 If an individual has a genetic defect in the enzyme that produces *N*-acetylglutamate, the most likely clinical finding would be hyperammonemia with

(A) elevated levels of argininosuccinate (the condensation product of citrulline and aspartate)
(B) no detectable citrulline
(C) elevated levels of arginine
(D) elevated levels of urea
(E) no detectable ornithine

26 Figure 9 from the color plate section depicts biopsy tissue from a raised brown nodule on the skin of a patient. The slide depicts cells containing

(A) iron
(B) lipofuscin
(C) melanin
(D) glycogen

27 Which one of the following clinical procedures best demonstrates damage to the cerebellum?

(A) Testing for voluntary weakness by having the patient grasp the examiner's fingers and squeeze as hard as possible
(B) Tapping the patellar tendon and observing the reflex response
(C) Having the patient flex the neck, touching the chin to the sternum, to determine if this action elicits pain
(D) Passively moving the patient's limbs to elicit an increased resistance to motion

28 Which of the following statements concerning the action potentials illustrated is correct?

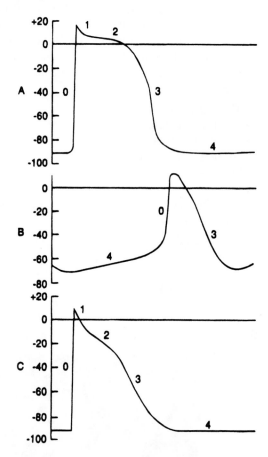

(A) *Trace B* represents the action potential from a myocardial cell in the left ventricle
(B) *Trace B* represents the action potential from a cell in the sinoatrial (SA) node
(C) *Trace C* represents the action potential from a cell in the atrioventricular (AV) node
(D) In *trace A*, concentration of the cells in the left ventricle correlates with *phase 4*
(E) In *trace A*, the cell can be further stimulated to generate another action potential during all of *phase 3*

29 Which of the following clinical conditions is not likely to be associated with or a cause of bronchiectasis?

(A) Alpha-1 antitrypsin deficiency
(B) Cystic fibrosis
(C) Necrotizing pneumonia
(D) Intralobular sequestration of the lung
(E) Kartagener's syndrome

30 A 39-year-old man presents for his regularly scheduled physical examination. During the cardiac portion of the examination, a palpable presystolic apical impulse is noted, and an S_4 is heard on auscultation. Which one of the following statements is most likely correct?

(A) The patient may have hypertrophic left ventricle secondary to aortic stenosis

(B) The patient likely has some form of underlying heart disease (e.g., myocardial infarction, mitral regurgitation)

(C) The patient has increased ventricular compliance

(D) The patient has aggravated hypotension

(E) The patient is undergoing atrial fibrillation

31 The upstroke of the ventricular action potential is primarily due to which one of the following actions?

(A) An inward flux of Ca^{2+}

(B) An inward K^+ current

(C) An outward K^+ current

(D) An outward Na^+ current

(E) An inward Na^+ current

32 Figure 10 from the color plate section depicts biopsy tissue from a patient with a saddle nose deformity, otalgia, and cavitating pulmonary nodules. Which of the following laboratory results would be expected from this patient?

(A) A decreased sedimentation rate

(B) Antineutrophil antibodies

(C) Hypercholesterolemia

(D) Antimitochondrial antibodies

33 A patient with previously suspected cholelithiasis presents with a fever of 39.4°C and an elevated serum white blood cell count (12,400/mm^3). Which of the following is a common pathogen in acute cholecystitis?

(A) Staphylococci

(B) Streptococci

(C) *Pseudomonas* species

(D) *Clostridium* species

(E) *Neisseria* species

34 Which of the following is a known predisposing factor for cholesterol and mixed stone formation?

(A) Chronic use of nonsteroidal anti-inflammatory drugs (NSAIDs)

(B) Obesity

(C) Excessive intake of vitamins

(D) Alcoholic cirrhosis

(E) Low-fiber diet

35 Which of the following statements correctly characterizes important contributors to the pathogenesis of cholelithiasis?

(A) Gallbladder hypomotility leads to the accumulation of biliary sludge, which is an important precursor of stone formation

(B) Decreased hydroxymethylglutaryl coenzyme A (HMG CoA) reductase activity and increased secretion of bile acids can greatly increase the stone-forming potential of bile

(C) Conjugated bilirubin associated with chronic hemolysis leads to the formation of pigmented stones

(D) Chronic infection of the biliary tree leads to nonpigmented stone formation by increasing the amount of conjugate bilirubin

(E) Decreased lecithin or bile acid synthesis results in an increased capacity for solubilizing biliary cholesterol

36 A 32-year-old woman visits her physician because of agitation, weight loss, and inability to sleep. When questioned further, she reveals an increased appetite and increased frequency of bowel movements. Previously, she had regular menstrual periods, but now they are less frequent and irregular. During the physical examination, the physician notes that her skin is warm and moist and that she has a fine tremor of the fingers, hyperreflexia, and lid lag. The woman has moderately severe exophthalmos, and her upward gaze seems weak and uncoordinated. Which one of the following disease processes is most likely manifesting itself?

(A) A thyroid adenoma that is secreting thyroxine

(B) Inappropriate hypothalamic secretion of thyrotropin-releasing hormone (TRH)

(C) Graves' disease

(D) Hashimoto's disease

(E) Sick euthyroid syndrome

37 Deficiency of alpha-L-iduronidase with accumulations of dermatan sulfate and heparan sulfate is characteristic of which disease?

(A) Mucopolysaccharidosis I

(B) Mucopolysaccharidosis II

(C) Gaucher's disease

(D) Fabry's disease

(E) Nieman–Pick disease type A

38 Bronchiolitis obliterans organizing pneumonia is histologically described as

- (A) a solid zone of inflammation with isolated multinucleated giant cells
- (B) a honeycomb pattern of lung with marked interstitial fibrosis and cystic transformation of pulmonary parenchyma
- (C) an exudative interstitial reaction with common intra-arterial thrombosis
- (D) a protein-rich, intra-alveolar edema with giant cells, chronic inflammatory cells, and eosinophils
- (E) replacement of terminal bronchioles with loose connective tissue, mild chronic inflammation of the alveolar septa, and alveolar collapse

39 Which of the following environmental insults is the most important risk factor for urothelial carcinoma?

- (A) Cigarette smoking
- (B) Exposure to automobile exhaust fumes
- (C) Intermittent catheterization
- (D) Nitrate consumption
- (E) Radon gas

40 Which of the following statements correctly pairs a useful medication for the treatment of Graves' disease and hyperthyroidism with its mechanism of action?

- (A) Propylthiouracil blocks the coupling reaction in thyroxine (T_4) synthesis
- (B) Methimazole reduces peripheral conversion of T_4 to tri-iodothyronine (T_3)
- (C) Radioactive iodine destroys follicular cells in the thyroid but is no longer used because of its carcinogenic effects
- (D) Prednisone blocks the sympathetic components of thyrotoxicosis
- (E) Propranolol may relieve mechanical exophthalmos and opthalmoplegia by reducing inflammation

41 Which of the following statements does not describe the epidemiology of the adrenal neoplasm pictured in Figure 11 from the color plate section?

- (A) 10% are malignant
- (B) 10% are pigmented
- (C) 10% are bilateral
- (D) 10% are familial

42 Which of the following types of proteins exhibit a structure that is common for physiologic components of cellular signal transduction systems?

- (A) Cytoskeleton proteins, such as actin
- (B) Lysosomal proteins
- (C) Mitochondrial proteins, such as cytochrome oxidase
- (D) GTP-binding proteins (or G-proteins)
- (E) Metallothioneins

43 Which of the following statements correctly describes the genetic code?

- (A) It is distinctly different for each organism
- (B) It consists of nucleotides that form codons of variable length
- (C) It represents all of the nucleotide sequence information within a transcription unit
- (D) It contains transcription start and stop sequences
- (E) It contains only one codon for each amino acid

44 Figure 12 from the color plate section depicts tissue from a needle biopsy of the prostate. Which of the following conditions is demonstrated?

- (A) Adenosis
- (B) Nodular hyperplasia
- (C) Adenocarcinoma
- (D) Chronic prostatitis with glandular atrophy

45 Which of the following supports biologic theory?

- (A) The effects of certain medications on the symptoms of schizophrenia
- (B) Normal ventricular size in significant numbers of patients with schizophrenia
- (C) No family history in many cases of bipolar disorder
- (D) The lack of effect of stimulant medication on the symptoms of attention deficit disorder in some children
- (E) Monozygotic twins discordant for schizophrenia

46 Which one of the following statements best describes the regulation of vascular smooth muscle during exercise?

(A) There is vasoconstriction in all vessels due to the increased sympathetic outflow that occurs during exercise

(B) Increased circulating levels of metabolic products such as H^1, CO_2, and adenosine cause vasodilation in all vessels

(C) Increased blood flow during exercise causes a cascade of events leading to release of nitric oxide and vasoconstriction

(D) Local metabolic vasodilator signals in the vessels of active skeletal muscle can overcome the vasoconstrictor signals of increased sympathetic outflow and cause a net vasodilation and increased perfusion of those muscles

(E) The ability of muscles to extract a higher percentage of the delivered oxygen makes it unnecessary for any changes in vascular smooth muscle activity to occur

47 The kidney tumor depicted in Figure 13 from the color plate section is sometimes associated with which one of the following conditions?

(A) Adrenal cortical carcinoma

(B) Tuberous sclerosis

(C) Seminomas of the testes

(D) Erythrocythemia

48 Which of the following nephritides is associated with normal complement levels?

(A) Immunoglobulin A (IgA) nephropathy

(B) Mesangioproliferative glomerulonephropathy

(C) Serum sickness

(D) Systemic lupus erythematosus (SLE)

(E) Vasculitis

49 Which of the following statements describing cell–extracellular matrix interactions is correct?

(A) Integrins are soluble nuclear proteins that directly alter gene transcription

(B) Tubulins, which are found in basement membranes, stimulate endothelial cells to organize into tube-like structures

(C) Fibronectin fragments play a pivotal role in wound healing by promoting migration of endothelial cells and fibroblasts to the damaged area

(D) Osteogenesis imperfecta is caused by inherited defects in laminin

(E) Receptor cholesterols on the surface of platelets are crucial to platelet aggregation at sites of exposed subendothelium

50 Which of the following human leukocyte antigen (HLA) associations is correctly paired?

(A) Rheumatoid arthritis—HLA-DR3

(B) Primary Sjögren's syndrome—HLA-DR4

(C) 21-Hydroxylase deficiency—HLA-DR4

(D) Postgonococcal arthritis—HLA-B27

(E) Chronic active hepatitis—HLA-DR1

Answer Key

1-A	11-B	21-C	31-E	41-B
2-B	12-C	22-A	32-B	42-D
3-C	13-B	23-C	33-D	43-D
4-D	14-C	24-D	34-B	44-C
5-A	15-C	25-B	35-A	45-A
6-B	16-B	26-C	36-C	46-D
7-B	17-A	27-B	37-A	47-B
8-C	18-B	28-C	38-E	48-A
9-C	19-E	29-A	39-A	49-C
10-E	20-B	30-A	40-A	50-D

Answers and Explanations

1 **The answer is A** *General principles / Pharmacology / Pharmacokinetics*

The volume of distribution (V_d) is the ratio of the amount injected to the extrapolated concentration (C_0) at time zero. Because equal amounts of X, Y, and Z were injected, V_d is inversely related to C_0. Therefore, X and Z have an identical V_d, and V_d Y > V_d X or V_d Z. Clearance is proportional to the ratio of V_d to $t_{1/2}$ Y), clearance of Z < clearance of X.

2 **The answer is B** *Cardiovascular system / Physiology / Capillary water and solute exchange*

According to Starling's forces, net filtration pressure is proportional to the difference in hydrostatic pressure between capillaries and interstitium minus the difference between oncotic pressure between capillaries and interstitium. The interstitial edema in patients with protein malnutrition results in the swollen belly appearance. This is most likely due to decreased plasma oncotic pressure secondary to malnutrition (kwashiorkor) that results in decreased manufacture of plasma proteins. Although these patients may have decreased hydrostatic pressure (or elevated interstitial hydrostatic pressure), these would result in decreased net filtration of fluids. Increased contraction of lymphatic smooth muscle (perhaps secondary to sympathetic stimulation) would be expected to ameliorate interstitial edema by hastening the removal of fluid and protein from the interstitium.

3 **The answer is C** *General principles / Behavioral science / Medical ethics*

The man's highly emotional state indicates that he may not be competent. Providing counseling and educating him about his options make a reasoned decision possible. Until he appears competent, his demand for testing is overridden by the physician's duty to prevent a suicide (beneficence). Lying to him about test results would disrespect his autonomy, as would refusing to test him without attempting to facilitate a state of mind in which he could make a reasoned decision. Testing for other diseases would be irrelevant as well as impractical.

4 **The answer is D** *Cardiovascular system / Pathology / Coronary artery disease*

The risk factors for coronary artery disease include hypertension, hyperlipidemia, smoking, and diabetes mellitus. Angina is a symptom of the disease. Assessment of a patient for coronary artery disease is aided by an exercise test because the clinically detectable manifestations of this disease often are not present at rest. Such an assessment is important before either performing surgery or releasing someone at high risk for sudden death. Dipyridamole is a vasodilator that acts by inhibiting adenosine metabolism. It causes increased coronary blood flow and can be used to assess coronary artery blockage. Thus, more invasive techniques may be put on hold.

5 **The answer is A** *Respiratory system / Physiology / Pulmonary mechanics*

Pleural pressure is not equally distributed from the base to the apex. For a variety of reasons, the pleural pressure is more negative at the apex, and therefore the transpulmonary pressure (i.e., alveolar–pleural pressure) is greater at the apex. The pressure–volume relationship depends on the lung's elastic properties, which are constant from base to apex. If it is correctly interpreted, the graph answers the question. The alveoli at different places in the lungs are subject to different pressures and thus have different volumes. At lung volumes close to FRC, which is the resting lung volume, the pressure–volume relationship is steep. Thus, the alveoli at the base, which have slightly smaller pressures, have much smaller volumes. At volumes close to VC, the transluminal pressure has reached the flat portion of the curve, so that the small pressure differences from base to apex no longer matter; alveoli are uniformly inflated. The transluminal pressure is actually negative (therefore closing the alveoli) at the base when the lungs are near residual volume. Not until the lungs have begun filling elsewhere do these alveoli open up again. Alveoli in the apex are nearer full at FRC than are alveoli at the base; therefore, they receive less ventilation than the alveoli at the base. In other words, alveoli that are already full do not have much room for more ventilation.

6 **The answer is B** *General principles / Pharmacology / Pharmacokinetics; pH partitioning*

A weak acid such as phenobarbital tends to be in its ionized form at a higher pH. Therefore, alkalinizing the urine with $NaHCO_3$ has the desired effect of hastening renal elimination. In addition, urine flow increases in the presence of alkali, further increasing the amount of phenobarbital that is eliminated. Alkalinization of plasma also tends to move un-ionized phenobarbital out of the CNS and into the plasma by creating a transient gradient in which movement can occur. Phenobarbital and other barbiturates tend to induce P_{450} enzymes, which should aid the elimination of these drugs. However, the induction of P_{450} enzymes is somewhat slower than desired in an emergency.

7 **The answer is B** *General principles / Microbiology / Staining techniques*

Acid-fast stains are used to demonstrate mycobacteria. They characteristically stain the mycolic acids within the cell wall of the mycobacteria, resulting in a red beaded appearance of the bacillary forms. This has led to the colloquial designation of mycobacterial agents as red snappers. Acid-fast stain morphology of the bacteria cannot discriminate among species. Variations of this stain can also demonstrate *Nocardia* and *Rhodococcus* species.

8 **The answer is C** *Central and peripheral nervous system / Physiology / Neuromuscular transmission*

Motor neurons innervate many skeletal muscle fibers. In large muscles, thousands of fibers may be innervated by one neuron. However, each fiber receives only one axon terminal. Depolarization of the nerve terminal releases ACh into the synaptic cleft, where it binds directly to Na^1 channels, causing an end-plate potential. The end plate itself is not electrically excitable, but passive spreading of end-plate potential to a nearby membrane leads to propagation of the action potential and contraction of all muscle fibers innervated by the motoneuron. When ACh is the neurotransmitter, termination of transmission is accomplished by hydrolysis via acetylcholinesterase.

9 **The answer is C** *Central and peripheral nervous system / Microbiology; anatomy / Herpes simplex virus of the nervous system*

Cold sores are caused by the herpes simplex virus (HSV), which usually infects the lips, philtrum, and the areas around the nares of affected individuals. After the primary infection, HSV establishes a latent state in the ganglia of CN V where the second (CN V_2) and third (CN V_3) branches of this nerve innervate the described areas. CN VII is not infected by this virus.

10 **The answer is E** *General principles / Genetics / DNA replication*

DNA replication begins at specific sites. In *Escherichia coli*, DNA replication starts at a unique origin and proceeds sequentially in opposite directions. Because of the size of the eukaryotic genome, multiple replication origins are important for timely DNA replication. DNA polymerase cannot start chains de novo; all known DNA polymerases add mononucleotides to the 39 hydroxyl end of an RNA primer, or as in the case of adenovirus replication, DNA synthesis begins from a serine residue on a protein primer. DNA replication occurs during the S phase of the cell cycle.

11 **The answer is B** *Respiratory system / Physiology / Pulmonary mechanics*

Compliance is defined as a change in volume over change in pressure. The steeper the curves of the static volume–pressure relationships shown in the figure, the more compliant the lungs. A compliant, or flabby, lung is typical of emphysema, in which recoil pressures are lower at any given lung volume and the functional residual capacity tends to be higher. In contrast, a fibrotic, stiff lung (subject C) has decreased compliance and increased elastic recoil and tends to have a lower functional residual capacity. This increased elastic recoil pulls the chest wall in until the outward recoil of the chest wall equals (but is opposite) the inward recoil of the lung, which lowers functional residual capacity.

12 **The answer is C** *Respiratory system / Pathology; microbiology / Diagnosis of syphilis*

A VDRL test and dark-field examination would be the most appropriate combination of tests for determining the cause of the penile lesion. A painless penile lesion that is crateriform, moist, and indurated suggests primary syphilis. The organism responsible, *T. pallidum,* cannot be cultured or detected by Gram stain. It can, however, be visualized by dark-field observation of scrapings from the lesion. Some but not all patients with primary syphilis have serologic evidence of infection, readily detected by the VDRL test. The FTA-ABS test is used only to confirm diagnosis and is not appropriate here.

13 **The answer is B** *General principles / Genetics / Radiolabeled nucleic acid utilization*

One of the best methods for measuring cellular proliferation is measuring the uptake of radiolabeled nucleic acid. Dividing cells require nucleotides for DNA synthesis, and the uptake of labeled thymidine and its incorporation in DNA are excellent indicators of cell proliferation. Uracil, which (except for some that is reconstituted through a salvage pathway) is used only in RNA synthesis, does not indicate cell division, only messenger RNA (mRNA) synthesis. Likewise, uptake and incorporation of radiolabeled methionine entails protein synthesis, not cell division. Trypan blue exclusion is used for quantitating viability and would not be useful in this experiment.

14 **The answer is C** *Respiratory system / Physiology / Pulmonary mechanics*

According to the equal pressure point theory, expiratory effort increases flow until airways are actually closed off by the pressure of the effort. Inspiratory efforts that lead to vital capacity inflate the lungs to a large end-inspiratory pressure. Therefore, positive alveolar pressure is sufficient to maintain patency through all airways, even with a large expiratory effort. Thus, from VC, increased expiratory efforts (i.e., increased positive pleural pressures) are rewarded with increased flow. However, at 50% of VC, increased expiratory efforts only increase the resistance of the airways because the pleural pressure exceeds the alveolar pressure and closes the airways. Because airway resistance decreases with increasing size of the airway, resistance is lowest at vital capacity, where the airways are at their largest caliber. At residual volume, the elastic properties of the chest wall are directed outward. (Try holding your lungs at residual volume for a moment to see how much elastic recoil exists.)

15 **The answer is C** *Cardiovascular system / Pathology; physiology / Congestive heart failure; cardiac mechanics*

The major signs of congestive heart failure are fatigue and dyspnea. Vascular congestion confirmed by physical examination (i.e., neck veins, rales) and third heart sounds due to abnormally high diastolic flow to a normal ventricle or normal flow into a dilated ventricle are also consistent with congestive heart failure. The enlarged cardiac silhouette with pulmonary vascular markings strongly suggests left-sided heart failure. Neither the heart rate nor blood pressure is elevated enough to consider this a malignant arrhythmia or emergency hypertensive crisis.

16 **The answer is B** *Cardiovascular system / Physiology / Congestive heart failure; cardiac mechanics*

In the control subject (X), end-diastolic pressure is low, and ejection is well maintained during systole. In the failing heart, end-diastolic pressure and volume are greatly elevated, and ejection is poorly maintained (stroke volume is reduced). Digitalis (Y) exerts a positive inotropic effect by inhibiting Na^+-K^+ adenosine triphosphatase (ATPase) and indirectly elevating intracellular Ca^{2+}. The effect is to decrease diastolic pressures and volumes and increase stroke volume.

17 **The answer is A** *Skin and related connective tissue / Pathology / Vascular sarcomas*

Kaposi's sarcoma is a presumed neoplasm that occurs frequently in the HIV-positive homosexual population. It is characterized by a proliferation of spindle cells thought to derive from endothelium. The spindle cell proliferation is associated with abundant extravasated red blood cells, which account for the purple discoloration of the overlying skin. Sporadic forms of Kaposi's sarcoma do occur on the distal extremities of non-HIV-positive patients, particularly older individuals.

18 **The answer is B** *Central and peripheral nervous system / Neuroanatomy / Structures of the brain*

The limbic system is concerned with unconscious biologic drives and emotions and therefore is considered the most primitive part of the brain. It contains the limbic lobe, hippocampus, anterior thalamic nucleus, hypothalamus, and the amygdala.

19 **The answer is E** *General principles / Biochemistry / RNA structure and function*

In eukaryotes, mRNA is formed in the nucleus and must be exported to the cytosol for translation. The initial product of transcription includes all of the introns and flanking regions, which must be removed by splicing before correct translation can occur. The splicing reaction involves hydrolysis of phosphodiester bonds and formation of new phosphodiester bonds within the mRNA molecule. Other processing reactions include additions at both the 59 and 39 ends. A guanosine triphosphate (GTP) molecule is added in reverse orientation to form a cap at the 59 end, and the cap is further modified by the addition of methyl groups. A polyadenylate tail is added at the 39 end.

20 **The answer is B** *General principles / Microbiology; pharmacology / Lyme disease*

Lyme disease is a recently described, tickborne disease in which the infectious agent is a spriochete, *Borrelia burgdorferi*. Erythema chronicum migrans and positive antibody to the spirochete are presumed to be diagnostic for this condition, which may be manifested by flu-like symptoms that may ultimately process toward arthritic, cardiac, and CNS symptoms.

21 **The answer is C** *General principles / Pathology / Histamine*

Histamine increases the vascular permeability of venules. It also causes arterioles to dilate and large arteries to constrict but causes no marked change in permeability of these vessels.

22 **The answer is A** *General principles / Biochemistry / Structure and function of amino acids in proteins*

The physical and chemical properties of the peptide reflect the properties of the constituent amino acids. At pH 7.4, the positive and negative charges of the a-amino and a-carboxyl terminal groups cancel one another. The side chains of the two aspartate and one glutamate residues are negatively charged; the side chain of arginine is positively charged. Cysteine and methionine both contain sulfur atoms. Any of the amino acids that contain a hydrogen atom attached to a sulfur, nitrogen, or oxygen atom or that contain an atom with an unshared pair of electrons can form hydrogen bonds. The amino acids valine, phenylalanine, methionine, and cysteine contribute hydrophobic character to the peptide. The specificity of chymotrypsin is for peptide bonds in which the carboxyl group is donated by an aromatic amino acid.

23 **The answer is C** *Cardiovascular system / Pharmacology / Treatment of arrhythmias*

Lidocaine is often the drug of choice for the treatment of ventricular arrhythmia. It suppresses Na^1 currents in the infarct area that have abnormal resting membrane potentials and elevated K^1 levels. If lidocaine fails, the most frequently chosen agent is another Na^1 channel blocker, procainamide. The Ca^{21} channel blockers (diltiazem, verapamil) and b-blockers (propranolol) have a greater effect on supraventricular disturbances in which slow Ca^{21} channels are involved more significantly than Na^1 channels.

24 **The answer is D** *Renal/urinary system / Pathology / Renal cell carcinoma*

The renal mass pictured is classic clear cell carcinoma of the kidney. The cells have round to oval nuclei and inconspicuous nucleoli. The cytoplasm is abundant; it is clear because of the large amounts of glycogen and lipid within these cells (the glycogen accounts for the yellow color). Renal cell carcinomas may be hemorrhagic, and they tend to invade the renal veins and inferior vena cava, from which they may metastasize to the bones and lungs.

25 **The answer is B** *General principles / Biochemistry / Urea cycle*

Urea is the principal compound by which ammonia is excreted from the body. The nitrogens in urea come from ammonia and aspartate. Ammonia reacts with carbon dioxide and adenosine triphosphate (ATP) to form carbamoyl phosphate in a reaction catalyzed by carbamoyl phosphate synthetase (ammonia). This enzyme requires *N*-acetylglutamate as a positive allosteric effector. Without this reaction, urea would not be formed, and ammonia levels would be high. The next step in the urea cycle is the reaction of carbamoyl phosphate with ornithine to form citrulline. In the absence of carbamoyl phosphate, ornithine levels are high, citrulline is undetectable, and neither argininosuccinate nor arginine is formed.

26 **The answer is C** *Skin and related connective tissue / Histology / Melanoma*

This slide demonstrates the classic morphology of a nodular melanoma. There is a proliferation of malignant cells with nuclei of variable size. Several of these nuclei have intranuclear cytoplasmic invaginations, and most of the nuclei have prominent eosinophilic nucleoli, a characteristic of malignant melanoma. The most striking aspect of this neoplastic proliferation is the brown pigment within the cytoplasm of the cells and within melanophages in the adjacent stroma. This pigment is melanin produced by the neoplastic cells themselves. It accounts both for the brown appearance of these nodules in the skin and for the brown appearance of metastatic lesions in the viscera.

27 **The answer is B** *Central and peripheral nervous system / Neuroanatomy / Assessment*

Cerebellar disease manifests as dystonia to palpation but does not alter grip strength. Pain elicited by touching the chin to the chest is known as Brudzinski's sign and usually indicates inflammation of the meninges. Cerebellar disease is indicated by decreased resistance of the limbs to passive movement. Deep tendon reflexes continue for longer than usual; in the patellar tendon this is known as the pendular knee jerk because of the motion of the limb when the reflex is elicited. Patients with cerebellar disease also show voluntary ataxia, dysdiadochokinesia, nystagmus, and dysarthria of the larynx. Cerebellar lesions usually affect the ipsilateral body.

28 The answer is C *Cardiovascular system / Physiology / Electrical activity of the heart*

The traces shown in *A, B,* and *C* are of cells from the left ventricle, SA node, and left atrium, respectively. The refractory period, during which the cell cannot fire another action potential, occurs during the first half to two thirds of *phase 3* in each of the traces. Contraction of the left ventricle occurs during the calcium plateau *(phase 2)* of myocytes in the left ventricle.

Phase 0 cells in the ventricles and atria are marked by the opening of voltage-gated tetrodotoxin-sensitive sodium channels. These "fast" sodium channels are responsible for the rapid upstroke of action potentials in the contractile cells; however, these channels do not seem to play a role in the action potentials of cells in the SA or AV nodes where Ca^{2+} channels conduct *phase 0* of depolarization. The fast sodium channels inactivate almost as rapidly as they activate, so that the increase in sodium conductance, which leads to depolarization, is soon terminated. No sodium currents are activated until the next action potential. The resting potential of contractile myocytes is maintained by a large potassium conductance. An increase in the potassium conductance does not result in rapid depolarization but, rather, mild hyperpolarization caused by a small potassium efflux. However, during the action potential, repolarization (*phase 3* of both traces *A* and *B*) is characterized by an increase in the potassium conductance, leading to an outward potassium current (efflux). Because the cell is depolarized at this time, the increase in potassium current quickly moves the cell toward the resting potential. Calcium-activated potassium currents seem to be particularly important in the ventricular repolarization (*phase 3*); these currents may be the site at which the calcium increases result in an increased heart rate (staircase effect). SA node automaticity (the unique pacemaker potential) occurs in *phase 4* (slow depolarization).

29 The answer is A *Respiratory system / Pathology / Bronchiectasis*

Bronchiectasis is a result of a chronic necrotizing infection of bronchi and bronchioles leading to abnormal dilatation of these airways, which is permanent. It is caused by bronchial obstruction (tumor, mucous impaction, foreign bodies), conditions that lead to a reduction in immune clearance of potential infections, and necrotizing pneumonia. Its pathogenesis is believed to be due to resorption of air distal to the insult and the collection of intraluminal secretions that lead to dilatation. Infection amplifies this expansion by weakening the bronchiolar walls through inflammation and infective insult leading to greater dilatation.

30 The answer is A *Cardiovascular system / Pathology / Fourth heart sound*

Under certain pathologic conditions, the fourth heart sound (S_4) is a low-frequency, presystolic sound that is produced in the ventricle during filling. It occurs on atrial contraction with the flow of blood into a stiffened, noncompliant ventricle. An S_4 is almost never heard during atrial fibrillation. An S_4 is commonly associated with ischemic heart disease, severe hypertension, aortic stenosis, and hypertrophic cardiomyopathies. However, the incidence of S_4 sounds increases with age, and S_4 sounds are often benign findings in a healthy, athletic person. Therefore, whether audible S_4 sounds are in themselves abnormal remains unclear.

31 The answer is E *Cardiovascular system / Physiology / Cardiac physiology*

The upstroke of the ventricular action potential is primarily due to a fast inward Na^+ current. Blockage of the rapid upstroke by tetrodotoxin and other studies have demonstrated this point. The plateau phase of the action potential is maintained by a combination of K^+, Ca^{2+}, and Na^+ currents, whereas repolarization is mainly due to increased K^+ conductance.

32 The answer is B *Respiratory system / Pathology / Wegener's granulomatosis*

This case history is classic for Wegener's granulomatosis, which, in its typical presentation, combines necrotizing granulomas and vasculitis of the upper and lower respiratory tracts with glomerulonephritis. The slide demonstrates areas of necrosis with a palisaded histiocytic reaction and segmental vasculitis. This triad of histologic abnormalities characterizes Wegener's granulomatosis. The presence of cytoplasmic antineutrophil antibodies has recently been noted to be very sensitive for the diagnosis of Wegener's granulomatosis. These autoantibodies are directed at proteinase 3, a serine protease. An elevated sedimentation rate may be seen. No alterations in cholesterol metabolism have been reported.

33 **The answer is D** *General principles / Pathology / Cholecystitis and cholelithiasis*

"Fat, forty, and female" are the features of a patient with a classic case of symptomatic gallstone disease. The pain is correctly described as biliary colic (i.e., severe pain lasting for up to 20 minutes and then subsiding, only to return several more times in the following hours). Such a characterization is highly specific to cholelithiasis. Nausea and vomiting often accompany biliary colic, and mild elevation of serum bilirubin occurs in 25% of these patients. However, none of these is a specific sign for biliary calculi. Ultrasonic radiography is diagnostic in more than 90% of cases and, if available, it is the evaluation of choice. Abdominal rigidity and rebound tenderness are the signs of an acute abdomen, a surgical emergency that is often the result of visceral perforation. Hemoccult-positive stool is a nonspecific indicator of a more urgent problem that requires additional workup. Excessive postprandial flatulence should be evaluated with other more specific signs of abdominal disease. Steatorrhea and lactose intolerance are two fairly common conditions that are associated with a tremendous amount of abdominal gas.

The fever and elevated white blood cell count are explained by an acute infection in the patient's gallbladder. Enterococci, *Escherichia coli, Klebsiella,* and *Clostridium* are commonly occurring enteric pathogens. *Neisseria* are not commonly found in the gut but, rather, cause urinary tract infections and meningitis. Staphylococci and streptococci cause many common infections but are not common causes of cholecystitis.

34 **The answer is B** *Gastrointestinal system / Pathology / Cholecystitis and cholelithiasis*

Cholesterol and mixed stones account for more than 80% of biliary calculi, with the remaining 20% being pigment stones. The risk factors for the more common cholesterol stones fall into two groups: (1) factors that increase cholesterol output, and (2) factors that decrease bile salt secretion. Clofibrate therapy, obesity, pregnancy, and diabetes mellitus all tend to increase cholesterol output. Oral contraceptive use and ileal disease or resection result in fewer bile salt secretions (the ileum is the principal site of bile salt recycling, which is a major source of secreted bile salts). Alcoholic cirrhosis and chronic hemolysis are examples of disease processes that result in elevations of unconjugated serum bilirubin. Insoluble bilirubin can be converted to calcium bilirubinate, the major component of pigment stones.

35 **The answer is A** *Gastrointestinal system / Pathology / Cholecystitis and cholelithiasis*

Cholesterol stones are formed when an imbalance between bile acid secretion and cholesterol output occurs. Increases in cholesterol output or decreases in the cholesterol-solubilizing bile acids result in an increased likelihood of stone formation. HMG CoA reductase performs the rate-limiting step in cholesterol synthesis and, therefore, it is the target of a family of cholesterol-reducing drugs (e.g., lovastatin). Hence, decreases in the activity of HMG CoA, combined with increased bile acid secretion, greatly decrease the stone-forming potential. Gallbladder hypomotility associated with severe trauma, total parenteral nutrition, and oral contraceptives is an important factor in the genesis of bile calculi. Infection of the biliary tree with certain pathogens can result in cleavage of the conjugation moieties, turning soluble conjugated bilirubin into insoluble unconjugated forms.

36 **The answer is C** *Endocrine system / Pathology; pharmacology / Graves' disease and hyperthyroidism*

Severe illness or physical trauma can cause changes in the thyroid hormone regulation, which are referred to as sick euthyroid syndrome (SES). Euthyroid indicates that the patient has sufficient but not excess thyroid hormone function. Clinically, the patient appears normal; however, the thyroid laboratory tests return values that indicate hypothyroidism or hyperthyroidism, depending on the variant of SES. Hashimoto's thyroiditis is characterized in the chronic phase by thyroid insufficiency. Symptoms common in hypothyroidism include lethargy, constipation, cold intolerance, hemorrhage, and weight gain. Dry skin and patchy hair loss emerge as the disease progresses. Graves' disease, thyroid adenomas, and the extremely rare overproduction of TRH by the hypothalamus all result in the hyperthyroid symptoms described. However, the ocular signs (i.e., exophthalmos, extraocular ophthalmoplegia) are characteristic of the disease. The inflammatory reaction against the muscles and connective tissue in the orbit causes edema, muscular weakness, and fibrosis leading to the described symptoms.

37 **The answer is A** *General principles / Pathology / Metabolic disorders*

Deficiency of alpha-L-iduronidase with accumulations of dermatan sulfate and heparan sulfate is characteristic of mucopolysaccharidosis I (MPS I) or Hurler's disease. MPS II or Hunter's disease is associated with a deficiency in L-iduronate sulfatase. Gaucher's disease (autosomal recessive) is characterized by a deficiency in glucocerebrosidase, which results in distended phagocytic cells found in the spleen, liver, bone marrow, lymph node, tonsils, thymus, Peyer's patches, and alveolar septa. Most commonly it is associated with pancytopenia or thrombocytopenia due to hypersplenism. Diagnosis can be made by measurement of glucocerebrosidase activity in peripheral blood leukocytes or cultured fibroblasts. Fabry's disease is characterized by a deficiency in alpha-galactosidase A. Niemann–Pick disease is characterized by a deficiency in sphingomyelinase; type A is a severe deficiency that leads to early death, but type B is a more mild disease with life expectancy extended into adulthood.

38 **The answer is E** *Respiratory system / Pathology / Bronchiolitis obliterans*

Bronchiolitis obliterans is an inflammatory reaction in the terminal bronchioles and alveolar ducts caused most commonly by infectious agents, noxious fumes, or a preexisting collagen disease. Answer D describes chronic eosinophilic pneumonia. Answer C describes diffuse alveolar damage. Answer B describes honeycomb lung. Answer A describes extrinsic allergic alveolitis.

39 **The answer is A** *Renal/urinary system / Pathology / Carcinogenesis*

Cigarette smoking is the most important risk factor for the development of urothelial carcinoma, given the large number of smokers. Arylamines, schistosoma infections, and long-term analgesic use have also been implicated, whereas the other environmental insults have not been strongly linked to urothelial carcinoma carcinogenesis. Radon gas has been linked to the development of cancers of the lung, and nitrate consumption has been associated with development of cancers of the digestive tract.

40 **The answer is A** *Endocrine system / Pathology; pharmacology / Graves' disease and hyperthyroidism*

Propylthiouracil (PTU) and methimazole share a common mechanism of action in inhibiting the synthesis of thyroxine, but methimazole is more potent. However, PTU offers the advantage of reducing the peripheral conversion of T_4 to T_3. PTU is therefore equipped to give faster relief from the symptoms of thyrotoxicosis, because T_3 has substantially more biologic activity. Radioactive iodine is a useful alternative to surgery in the patient who may have preoperative complications (e.g., the elderly, those with severe thyrotoxicosis). No carcinogenic effects have been documented, but radioactive iodine may be contraindicated in women who want to become pregnant in the future. Because the mechanical components of the ocular signs of Graves' disease are inflammatory, they are relieved with large doses of glucocorticoid (2 mg/6 hours). Propranolol (120 mg/day) provides the fastest symptomatic relief of the nervousness, tachycardia, lid lag, and other symptomatic manifestations.

41 **The answer is B** *Endocrine system / Pathology / Pheochromocytoma*

This slide demonstrates classic features of pheochromocytoma, a neoplasm derived from the cells of the adrenal medulla. Pheochromocytoma is frequently accompanied by a history of facial flushing and systemic hypertension. These clinical symptoms are caused by the production of norepinephrine by the tumor cells. Pheochromocytomas are almost always brown or mahogany-colored neoplasms. They have been labeled the 10% tumor—roughly 10% are malignant, 10% are bilateral, 10% are familial, and 10% are extra-adrenal. Histologically, they are characterized by a grape-like clustering of the neoplastic cells accompanied by a delicate, branching vascular network. The cells contain granular cytoplasmic contents that correspond to neurosecretory granules containing norepinephrine.

42 **The answer is D** *General principles / Histology / Protein structure; receptors*

Known receptors for physiologic growth factors and effectors display a small group of structures that are shared among different proteins and are found on either the external or internal domain of the protein. These structures are recognizable at a primary amino acid sequence level. This allows receptors to be classified into groups that resemble ion channels; groups that resemble kinases (especially tyrosine), serine, and threonine kinases; and cyclases. Several plasma membrane receptors require interactions with GTP-binding proteins to function in signal transduction. Metallothioneins are good acceptors for zinc and heavy metal, but they have not been reported to be receptors or elements in signal transduction systems.

Cytoskeleton proteins can provide the physical support for signal transduction systems but seldom are the physiologic transducing systems. Lysosomal proteins participate in protein degradation, whereas mitochondrial proteins often are involved in energy generation (although they can participate in cell death processes).

43 **The answer is D** *General principles / Biochemistry / Nucleotides*

Three nucleotides are required to specify an amino acid, which is inserted into a growing polypeptide chain. These groups of three nucleotides make up a codon that is represented in the 5′ to 3′ direction. Because there are four bases in RNA, the maximum number of codons is 64; 61 of these codons specify the 20 amino acids, and some amino acids have more than one. The triplet AUG serves as a start signal, and three triplets that do not code for any amino acid serve as stop signals. The genetic code is virtually universal; all organisms use the same codons to translate their genomes into proteins. A transcription unit can be influenced by promoter and enhancer elements as well as methylation of nucleotides.

44 **The answer is C** *Reproductive system / Pathology / Prostatic adenocarcinoma*

The histologic appearance of prostatic adenocarcinoma is characterized by small glands in a tightly compact architectural configuration. The glands are lined by a single cell, and the cells contain large nuclei with eosinophilic nucleoli. Occasional intraluminal crystalloids are also seen. Prostatic adenocarcinomas are frequently associated with elevation of serum prostate-specific antigen and prostatic acid phosphatase.

45 **The answer is A** *Central and peripheral nervous system / Behavioral science / Biologic theory*

Biologic theory proposes some alteration of brain function as underlying a mental disorder. Concordance in monozygotic twins, strong family history, morphologic changes in brain structure, and effects of medications on symptoms of mental disorders would all support biologic theory.

46 **The answer is D** *Musculoskeletal system / Physiology / Regulation of blood flow*

The muscles have a much higher oxygen demand during exercise than they do at rest. Although active muscles are able to extract a higher proportion of the delivered oxygen, increased perfusion is also required to satisfy the enormous demand for oxygen. Metabolic byproducts such as $H+$, CO_2, adenosine, phosphate, and prostaglandins act as signals within the exercising muscles to cause vasodilation. These metabolic signals can even overcome the vasoconstrictive signal of increased sympathetic outflow; however, the sympathetic outflow does result in vasoconstriction of the vascular beds that are not directly involved with the exercise (e.g., the vessels in the arms of someone on a stationary bicycle). Another signal mechanism is the release of nitric oxide from endothelial cells when blood flow is increased because of the metabolic signals. Nitric oxide is an inhibitor of smooth muscle contraction; therefore, it further decreases the resistance and increases perfusion in the vessels leading to the active skeletal muscles.

47 **The answer is B** *Renal/urinary system / Pathology / Renal neoplasm*

This slide shows a rare renal neoplasm called an angiomyolipoma. Angiomyolipomas contain adipose tissue, a vascular component composed of tortuous blood vessels that frequently lack elastic laminae, and a smooth muscle component that consists of spindle-shaped smooth muscle cells that exhibit pleomorphism and mitotic activity. The presence of fat and the prominent vascularity make the tumor readily recognizable on ultrasonography and CT. In approximately one third of patients, neurologic and/or cutaneous findings suggesting tuberous sclerosis are also present. These tumors can cause massive and sometimes fatal hemorrhage and may be locally aggressive. For the most part, however, they behave in a benign fashion.

48 **The answer is A** *Renal/urinary system / Pathology / Hypocomplementemia-associated renal disease*

Complement levels are normal in IgA nephropathy and diffuse proliferative glomerulonephritis (poststreptococcal glomerulonephritis). Nephritides associated with hypocomplementemia include cryoglobulinemia, membranoproliferative glomerulonephropathy, and various visceral infections, including infections of peritoneal and CNS shunts (shunt nephritis).

49 **The answer is C** *General principles / Biochemistry / Extracellular matrix*

Cell–cell interactions and cell–matrix interactions are essential for normal development and wound healing. The integrins are part of the supergene family, which also includes leukocyte adhesion molecules and receptors on the platelet membrane surface. These transmembrane glycoproteins have extracellular domains that bind matrix molecules (e.g., fibronectin) and intracellular domains that interact with cytoskeletal elements to activate signals in the cytosol and nucleus. The integrins stimulate gene transcription indirectly as a result of their mobilization of cytosolic signal-transducing pathways. Tubulins are globular proteins that polymerize into microtubules, which are important components of the cytoskeleton. Platelet aggregation requires a fibrinogen bridge between two transmembrane receptors. Adhesion to the damaged surface requires that a different receptor interact with von Willebrand's factor and the subendothelium. Laminin is thought to be important in the developing nervous system, and several extracellular matrix molecules, including type IV collagen, are crucial to the formation of proper relationships between cells (e.g., endothelial cells making tubes). Osteogenesis imperfecta, also called brittle bone disease, is caused by defects in collagen. The bones of patients with this disease are easily bent and fractured because they lack normal collagen.

50 **The answer is D** *General principles / Immunology / HLA-associated disorders*

The major histocompatibility complex (HLA complex) has been associated with a variety of diseases. Probably the best-known association is the one between HLA-B27 and ankylosing spondylitis. HLA-B27 is also associated with postgonococcal arthritis. Rheumatoid arthritis is associated with HLA-DR4. Primary Sjögren's syndrome is associated with HLA-DR3. 21-Hydroxylase deficiency is associated with HLA-BW47. Chronic active hepatitis is associated with HLA-DR3.

test **3**

Questions

Directions: *Single best answer questions consist of numbered items or incomplete statements followed by answers or by completions of the statement. Select the ONE lettered answer or completion that is BEST in each case.*

1 A 64-year-old man with a 40-year history of smoking one and one-half packs of cigarettes per day visits his physician's office complaining of an unproductive cough of 6 months' duration. When questioned further, the patient discloses hoarseness and generalized muscle weakness. Previously active sexually, he says that he has "lost interest" lately. During a physical examination, the physician notes muscle wasting, an unusual pattern of weight gain in the face and back, and abdominal stria. His serum glucose is 180 mg/dL. Which single set of laboratory tests is best suited to establish a tentative diagnosis?

(A) Serum thyroxin, tri-iodothyronine resin uptake, and cervical ultrasound
(B) Urinary glucocorticoids, abdominal CT, and chest radiograph
(C) Dexamethasone suppression test and chest radiograph
(D) Inpatient hospitalization with water restriction, CT of the head, and chest radiograph
(E) Glucose tolerance, urinary ketones, abdominal ultrasound, and chest radiograph

2 A patient is asked to lower a fully abducted limb and, at 90-degrees abduction, the limb suddenly drops uncontrollably. This patient may have

(A) supraspinitus muscle tear
(B) elbow tendonitis
(C) brachial plexus injury
(D) injury to the long thoracic nerve
(E) radial nerve injury

3 Propylthiouracil is the prototype of antithyroid drugs of the thiamide type. It

(A) is contraindicated in the therapy of Graves' disease
(B) is not used in thyrotoxicosis in pregnancy
(C) inhibits the active transport of iodide in the thyroid gland
(D) interferes with the incorporation of iodine into tyrosyl residues of thyroglobulin
(E) is without significant effect on peripheral deiodination of thryoxine to tri-idothyronine

4 Which of the following statements correctly describes evidence that relates cigarette smoking to bronchogenic carcinomas?

(A) Occasional smokers (i.e., five cigarettes a week) have a 100-fold greater lifetime risk of developing bronchogenic carcinoma than nonsmokers
(B) Individuals with a 15-year, two pack/day smoking habit who cease smoking for 6 months can expect to have a cancer risk equivalent to nonsmokers
(C) The bronchial epithelium in more than 10% of cigarette smokers shows atypical or hyperplastic changes on autopsy
(D) Individuals who smoke more than one pack/day for 30 years uniformly develop bronchogenic carcinomas
(E) Lung cancer runs in families in which cigarette smoking is common

5 Which of the following is a possible paraneoplastic syndrome associated with bronchogenic tumors?

(A) Hypokalemia
(B) Hyperaldosteronism
(C) Hypercalcemia
(D) Hypermagnesemia
(E) Hypocortisolism

6 Asthma is characterized by increased responsiveness of the trachea and bronchi to various stimuli and is manifested by widespread narrowing of the airway. Which of the following results of pulmonary function tests during an acute asthma attack will be demonstrated?

(A) Increased forced expiratory volume in 1 second (FEV_1)
(B) Increased forced vital capacity (FVC)
(C) Decreased FEV_1/FVC
(D) Decreased total lung capacity (TLC)

7 Which of the following statements about the influence of cardiovascular disease on sexuality is true?

(A) Some patients have impaired sexual functioning after a myocardial infarction
(B) Myocardial infarctions that occur during intercourse are rarely associated with unusual and stressful circumstances
(C) Exercise is not helpful in restoring normal sexual function in these patients
(D) It is not important to involve the partner in rehabilitation

8 Which of the following thalamic nuclei is connected with the superior colliculus and projects to visual cortical areas 18 and 19?

(A) Ventrolateral
(B) Medial central
(C) Pulvinar
(D) Ventroanterior

9 A 50-year-old woman complains of increasing fatigue during the past 2 weeks. She has a history of ovarian carcinoma and has been treated with several courses of cyclophosphamide therapy during the past 3 years; her last course of treatment was given 1 month previously. The physical examination shows slight hepatic enlargement. One examiner thinks the patient has some excess abdominal fluid. Laboratory examination reveals a white blood cell count of 2,000/μL, with 10% polymorph nuclear leukocytes and 90% lymphocytes. The hemoglobin concentration is 9 g/dL, and the platelet count is 50,000/μL. Which of the following statements about this patient is true?

(A) The differential diagnosis of the patient's pancytopenia includes chronic lymphocytic leukemia, cyclophosphamide toxicity, and recurrent ovarian carcinoma
(B) The differential diagnosis of the patient's pancytopenia includes acute myelogenous leukemia, cyclophosphamide toxicity, and recurrent ovarian carcinoma
(C) Further evaluation should include cytologic examination of ascites, radiographic studies of the abdomen, bone marrow aspiration and biopsy, and immunoglobulin gene rearrangement studies
(D) Further evaluation should include immunoglobulin gene rearrangement studies, radiographic studies of the abdomen, bone marrow aspiration and biopsy, and liver function studies
(E) Lymphocytes usually represent 80% of the total white blood cell count

10 Which of the following statements about cyclophosphamide is true?

(A) It is given intravenously only
(B) It is an antimicrotubule agent
(C) It is metabolized in the kidney
(D) Side effects include myelosuppression and hemorrhagic cystitis

11 An elderly woman presented with an area of persistent ulceration of the nipple of the breast. The ulceration was unresponsive to multiple topical steroid creams, and a biopsy was performed. The biopsy tissue in Figure 14 from the color plate section is characteristic of which one of the following conditions?

(A) Seborrheic keratosis
(B) Verruca vulgaris
(C) Paget's disease
(D) Neurodermatitis

12 A 62-year-old man has crushing substernal chest pain. After 4 days of circulatory support in the intensive care unit, he dies. Which of the following findings would be shown after a histologic study of his heart?

(A) Coagulative necrosis
(B) Liquefactive necrosis
(C) Hyperbasophilic wavy fibers
(D) Natural killer cell infiltrate

13 Which of the following descriptions best characterizes chronic type B (antral) gastritis?

(A) Circulating antibodies to parietal cells and intrinsic factor
(B) Glandular atrophy with very few short, cystically dilated glands
(C) Commonly found in individuals with pernicious anemia
(D) Associated with high serum gastrin levels
(E) Normal rugal folds

14 Which of the following statements concerning the contraction of myofibrils in skeletal muscle is true?

(A) The size of the A band decreases
(B) The size of the H band increases
(C) The size of the I band does not change
(D) Thin filaments penetrate the A band
(E) Z disks are pulled away from the A band

15 Which of the following statements concerning intercostal nerves is correct?

(A) They are the ventral rami of the thoracic spinal nerves
(B) There are 11 pairs of thoracic spinal nerves
(C) The thoracic spinal nerves are commonly called subcostal nerves
(D) The ventral rami of the thoracic spinal nerves supply muscle, bone, joint, and skin of the back
(E) They supply the parietal pleura and are mainly sensory nerves

16 Which of the following statements concerning mammalian chromosomes is correct?

(A) In higher eukaryotic genomes, cytosine is methylated at cytosine-guanine (CG) islands in inactive segments of DNA
(B) Of the sequences contained in the eukaryotic genome, 37% are copied into RNA
(C) Euchromatin is a term used for inactive DNA, and heterochromatin is a term used for those regions of DNA that are transcriptionally active
(D) DNase I can be used to treat chromosomes to determine inactive regions of DNA

17 A 6-year-old boy is brought to the physician's office by his mother. His mother is concerned that he can no longer keep up with his friends, and she notes that he is using his hands to pull himself up from the floor. Medical history reveals that an uncle on her side of the family died in his late teens. During the physical examination, the physician notes that the boy's calf muscles appear enlarged and that his heel tendon is unusually taut. His muscle strength is extremely impaired. Which of the following is most likely to account for the patient's findings?

(A) Friedreich's ataxia
(B) Guillain–Barré syndrome
(C) Amyotrophic lateral sclerosis (ALS; Lou Gehrig's disease)
(D) Myasthenia gravis
(E) Duchenne's muscular dystrophy

18 What is the most common complication in a patient who has just suffered an acute myocardial infarction?

(A) Cardiac tamponade
(B) Cardiac arrhythmia
(C) Cystic medial necrosis
(D) Aortic aneurysm
(E) Rupture of the ventricular septum

19 Which of the following associations regarding diseases and their signs is most correct?

(A) Strawberry tongue—parvovirus
(B) Tetanic contraction—botulism
(C) "Slapped-cheek"—streptococcus
(D) Rose spots on the abdomen—typhoid fever

20 Which of the following associations regarding neural tube development is most correct?

(A) Telencephalon—aqueduct
(B) Myelencephalon—cerebellum
(C) Mesencephalon—third ventricle
(D) Metencephalon—midbrain
(E) Diencephalon—thalamus

21 Which one of the following families of viruses is paired with the form of nucleic acids that constitute its genome?

(A) Parvoviruses—circular double-stranded DNA

(B) Papovaviruses—single-stranded RNA

(C) Adenoviruses—linear double-stranded DNA

(D) Retroviruses—two linked segments of linear double-stranded DNA

(E) Coronaviruses—linear, segmented double-stranded RNA

(F) Herpesvirus—triplex DNA

22 Immunologic memory is the name given to the body's improved ability to fight pathogens that it has encountered previously. Antibodies play a large role in mounting an immune response to a new antigen (primary antibody response) as well as a previously encountered antigen (secondary antibody response). Which of the following differences between the primary antibody response and the secondary antibody response is correct?

(A) The amount of antibody made in the primary response is greater than the amount made in the secondary response

(B) Immunoglobulin (Ig) G is the predominant class of antibody made during the initial antigen encounter

(C) IgM is the predominant class of antibody made during the secondary antigen encounter

(D) Antibodies are produced more quickly during the primary antibody response than during the secondary response

(E) Antibody affinity for the antigen is greater in the secondary antibody response than in the primary response

23 During the past year, Andrew, age 17, has retreated more and more often to his room. He has few friends and never calls anyone. His school performance has deteriorated during this time. His mother finds pieces of paper in his trash can with unintelligible poems written on them. Which of the following most likely describes his disorder?

(A) Narcissistic personality disorder

(B) Phencyclidine (PCP) ingestion

(C) Schizophrenia

(D) Borderline personality disorder

(E) Bipolar illness

24 A 28-year-old man is taken to the emergency department after being lost in the desert for 2 days. The patient complains of a headache and pain from multiple wounds. On examination, the patient has a fever and is severely dehydrated. Which one of the following statements is most likely correct?

(A) The patient should be given a nonsteroidal anti-inflammatory drug to relieve his headache and fever

(B) The patient's levels of angiotensin II are low

(C) The patient's antidiuretic hormone levels are below normal

(D) The patient's kidneys are producing higher levels of prostaglandins than normal

(E) The patient has reduced serum sodium levels and bradycardia

25 The skin lesion depicted in Figure 15 from the color plate section is characteristically associated with

(A) exposure to drugs

(B) vulvar abnormalities

(C) pruritus

(D) microabscesses

26 The cystic ovary depicted in Figure 16 from the color plate section exuded a clear, yellow fluid upon opening. The inner lining demonstrates which one of the following conditions?

(A) Teratoma

(B) Serous intermediate tumor

(C) Tubal pregnancy

(D) High-grade ovarian carcinoma

27 Which one of the following descriptions is typically associated with a nephrotic syndrome?

(A) Red blood cell casts, a low level of proteinuria, and granular casts

(B) Heavy proteinuria, oval fat bodies, and fatty casts

(C) Hematuria, granular casts, and broad waxy casts

(D) Proliferative glomerulonephritis on renal biopsy

(E) Hematuria, oval fat bodies, and proliferative glomerulonephritis on renal biopsy

28 A renal biopsy has been performed on an elderly woman with chronic renal failure and edema. Ultrasound demonstrated that the patient's kidneys were enlarged. On light microscopy, the glomeruli have normal cellularity but have a waxy material that expands the mesangium and basement membrane. Congo red stain reveals areas of apple-green birefringence under polarized light. Which one of the following is most likely true?

(A) An immunofluorescence stain for IgA would show a linear pattern of fluorescence

(B) An immunofluorescence stain for IgE would show a linear pattern of fluorescence

(C) The Congo red stain is binding to the cross-β-pleated configuration of amyloid fibrils

(D) The patient should be informed that she has amyloidosis and that it will likely respond to immunostimulatory agents

(E) The patient should be informed that she has sarcoidosis and that it will likely respond to treatment with steroids

(F) Electron microscopy would not be helpful in confirming a diagnosis

29 A 55-year-old man with no previous medical problems visits a physician because his arms have become progressively weaker during the past 2 months. He is divorced and has been sexually active with more than one partner. The weakness and fatigue began first in one arm and developed later in the other arm. During the physical examination, the physician notes hyperreflexia and generalized muscle weakness in all four extremities. The man has no sensory dysfunction, and his gait is normal, considering his weakness. Which of the following diagnoses is most likely to account for the patient's findings?

(A) Cerebrovascular accident in the motor cortex

(B) Guillain–Barré syndrome

(C) ALS

(D) Neurosyphilis

(E) Friedreich's ataxia

30 Which one of the following statements about the replication cycle of viruses is correct?

(A) During the eclipse period, infectious virus particles accumulate within the cell, but none are released

(B) During the latent period, the infecting viral particles are completely inactive and waiting for an opportunity to produce new viral particles

(C) The elevated period is the time when infectious viral particles accumulate intracellularly but none have been released from the cell

(D) Cell lysis is always the final step of a viral infection

(E) During the eclipse period, no infectious viral particles have been made

31 George is indignant when his graduate school thesis committee refuses to approve his project. "They're just jealous of me because they know I'll be the most brilliant anthropologist in history," he says. He has had this attitude throughout his life. Which of the following most likely describes his disorder?

(A) Narcissistic personality disorder
(B) Histrionic personality disorder
(C) Antisocial personality disorder
(D) Schizoid personality disorder
(E) Schizotypal personality disorder

32 Agammaglobulinemias result from the absence of antibodies due to mutations of B lymphocytes. People who lack antibodies have an increased risk for

(A) recurrent viral infections
(B) recurrent infections by extracellular bacteria
(C) recurrent viral infections and infections caused by extracellular bacteria
(D) recurrent infections by fungi and viruses
(E) nothing, because the immune system has redundant mechanisms that make up for the lack of antibodies

33 A 24-year-old man who returned from India a few weeks ago has a mild fever and is noticeably jaundiced. The patient has not been feeling well for approximately 10 days. The patient's symptoms are vomiting, anorexia, fatigue, a sore throat, and joint pain. Laboratory results are significant for elevated aspartate aminotransferase (AST), alanine aminotransferase (ALT), and bilirubin. Test results are positive for antihepatitis A virus (HAV) IgG. Which of the following statements is correct?

(A) The most common mode of transmission of the causative organism is parenterally
(B) The prognosis for this patient is poor because his condition frequently progresses to a chronic disease
(C) Prophylactic measures are not available for this disease
(D) This patient does not require treatment and should recover completely during the next couple of weeks
(E) HAV IgG is never found in people who do not have a history of severe hepatitis

34 The following radiograph and CT of a femoral joint depicts a 40-year-old mail carrier. These images show significant osteophyte formation. Which of the following diagnoses is correct?

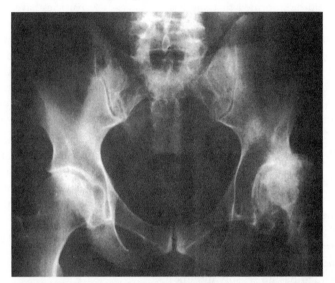

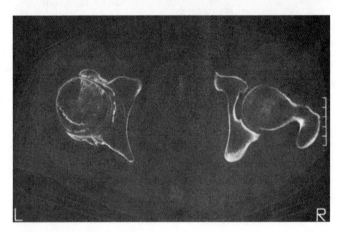

(A) Septic arthritis
(B) Osteoarthritis (degenerative joint disease)
(C) Rheumatoid arthritis
(D) Lyme disease
(E) Gout

35 A synovial biopsy of a wrist from a 50-year-old woman shows invasive pannus tissue eroding the cartilage. Which of the following diagnoses is correct?

(A) Osteoarthritis (degenerative joint disease)
(B) Septic arthritis
(C) Rheumatoid arthritis
(D) Systemic sclerosis
(E) Reiter's syndrome

36 The gallbladder in Figure 17 from the color plate section demonstrates which one of the following conditions?

(A) Vasculitis
(B) Invasive carcinoma
(C) Choledocholithiasis
(D) Cholesterolosis

37 A 26-year-old man develops arthritis after an episode of urethritis. HLA typing of the patient shows that the patient tests positive for HLA-B27. Which of the following is the most likely diagnosis?

(A) Rheumatoid arthritis
(B) Lyme disease
(C) Systemic sclerosis
(D) Gout
(E) Reiter's syndrome

38 A 44-year-old African American woman presents to her physician in Tempe, Arizona, with the following symptoms: chest pain, fever, cough, and malaise. A few weeks ago, this fourth-grade teacher took her class on a rock-hunting trip. A few of the students have also recently become ill. A chest radiograph showed hilar adenopathy, and a biopsy contained spherules. Which one of the following is the most likely diagnosis?

(A) Candidiasis
(B) Aspergillosis
(C) Coccidioidomycosis
(D) Histoplasmosis
(E) Blastomycosis

39 Which of the following inflammatory bowel diseases is most likely represented in Figure 18 from the color plate section?

(A) Crohn's disease
(B) Ulcerative colitis
(C) Ischemic colitis
(D) Pseudomembranous colitis

40 Which one of the following statements about leprosy is true?

(A) It is caused by *Mycobacterium leprae,* an extremely fast-growing organism that is easily cultured
(B) It is one of the most contagious diseases known
(C) Affected patients usually die because there is no effective treatment
(D) The disease-causing organism is able to survive being phagocytosed by a macrophage
(E) The disease exists in two distinct forms, lepromatous and tuberculoid, and there is no crossover of these typical patterns within one individual

41 A 39-year-old man presents to his physician because of progressive muscle weakness of 1 week's duration. His medical history is unremarkable, although he reports having had an influenza-like episode approximately 2 weeks ago. He has been sexually active since age 16. During the physical examination, the physician notes a marked decrease in reflexes and a loss of light touch and vibration sensation in the distal extremities. Which of the following diagnoses is most likely to account for the patient's findings?

(A) Cerebrovascular accident in the motor cortex
(B) Guillain–Barré syndrome
(C) ALS
(D) Neurosyphilis
(E) Friedreich's ataxia

42 The testis depicted in Figure 19 from the color plate section demonstrates which one of the following conditions?

(A) Embryonal carcinoma
(B) Teratoma
(C) Seminoma
(D) Epidermal inclusion cyst

43 Cloudy synovial fluid with a leukocyte count of 110,000/mm³ (95% polymorphonuclears) was drained from the hip of an elderly woman who had acute warmth and tenderness in the joint. Which of the following is the most likely diagnosis?

(A) Septic arthritis
(B) Rheumatoid arthritis
(C) Osteoarthritis (degenerative joint disease)
(D) Lyme disease
(E) Gout

44 A 9-year-old girl presents to her physician with a 1-month history of pain in her knees. Before she had this pain, she developed a maculopapular erythematous rash on the back of her left leg that later spread to multiple locations on her body. Which of the following is the most likely diagnosis?

(A) Rheumatoid arthritis
(B) Reiter's syndrome
(C) Septic arthritis
(D) Lyme disease
(E) Systemic sclerosis

45 The section of spleen depicted in Figure 20 from the color plate section demonstrates which one of the following conditions?

(A) Gaucher's disease
(B) Acute myelogenous leukemia
(C) Hereditary spherocytosis
(D) Malignant lymphoma

46 Which of the following conditions would result in focusing of light rays behind the retina?

(A) Emmetropia
(B) Myopia
(C) Presbyopia
(D) Astigmatism
(E) Hyperopia

47 A drug experiment was conducted, and the results have been plotted in two different ways. Which of the following labeled points corresponds with the K_D of this particular drug?

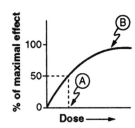 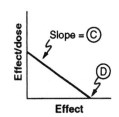

48 A patient is given a constant infusion of two drugs, A and B, whose pharmacokinetic profiles follow first-order kinetics and are completely independent of each other. Both A and B reach steady state plasma levels, and it is later decided that they should be withdrawn simultaneously. Given that the half-life of drug A is 4 hours and the half-life of drug B is 8 hours, which of the following statements is correct?

(A) After 8 hours, 50% of drug A remains and 50% of drug B remains
(B) After 24 hours, less than 5% of drug A remains and more than 10% of drug B remains
(C) After 8 hours, 25% of drug A remains and 75% of drug B remains
(D) After 24 hours, more than 5% of drug A remains and more than 10% of drug B remains
(E) After 16 hours, more than 5% of drug A remains and less than 10% of drug B remains

49 Which of the following statements regarding the effects of a noncompetitive inhibitor on the enzyme kinetic parameters K_m and V_{max} is true?

(A) K_m is decreased and V_{max} remains the same
(B) K_m is increased and V_{max} remains the same
(C) K_m remains the same and V_{max} decreases
(D) K_m remains the same and V_{max} increases
(E) Only competitive inhibitors affect K_m or V_{max}

Answer Key

1-C	11-C	21-C	31-A	41-B
2-A	12-A	22-E	32-B	42-C
3-D	13-B	23-C	33-D	43-A
4-C	14-D	24-D	34-B	44-D
5-C	15-A	25-A	35-C	45-D
6-C	16-A	26-B	36-D	46-E
7-A	17-E	27-B	37-E	47-A
8-C	18-B	28-C	38-C	48-B
9-B	19-D	29-C	39-A	49-C
10-D	20-E	30-E	40-D	

Answers and Explanations

1 The answer is C *Endocrine system / Pathology; endocrinology / Paraneoplastic syndromes*

Paraneoplastic syndromes are an important source of morbidity in the spectrum of cancer path physiology. The varied signs and symptoms that fall into this category cannot be directly related to the physical tumor, but are instead a result of the tumor's presence in the body. Although the mechanisms involved are not completely understood, in some cases the tumor produces a substance, and in other cases, the signs and symptoms are probably related to the body's immunologic reaction against the tumor.

This patient has the classic symptoms of Cushing's syndrome, which is indicated by an excess of corticosteroids. In this case, the lack of libido is the result of cortical suppression of the pituitary's secretion of protein metabolism, which results in degradation of the connective tissue. The characteristic patterns of weight gain (e.g., buffalo hump, moon facies) are due to ill-defined effects of excess steroids on lipid metabolism. The signs and symptoms of a paraneoplastic syndrome often begin at the same time as or earlier than the symptoms associated with the tumor (e.g., hoarseness, cough). The two sets of signs together are a strong indicator of a bronchogenic tumor.

The best confirming tests are a chest radiography and dexamethasone suppression test. The suppression test helps to differentiate between endocrine dysregulation and completely autonomous steroid production (i.e., no regulation). Although urinary glucocorticoids can indicate that steroids are being produced in excess, physical examination is needed to confirm a diagnosis. The water restriction is useful for diagnosing syndrome of inappropriate and diuretic hormone secretion (SIADH), which is characterized by hyponatremia and water retention. The other tests are useful for diagnosing primary thyroid and glucose abnormalities, which are not likely given this clinical scenario.

2 The answer is A *Musculoskeletal system / Anatomy / Upper limb*

The superspinitus muscle, along with infraspinitus, teres minor, and subscapularis muscles, comprise the rotator cuff. The rotator cuff stabilizes the shoulder joint and gives it mobility. Injury or degeneration to these muscles, especially the supraspinitus, will result in instability during a maneuver after abduction. Injury of the long thoracic nerve may paralyze the serratus anterior. In this patient, raising the arm results in the scapula pulling away from the thoracic wall (e.g., winged scapula). Injury to the superior trunk of the brachial plexus may give rise to the so-called waiter's tip position in which the limb hangs by the side in medial rotation. Injury to the radial nerve may give rise to characteristic wrist drop.

3 The answer is D *Endocrine system / Pharmacology / Thyroid*

Propylthiouracil, methimazole, and carbimazole are in a class of antithyroid drugs that interfere with the incorporation of iodine into tyrosyl residues of thryoglobulin. The molecular determinant appears to involve inhibiton of peroxidase enzyme. Propylthiouracil has some of its therapeutic effect by inhibiting peripheral deiodination of thyroxine to tri-iodothyronine, and this adds to its utility in treatment of severe hyperthyroidism such as thyrotoxicosis. In contrast to the other available agents in this class, propylthiouracil does not penetrate the placental barrier very efficiently, and thus may be useful in the treatment of thyrotoxicosis in pregnancy. Propylthiouracil is useful for the control of hyperthyroidism in Graves' disease in anticipation of spontaneous remission or in combination with radiotherapy and/or surgery.

4 **The answer is C** *Respiratory system / Pathology; endocrinology / Paraneoplastic syndromes*

Lung cancer in families with members who smoke is not definitive epidemiologic evidence for either a genetic or an environmental hypothesis of lung carcinoma. When trying to establish a correlation between a variable (cigarette smoking) and a disease (lung cancer), one must look for a confounding relationship (i.e., a positive family history for both). Heavy smokers (i.e., more than one pack/day) have a 20-fold greater lifetime risk of developing bronchogenic cancer. Cessation of smoking for 10 years or more is required to reduce the cancer risk of an individual to that of a nonsmoker. Not all smokers develop bronchogenic carcinoma. Lung cancer in families with members who smoke is not definitive epidemiologic evidence for either a genetic or an environmental hypothesis of lung carcinoma.

5 **The answer is C** *Respiratory system / Pathology / Paraneoplastic syndromes*

Hypercalcemia is a common paraneoplastic syndrome that is seen with bronchogenic tumors, especially with squamous cell carcinomas. Hypokalemia, hyperaldosteronism, and hypermagnesemia are not conditions that are commonly associated with cancer. Cortisol levels are often elevated (e.g., Cushing's syndrome) and are not decreased in small cell carcinoma of the lung.

6 **The answer is C** *Respiratory system / Physiology; pulmonology / Asthma, pulmonary mechanics*

The FVC is unchanged or decreased during an acute asthma attack. An important spirometric manifestation of asthma is a decrease in FEV_1 by itself or normalized to FVC. The TLC will be normal or possibly elevated because of loss of elastic recoil.

7 **The answer is A** *Respiratory system / Neuroanatomy / Thalamic connections*

The most common reasons for decreased frequency of sexual intercourse after a myocardial infarction are psychological. Patients who have had a myocardial infarction can have decreased self-esteem and concerns about impotence. The stress associated with an unusual circumstance (e.g., an atypical sexual activity, inebriation, a new sexual partner) is often responsible for myocardial infarction during intercourse. Exercise and educational programs have been effective in helping cardiac patients resume a normal life, but the involvement of the partner in these programs is important.

8 **The answer is C** *Central and peripheral nervous system / Neuroanatomy / Thalamic connections*

The pulvinar nucleus receives input from the superior colliculus and pretectal areas and projects to visual cortex areas 18 and 19. It does not connect with the basal ganglia or the vagus.

9 **The answer is B** *Hematopoietic and lymphoreticular system / Pathology / Acute leukemia*

Pancytopenia is not associated with chronic lymphocytic leukemia. Patients with acute myelogenous leukemia, recurrent ovarian carcinoma, and aplastic anemia can have pancytopenia. Cyclophosphamide, which is used to treat some patients with ovarian carcinoma, does cause bone marrow depression, and recovery can be delayed. An immunoglobulin gene rearrangement analysis would not be useful for this patient unless she had shown evidence of a lymphoproliferative disorder. Radiographic and cytologic studies could confirm the presence of ascites and possible recurrent ovarian carcinoma. Bone marrow aspiration is essential to establish the diagnosis. With hepatic enlargement, it is necessary to evaluate the patient for evidence of liver damage. Some agents that damage the liver can also damage the bone marrow. Lymphocytes typically represent 20% to 40% of the total white blood cell count.

10 **The answer is D** *General principles / Pharmacology / Antineoplastic agents*

Cyclophosphamide is an alkylating agent that cross-links tumor cell DNA. It may be given intravenously or orally and is activated and metabolized in the liver. Its side effects include myelosuppression, hemorrhagic cystitis, ureteritis, nausea, and vomiting.

11 The answer is C *Respiratory system / Pathology / Paget's disease*

This slide shows a proliferation of pleomorphic malignant cells along the dermal–epidermal junction. These neoplastic cells have abundant clear cytoplasm and contain cytoplasmic mucin. They derive from the apocrine sweat glands of the breast or possibly from intraductal carcinomas of the breast whose cells have migrated up the major ducts to involve the overlying skin. Paget's disease of the nipple is a common cause of nonhealing ulcers, and clinical concern for this malignant condition should precipitate biopsy.

12 The answer is A *Cardiovascular system / Histology / Liquefactive necrosis*

Coagulative necrosis follows hypoxic death in most body tissues except those of the central nervous system (CNS). For example, the necrotic process that follows a myocardial infarction is coagulative necrosis due to occlusion of the coronary vessels. Liquefactive necrosis occurs only in the CNS and is the result of vascular occlusion. It is commonly caused by pyogenic bacterial infection or septic emboli. In addition to coagulative necrosis, histologic study of this man's heart would show hypereosinophilic wavy fibers and neutrophilic infiltrate.

13 The answer is B *Gastrointestinal system / Pathology / Chronic type B gastritis*

Chronic type B gastritis is four times as common as type A (fundal) gastritis, in which there are circulating antibodies to the parietal cells and intrinsic factor. *Helicobacter pylori* is the agent responsible for type B gastritis, which can be facilitated by chronic alcohol or aspirin use, bile reflux, ulcer disease, or postgastrectomy states. Chronic *H. pylori* gastritis leads to multifocal glandular atrophy with a few short, cystically dilated glands. Type A gastritis is found in elderly individuals and those with pernicious anemia. Levels of gastrin tend to be low, and there may be antibodies to gastrin-producing cells in type B gastritis, compared with type A gastritis. In type B gastritis, the stomach wall loses its rugal folds and becomes flattened, glazed, and red.

14 The answer is D *Musculoskeletal system / Physiology / Skeletal muscle contraction*

The length of the A band remains constant during the contraction of myofibrils in skeletal muscle. The sarcomere of the myofibril consists of thick and thin filaments. According to the sliding filament hypothesis, thick and thin filaments slide past one another during contraction, increasing the amount of overlap between them; their length does not change. The H band contains only thick filaments; the A band contains thin and thick filaments. The I band contains only thin filaments, which are anchored in the middle of the I band by components of the Z disk. During contraction, thin filaments slide into the A band, reducing the size of both the H band and I band and drawing the Z disks closer to the A band.

15 The answer is A *Central and peripheral nervous system / Neuroanatomy / Intercostal nerves*

Twelve pairs of thoracic nerves pass through the intervertebral foramina and then divide into ventral and dorsal primary rami. The ventral rami of T1 through T11 are called intercostal nerves, because they enter the intercostal space. T12 does not enter the intercostal space; it is the subcostal nerve. Dorsal rami pass posteriorly immediately lateral to the articular process of the vertebrae to supply muscle, bone, joint, and skin of the back.

16 The answer is A *General principles / Genetics / Transcriptional activation of chromosomes*

Mammalian DNA uses only about 7% of the genome to transcribe RNA. Inactive DNA, or heterochromatin, is tightly wound in an organized fashion in conjunction with nucleosomes. Inactive DNA is also methylated at CG islands, but the exact relation between inactivation and methylation is not clear. Active segments of DNA are called euchromatin. Euchromatin is not wound as tightly and is less protein-bound than heterochromatin. Because it is less organized, euchromatin also happens to be more sensitive to enzymatic digestion by DNase I, which can be used to determine active regions of DNA.

17 **The answer is E** *Musculoskeletal system / Pathology; neurobiology / Differential diagnosis of neuromuscular disease*

Duchenne's muscular dystrophy is a primary myopathy whose clinical course is severe, resulting in death from respiratory failure by the middle to late teens. The age of onset is usually 3 to 7 years. The mother observed all of the common symptoms of Duchenne's muscular dystrophy. Earlier difficulties are noticed in particularly active children (e.g., difficulty running, frequent tripping, difficulty climbing). The pseudohypertrophy, which is seen mainly in the calf, is nearly pathognomonic at 6 years of age, and biopsy reveals significant fibrosis with almost no normal muscle fibers. Most children are confined to a wheelchair by 12 years of age.

18 **The answer is B** *Cardiovascular system / Pathology / Acute myocardial infarction*

Cardiac arrhythmias account for 75% of complications in acute myocardial infarction. Cardiac tamponade, mitral valve incompetence, and rupture of the ventricular septum are serious complications following damage to the myocardial wall or the papillary muscles. Peripheral embolism can also occur as a result of mural thrombosis after infarctions involving the cardiac endothelium. Aortic aneurysm is usually related to peripheral atherosclerotic disease; therefore, it is related to coronary atherosclerotic disease. Cystic medial necrosis can cause a dissecting form of aortic damage without much aortic dilation. Syphilis can cause aneurysmal dilation, especially in the ascending aorta. However, there is no common relationship between acute myocardial infarction and any of these aortic diseases.

19 **The answer is D** *General principles / Microbiology / Bacterial infections*

Botulism is associated with flaccid, not tetanic, paralysis because it blocks acetylcholine (ACh) release at the neuromuscular junction. *Clostridium tetani* is associated with tetanic contraction, because tetanus toxin acts in the CNS to block the release of inhibitory neurotransmitters. *Salmonella typhi*, a gram-negative facultative rod, is the causative agent of typhoid fever; rose spots on the abdomen are associated with this disease. A strawberry tongue is a common symptom of group A streptococcal infection. This manifestation is caused by an erythrogenic toxin that also causes a red rash that starts on the chest and spreads. Parvovirus B19 causes a facial rash with a "slapped-cheek" appearance following a low-grade fever and minor upper respiratory symptoms.

20 **The answer is E** *Central and peripheral nervous system / Neuroanatomy / Neural tube development*

The diencephalon, which is also derived from the forebrain, develops into the thalamus and third ventricle. The telencephalon develops from the forebrain (prosencephalon) into the cerebral hemispheres and lateral ventricles. The mesencephalon develops into the midbrain and aqueduct. Finally, the pons and cerebellum are derived from the metencephalon, and the medulla is derived from the myelencephalon. The metencephalon and myelencephalon both originate from the hindbrain.

21 **The answer is C** *General principles / Microbiology / Viral genomes*

The adenoviruses have a linear double-stranded DNA genome with a molecular weight of approximately 20 to 30×10^6. Coronaviruses and papovaviruses are DNA, not RNA, viruses. Parvoviruses have a linear single-stranded genome and are the smallest of the DNA viruses. Retroviruses are RNA viruses with unlinked segments of single-stranded RNA. Herpesviruses have a linear double-stranded DNA genome.

22 **The answer is E** *General principles / Immunology / Primary versus secondary immune responses*

Approximately 5 days after the immune system encounters an antigen, the B lymphocytes begin producing antibodies. This lag time is required for the antigen to be recognized by the naive immune cells and for sufficient numbers of B cells to be activated to synthesize antibodies. The primary response consists of primarily IgM antibodies. During the initial antibody response, antibody affinity maturation occurs, so that memory B cells, which can make antibodies with a stronger affinity for the antigen, are formed. During subsequent encounters of the antigen, these memory B cells begin to synthesize IgG antibodies in only 1 to 2 days because they were previously activated. During this secondary antibody response, a much larger quantity of antibodies is produced.

23 **The answer is C** *Central and peripheral nervous system / Behavioral science / Personality disorders*

Andrew's deterioration in performance, his social withdrawal, and his apparent difficulties in cognition have lasted longer than 6 months. These symptoms, as well as his age, suggest a diagnosis of schizophrenia. A narcissistic personality disorder would be characterized by grandiosity and feelings of special entitlement with lack of empathy. Borderline personality disorders are typified by unstable behavior and mood, feelings of emptiness and loneliness, and even periods of minipsychosis. PCP ingestion is normally associated with violent behavior and vertical nystagmus. Finally, bipolar disorder is characterized by episodes of major depression and mania.

24 **The answer is D** *General principles / Physiology / Renal response to volume depletion*

Dehydration, as well as volume-depleted states due to other causes, induces the release of renin, which leads to an increase in angiotensin II. Antidiuretic hormone release is also stimulated by both the volume depletion and the angiotensin II. In an effort to maintain blood pressure, the angiotensin II functions as a vasoconstrictor, whereas the antidiuretic hormone acts in several ways to formulate concentrated urine and to minimize water loss. The vasoconstricting effects of angiotensin II in the afferent arterioles of the kidney cause a decrease in renal plasma flow. Increased prostaglandin synthesis counterbalances the decrease in renal plasma flow by causing afferent arteriole dilation. Thus, giving a volume-depleted patient a nonsteroidal anti-inflammatory drug, which works by blocking prostaglandin synthesis, could cause renal failure. The angiotensin II would cause the afferent arteriole to constrict, and renal plasma flow would decrease dramatically. Severe dehydration results in an increase in serum sodium and tachycardia.

25 **The answer is A** *Skin and related tissue / Pathology / Drug-induced disease*

The skin biopsy shows features of erythema multiforme, which frequently manifests as a generalized vesicobullous disease. Vesicobullous lesions are evaluated microscopically by observing the level of the plane of separation of the epidermis and by identifying the type of cellular infiltrates. This slide demonstrates a subepidermal split between the epidermis and dermis, which raises three major histologic differential diagnoses: bullous pemphigoid, dermatitis herpetiformis, and erythema multiforme. The features most characteristic of erythema multiforme are subepidermal edema, abundant nuclear dust in the dermis, and a superficial perivascular lymphoplasmacytic infiltrate. It is frequently associated with exposure to drugs and is presumably a result of immune complexes depositing along the basement membrane.

26 **The answer is B** *Reproductive system / Pathology / Ovarian tumors*

Serous intermediate tumors of the ovary are characterized grossly by a cauliflower-like proliferation of cytologically bland cuboidal cells, frequently accompanied by psammoma bodies. These papillary lesions are noninvasive and have an excellent prognosis in contrast to invasive serous carcinomas of the ovary. They occur in young women and may recur in the abdomen, causing small bowel obstruction.

27 **The answer is B** *Renal/urinary system / Pathology / Glomerulonephritis*

A nephrotic syndrome is normally associated with 3 to 4+ proteinuria, fatty casts, oval fat bodies, free fat droplets, and nonproliferative glomerulonephritis. Typically, hematuria and red blood cell casts indicate a nephritic syndrome and proliferative glomerulonephritis. Chronic glomerulonephritis is characterized by proteinuria, variable hematuria, broad waxy casts, and granular casts.

[28] The answer is C *Renal/urinary system / Pathology / Amyloidosis*

Amyloidosis is a life-threatening disease for which there is no effective treatment. It is characterized by large, pale kidneys on autopsy; apple-green birefringence with a Congo red stain under polarized light; autofluorescence with a thioflavin stain; immunoperoxidase staining for amyloid P and sometimes amyloid A; short, nonbranching rods on electron microscopy; and mesangial and glomerular basement membrane expansion, as well as deposits in the arteries. Congo red binds to amyloid fibrils. IgA or IgE deposition is not common. This disease typically affects multiple organs including the liver, heart, and blood vessels. There is no evidence that immunostimulation affects amyloidosis; however, recent clinical trials suggest that combinations of prednisone, colchicine, and melphalan can prolong the lives of these patients. Sarcoidosis is characterized by mononuclear cell granulomatous inflammation, which rarely affects the kidneys. The lungs are frequently affected, and sarcoidosis is usually responsive to glucocorticoids.

[29] The answer is C *Central and peripheral nervous system / Pathology / Differential diagnosis of neuromuscular disease*

The differential diagnosis of muscular weakness is an essential skill for both a neurologist and a general practitioner. In ascertaining a diagnosis, it is important to distinguish between purely motor difficulties and sensorimotor difficulties and to localize the problem (i.e., upper versus lower motor neuron disease, neuromuscular junction, muscular atrophy). Cerebrovascular accidents in the motor cortex almost always give rise to two distinct phases: flaccid paralysis of the affected areas, followed by distinct upper motor neuron signs (e.g., hyperreflexia, hypertonia, minimal muscular atrophy). Generally, the affected areas are well-demarcated, and most cerebrovascular accidents do not cause bilateral symptoms. Furthermore, only the 55-year-old man would be in the age range in which cerebrovascular accidents would be high in the differential diagnosis. ALS is slightly more common in men than in women and rarely has its onset before 50 years of age. It is a relentlessly degenerating disease that attacks both upper and lower motor neurons. One of the cardinal features of ALS, as is seen in this man, is that it occurs in the complete absence of any sensory loss. The cause of this disease is unknown, and no treatment is available. The clinical onset includes weakness and fatigue that generally begin in one extremity and progress to include the entire body. Hyperreflexia is usually apparent early and is a sign of upper motor neuron disease. Babinski's sign is often present (i.e., up-going). As the underlying disease progresses, the lower motor neuron degenerates so that areflexia and flaccid paralysis predominate in the later stages. Muscle wasting leads eventually to the amyotrophy that gives the disease its name.

[30] The answer is E *General principles / Microbiology / Viral replication*

The viral replication cycle begins with the eclipse phase, during which the viral genome is present within the cell but no infectious viral particles have been made. The second phase is the intracellular accumulation period, during which nucleocapsids are being made but are not released from the cell. There will be infectious viral particles only if the virus does not need to make its envelope from the plasma membrane of the cell. The latent period includes the eclipse phase and the intracellular accumulation period and ends when the first virus particle is released from the cell. When the latent period ends, the elevated period begins and continues as long as the extracellular virus particles continue to increase. Lysis of the infected cell may be the final step of an infection, but persistent infection and latent infection are two other options.

[31] The answer is A *Central and peripheral nervous system / Behavioral science / Personality disorders*

The type of reaction to major disappointments that is exhibited by George is typical of individuals with narcissistic personality disorders. These individuals have a sense of self-importance and entitlement. Fantasies concerning success and infinite capabilities are also characteristic. A histrionic personality disorder is characterized by extroverted, emotional, dramatic, and possibly sexually provocative behavior. Antisocial behavior is characterized by unwillingness to conform to social norms; this behavior is associated with conduct disorder in childhood and criminal activity in adulthood. Schizoid personality disorder is most commonly characterized by longstanding periods of voluntary social withdrawal, whereas schizotypal personality disorder is commonly characterized by peculiar appearance and odd thought patterns and behavior in the absence of psychosis.

32 **The answer is B** *General principles / Immunology / Agammaglobulinemia*

Antibodies are a main defense against extracellular bacteria. Antibodies bind the bacteria and enable phago-cytic cells (e.g., macrophages and neutrophils) to "get a grip" on the pathogen. This process is especially important for phagocytosis of bacteria that have antiphagocytic capsules. Intracellular pathogens (e.g., viruses) are eliminated primarily by the cell-mediated immune system, which contains natural killer cells and cytotoxic T lymphocytes. The immune system has many redundancies, but the lack of antibodies is not fully compensated for in patients with agammaglobulinemia. Thus, they are susceptible to infections by *Haemophilus influenzae*, *Streptococcus pneumoniae*, *Streptococcus pyogenes*, and *Staphylococcus aureus*. Treatment includes prophylactic antibiotics and γ-globulin.

33 **The answer is D** *Gastrointestinal system / Microbiology / Hepatitis A*

HAV is an acute infection that is most common in children and young adults. It is frequently transmitted by fecal–oral contamination. Although it is associated with a wide variety of symptoms, no treatment is required. The disease usually resolves completely within a few weeks. A vaccine is available, and Ig injections may also be used for prophylaxis in some cases. Anti-HAV IgG is present in many individuals who have not had a symptomatic episode of hepatitis A; however, the prevalence has been declining since the 1970s, leaving more adults susceptible.

34 **The answer is B** *Musculoskeletal system / Radiographic anatomy / Differential diagnosis of arthritis*

Osteoarthritis is a degenerative disease that most commonly affects the large, weight-bearing joints. Osteoar-thritis is related to use; therefore, mail carriers are more susceptible than office administrators. The radio-graph shows classic findings of osteoarthritis, including asymmetric involvement of joints (i.e., only the left), segmental narrowing of the medial and superior joint space, subchondral sclerosis of the bone, and osteophyte formation. The osteophyte formation is striking and can best be seen on CT—the normal femoral head has been completely dislodged from the joint space by the large femoral osteophyte, and the acetabulum is covered with its own distinct osteophyte. This is an advanced case, and these radiographs were taken immediately prior to total joint replacement. Generally speaking, inflammatory changes are not a feature of osteoarthritis.

35 **The answer is C** *Musculoskeletal system / Pathology; radiographic anatomy / Differential diagno-sis of arthritis*

Rheumatoid arthritis is an autoimmune disease in which cellular inflammation and antibody complex formation destroy normal synovial tissue and articular cartilage. It has a propensity to affect the small joints of the wrists, hands, ankles, and feet. The lymphokines and hydrolytic enzymes found in the synovial fluid of a patient with rheumatoid arthritis combine with activated inflammatory cells to destroy articular cartilage. Chronic rheumatoid arthritis is characterized by the formation of pannus, a form of granulation tissue with inflammatory cells, proliferating fibroblasts, and small blood vessels. This destructive tissue ultimately re-places articular cartilage with a fibrous scar, which frequently results in joint ankylosis. Two other histopatho-logic features of rheumatoid arthritis are large lacunae in the cartilage (the result of invasive pannus) and inflammatory cells in the marrow, which can destroy bone. Rheumatoid arthritis is associated with the DR4 haplotype of the human leukocyte antigen (HLA-DR4).

36 **The answer is D** *Gastrointestinal system / Pathology / Biliary/hepatic pathology*

The gross appearance of this gallbladder, indicative of cholesterolosis, is characteristic of the so-called strawberry gallbladder. This term derives from the mixture of bile-stained epithelium, which appears green in the slide, admixed with biliary epithelium that overlies submucosal aggregates of fat-laden macrophages. These aggregated macrophages impart the yellow, reticulated appearance to the gallbladder mucosa. Choles-terolosis is frequently associated with gallstones and is common in individuals who are obese or have hypercholesterolemia.

37 **The answer is E** *Musculoskeletal system / Pathology / Differential diagnosis of arthritis*

Reiter's syndrome is seronegative arthritis that follows an episode of infectious urethritis, cervicitis, or dysentery. When initially described, the complete triad also included noninfectious conjunctivitis. The inflammation associated with the ocular and joint symptoms is reactive and probably related to an autoimmune phenomenon triggered by urethritis. Other documented symptoms include hyperkeratotic lesions of the skin and painless shallow ulcers of the penis, urethral meatus, and mouth. HLA-B27 occurs in approximately 80% to 90% of all patients with Reiter's syndrome. The knee and ankle joints are commonly involved, and sacroiliitis occurs in approximately 25% of patients. Most episodes of Reiter's arthritis last for less than 6 months, and it is rarely debilitating.

38 **The answer is C** *General principles / Microbiology / Fungal infections*

Coccidioidomycosis is endemic to the American southwest and other arid climates. It is caused by the fungus *Coccidioides immitis,* which is found in soil. Often, several people become infected when soil is disturbed and the dust carries the fungus. Symptoms include those common to other pulmonary diseases along with possible hypersensitivity reactions and dissemination to the CNS, skin, and joints. Frequently the disease is progressive in African Americans, Native Americans, and Filipinos. Infiltrates, hilar adenopathy, and pleural effusion may be been seen on radiograph, and spherules may be seen on biopsy. Candidiasis and aspergillosis are rare in immunocompetent people. Histoplasmosis is endemic to regions with moist soil, such as the Midwest. Blastomyces is also rare in the Southwest; it is more common in the Southeast, Midwest, and in men rather than in women.

39 **The answer is A** *Gastrointestinal system / Pathology / Crohn's disease*

Crohn's disease is characterized by segmental involvement of the bowel, which contrasts with diffuse involvement of the bowel characteristic of ulcerative colitis. This photograph shows two strictures surrounding apparently normal mucosa. These strictures account for the frequent presence of fistulae between portions of the small and large bowel and reflect the transmural thickening and inflammation of the bowel wall, a common feature in Crohn's disease.

40 **The answer is D** *General principles / Microbiology / Leprosy*

Leprosy is caused by *Mycobacterium leprae,* a slow-growing, strict aerobe that is an obligate intracellular pathogen and is difficult to culture. It can survive being phagocytosed by a macrophage. In fact, macrophages may be the vehicles that enable spread of the disease through the body. Leprosy exists in two forms: lepromatous, which is characterized by ineffective cell-mediated immunity, and tuberculoid, which is characterized by an effective cell-mediated immunity. However, there is a great deal of overlap between these two forms, even within one individual. Transmission of the disease requires prolonged exposure to infected individuals, even those who are not receiving treatment. Effective treatments for leprosy are dapsone, rifampin, and clofazimine. In untreated patients, death is more commonly due to secondary infections than the leprosy itself.

41 **The answer is B** *Central and peripheral nervous system / Neurobiology / Differential diagnosis of neuromuscular disease*

Guillain–Barré syndrome is an autoimmune disorder that is frequently triggered by a preceding viral infection or surgery. Herpes-type viruses are thought to be involved in an unusually large number of cases. The principal feature of the disease is peripheral demyelination, and the clinical presentation is generally gradual at first, leading later to fulminant symptoms that require hospitalization (many patients need ventilatory support). Early clinical findings are related to the demyelination, including hyporeflexia, hypotonic paralysis (especially in the distal extremities), and loss of light touch and vibration sensation. Although the motor symptoms mimic upper motor neuron disease, the findings are actually related to the decreased muscle spindle fiber (i.e., inhibitory) input to the anterior horn cells. Recovery is usually complete within 1 month.

42 The answer is C *Reproductive system / Pathology / Testicular/germ cell tumor*

This testis contains a well-circumscribed, fleshy gray tumor nodule. The differential diagnosis of such white or gray tumor nodules in the testes is limited to two possibilities: seminoma and malignant lymphoma. Seminomas tend to be sharply circumscribed, whereas lymphomas are diffuse, infiltrative neoplasms. The sharp circumscription of this lesion should lead to a diagnosis of seminoma. The absence of hemorrhage and necrosis argues against embryonal carcinoma.

43 The answer is A *Musculoskeletal system / Pathology / Differential diagnosis of arthritis*

Septic arthritis is most common in elderly people and individuals who are immunocompromised. It is most frequently caused by *Staphylococcus aureus*, although *Staphylococcus epidermidis* and group A streptococci are also encountered. People with connective tissue diseases and those with chronic arthritis are more inclined to develop coincidental septic arthritis. Disseminated gonococcal infection is the most common bacterial arthritis in urban populations, complicating as many as 0.5% of all gonococcal infections. However, disseminated gonococcal infection is usually distinguished from other forms of septic arthritis because of its route of transmission. In general, infectious arthritis is characterized by the acute onset of a warm, swollen joint, most commonly the knee (involvement of more than one joint indicates disseminated gonococcal infection). A synovial leukocyte count greater than 50,000 with 80% or more polymorphonuclear leukocytes strongly suggests septic arthritis. Although other inflammatory arthritides can elevate synovial cell counts to that level, the high percentage of polymorphonuclear leukocytes is relatively specific to infections. A Gram stain or culture is necessary for a definitive diagnosis. Treatment of infectious arthritis requires immediate and complete drainage of the synovial fluid. Intravenous antibiotics administered without delay can help reduce the potentially irreversible joint damage associated with such a large inflammatory response. Even with prompt therapy, complete functional recovery following *S. aureus* arthritis is less than 60%, and infectious arthritis is a significant cause of joint deformity.

44 The answer is D *Musculoskeletal system / Pathology / Differential diagnosis of arthritis*

Lyme disease is an infectious process caused by the tickborne spirochete *Borrelia burgdorferi*. The first stage of the illness occurs within 1 month of exposure and is characterized by erythema migrans at the site of the tick bite. Flu-like symptoms can accompany the rash, and the rash frequently spreads to other sites. In approximately 10% of patients, neurologic or cardiac involvement occurs within weeks to months. As many as 67% of patients develop frank arthritis following the initial rash. Intermittent attacks of arthritis in the large joints, particularly the knee, are typical. The clinical symptoms of Lyme disease have a slower onset than do the symptoms of acute infectious arthritis. Lyme disease can cause irreversible damage if the disease is not discovered until the later stages (weeks to months after the initial rash). However, most patients respond to oral tetracycline in the early stages, and complete recovery is fairly common.

45 The answer is D *Gastrointestinal system / Pathology / Lymphomas involving the spleen*

Malignant lymphomas that involve the splenic parenchyma characteristically cause either large, white tumor nodules or small, pinpoint white tumor nodules. In most instances, low-grade malignant lymphomas cause small (2 to 4 mm in diameter) white nodules, such as those depicted in this slide. These nodules replace the normal malpighian bodies of the spleen. Low-grade lymphomas include small-cleaved cell lymphoma and small lymphocytic lymphoma. As a general rule, large, white nodules in the spleen indicate either Hodgkin's disease or high-grade large cell lymphoma.

46 The answer is E *Central and peripheral nervous system / Neurophysiology / Visual science*

In hyperopia, the eyes must continuously accommodate to see distant objects clearly. In the absence of this accommodation, the focusing point for rays of light falls behind the retina. Hyperopia can be corrected by using a converging lens. Emmetropia, or perfect vision, occurs when rays of light are focused perfectly on the retina. Myopia results from the focusing of light in front of the retina. Presbyopia arises from a decrease in the elasticity of the lens.

47 **The correct answer is A** *General principles / Pharmacology / Quantitative dose-response curves*

The figure on the *left* represents an ideal dose–response curve for a drug and shows the typical hyperbolic effect. The dose that gives the half-maximal effect (K_D) can be estimated from the figure, but the maximal effect cannot easily be determined because of the hyperbolic nature of the data. The figure on the *right* is a mathematical transformation of these data to a linear form that is more useful—a Scatchard plot that allows the maximal effect to be determined from the intercept at the x-axis. The concentration of K_D is the reciprocal of the slope.

48 **The answer is B** *General principles / Pharmacology / Half-life of drugs*

The amount of drug remaining in the plasma after its administration has ceased is a complex interplay of the drug's modality of distribution, metabolism, and excretion, all of which are characterized by its half-life. For drugs that follow first-order kinetics, this value is independent of dosage. Therefore, 50% remains after 1 half-time (4 hours for drug A and 8 hours for drug B), and 25% remains after 2 half-times, and so on.

49 **The answer is C** *General principles / Biochemistry / Enzyme kinetics*

Noncompetitive inhibitors do not affect substrate binding and therefore do not affect K_m. However, they do affect the efficiency of enzymatic action and therefore decrease V_{max}. Competitive inhibitors impair substrate-binding events, thus increasing the apparent K_m, but they have no effect on enzymatic activity, which is shown by no change in V_{max}.

test **4**

Questions

Directions: Single best answer questions consist of numbered items or incomplete statements followed by answers or by completions of the statement. Select the ONE lettered answer or completion that is BEST in each case.

1 Which of the following is true about the esophagus in a patient with Barrett's esophagus?

(A) Columnar epithelium replaces the squamous epithelium

(B) There is a loss of immature pluripotent stem cells

(C) There is decreased exposure to pepsin and lysolecithin

(D) There are no inflammatory processes

(E) It is a benign condition that is not associated with esophageal adenocarcinoma

2 Of the following effects, drug binding to plasma proteins generally

(A) limits glomerular filtration

(B) is highly drug-specific

(C) is an interaction between drug and immunoglobulins

(D) is irreversible

(E) limits renal tubular secretion

3 A 36-year-old woman is brought to the emergency department because a friend found her unresponsive on the floor at home. Her friend relates a recent history of depression. An empty prescription bottle for 30 100-mg amitriptyline tables was found nearby. The woman's amitriptyline level is 2,300 ng/mL. The physician's first step would be to

(A) prepare involuntary commitment documents

(B) order an immediate electroencephalogram

(C) insert a nasogastric tube

(D) administer physostigmine

(E) order a respirator

4 Which of the following clinical or environmental circumstances is least likely to be associated with secondarily amyloidosis?

(A) Renal cell carcinoma

(B) Heroin abuse

(C) Hodgkin's disease

(D) Hashimoto's thyroiditis

(E) Rheumatoid arthritis

5 Aspirin causes which of the following effects when taken at therapeutic doses?

(A) Lowers normal body temperature

(B) Alleviates severe pain of visceral origin

(C) Results in tolerance or physical dependence

(D) Affects cellular accumulation and/or proliferation associated with rheumatoid arthritis

(E) Leads to damage of the gastrointestinal epithelium

6 A patient presents with ataxia, leg weakness, sphincter disturbances, and peripheral neuropathy affecting both sensory and motor components. A vitamin B_{12} deficiency is suspected, but lab values show cobalamin levels to be within the normal range. What is the most likely environmental cause of these findings?

(A) Chronic cyanide exposure

(B) Prolonged carbon monoxide exposure

(C) Hexachlorophene toxicity

(D) Nitrous oxide toxicity

(E) Amphotericin B ingestion

7 The plasma membrane consists of lipids and proteins with the basic structure of a lipid bilayer. Which of the following statements regarding the structure and function of the plasma membrane is correct?

(A) Phospholipids are uncharged membrane components that reside within the bilayer

(B) Proteins penetrate only the hydrophobic portion of the bilayer

(C) Phospholipids promote free diffusion of ions and small water-soluble molecules

(D) Proteins are not amphipathic

(E) Some large proteins are free to diffuse laterally in the plane of the membrane

8 A polymerase chain reaction can increase the sensitivity of certain genetic tests. Which of the following characteristics applies to polymerase chain reactions?

(A) The sequence of the segment of DNA to which the primers will bind must be known

(B) Addition of a heat-resistant restriction endonuclease is required

(C) Multiple cycles lead to the rapid, linear amplification of the DNA

(D) The DNA to be amplified is denatured in the presence of an equimolar ratio of primers

9 Of the following statements about messenger RNA (mRNA) transcription, the most accurate is that it

(A) proceeds by synthesis of the RNA in the 3′ to 5′ direction

(B) involves the removal of internal regions of DNA from the genome

(C) occurs only in the cytoplasm of the human cell

(D) may be regulated by hormones

(E) involves the posttranscriptional addition of adenylate nucleotides to the 5′ end of the molecule

10 The presence of seborrheic keratosis and acanthosis nigricans may signify which of the following diseases?

(A) Paget's disease

(B) Gastric carcinoma

(C) Diabetes mellitus

(D) Hemophilia A

(E) Thrombotic thrombocytopenic purpura

11 The leather-bottle stomach depicted in Figure 21 from the color plate section reflects involvement by

(A) Ménétrier's disease

(B) adenomatous polyps

(C) reflux esophagitis

(D) signet ring adenocarcinoma

12 Which sequence below is the correct order of epidermal maturation?

(A) Stratum basale, stratum spinosum, stratum lucidum, stratum granulosum, stratum corneum

(B) Stratum basale, stratum spinosum, stratum granulosum, stratum lucidum, stratum corneum

(C) Stratum basale, stratum granulosum, stratum spinosum, stratum lucidum, stratum corneum

(D) Stratum basale, stratum lucidum, stratum spinosum, stratum granulosum, stratum corneum

(E) Stratum basale, stratum lucidum, stratum granulosum, stratum spinosum, stratum corneum

13 A 25-year-old sexually active woman is evaluated for her fourth acute urinary tract infection during the past 12 months. Her infections are characterized by frequency, urgency, dysuria, and *Escherichia coli* bacteriuria. Her recurrent infections are most likely due to

(A) overgrowth of highly resistant *E. coli* in her fecal reservoir

(B) passage of an infected renal calculus

(C) resistance of the bacteria to the drugs selected for treatment

(D) a foreign body within the genitourinary tract

(E) colonization of the vaginal introitus with fecal Enterobacteriaceae

14 A 2-year-old child is hospitalized with splenomegaly, anemia, hypersplenism, hepatomegaly, and progressive nervous system dysfunction. Enzyme studies show absence of glucocerebrosidase with an accumulation of β-glucosylceramide in macrophages and hepatocytes. The lipid storage disease most likely to be diagnosed in this child is

(A) Niemann–Pick disease

(B) Gaucher's disease, type II

(C) Krabbe's disease

(D) Tay–Sachs disease

15 Which of the following organs is pictured in this micrograph of the male reproductive system?

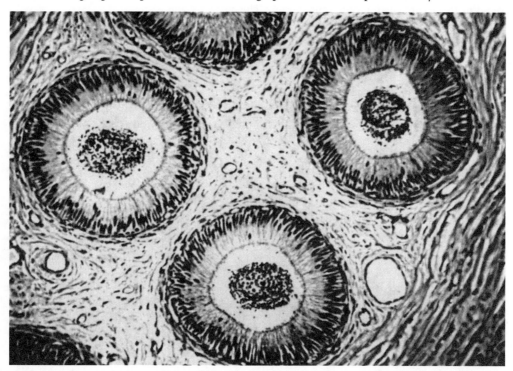

(A) Testis
(B) Epididymis
(C) Vas deferens
(D) Seminal vesicle
(E) Bulbourethral gland

16 A 55-year-old woman presents to a health clinic complaining of a resting tremor in her hand. Her son adds that she has really slowed down in the last 6 months and seems to move rigidly. A preliminary diagnosis of Parkinson's disease is explored. Which of the following statements concerning Parkinson's disease is correct?

(A) Average age of onset is 65 years
(B) Parkinson's disease does not affect personality
(C) Symptoms develop when about 10% of dopamineric neurons are affected
(D) Parkinson's disease is more common in women than men
(E) Lewy bodies are found in the substantia nigra in addition to dopaminergic neuron loss

17 A 25-year-old woman presents to her primary care physician with a primary complaint of "droopy eyelids." Upon further examination she is found to have limb weakness and some difficulty swallowing. Which of the following statements is true concerning this woman's diagnosis?

(A) Her illness may have been caused by infection with beta-hemolytic streptococcus as a child
(B) An MRI would show diffuse white matter changes within her brain
(C) Her symptoms are caused by a common antidepressant medication
(D) Her diagnosis could be confirmed by a single treatment of edrophonium
(E) Her present illness leaves her at increased risk for the development of Parkinson's disease

18 What condition is marked by formation of a malignant pustule?

(A) Enteritis necroticans
(B) Lockjaw
(C) Cutaneous anthrax
(D) Pseudomembranous colitis
(E) Woolsorter's disease

19 A 52-year-old man had painless swelling of his right testis. An orchiectomy was performed. A sample of the tissue is pictured in the accompanying photomicrograph. The correct diagnosis is

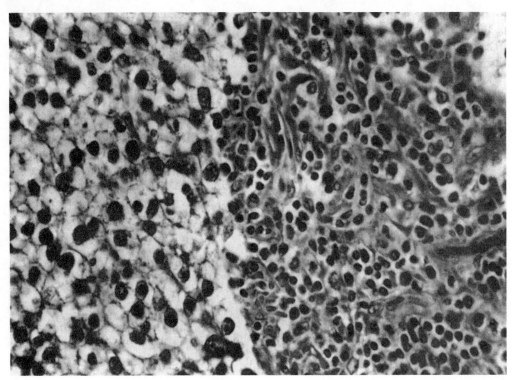

(A) seminoma
(B) mumps orchitis
(C) immature teratoma
(D) choriocarcinoma

20 A patient must be evaluated because of thrombocytopenia. The patient is a 55-year-old, previously well man who was admitted to the hospital yesterday because of pneumonia. Antibiotic therapy was started; although his temperature continues to spike, it is lower than it was on admission. On admission, his hemoglobin was reported to be 13 g/dL, his white blood cell count was 9,000/μL, and his platelet count was 70,000/μL. The next laboratory study that should be done is

(A) bone marrow examination
(B) bleeding time
(C) examination of the peripheral smear
(D) platelet aggregation studies
(E) antiplatelet antibody detection tests

21 An infant is brought to the emergency department with severe oral thrush and hypocalcemia. A complete blood count shows a white cell count within normal limits. The mother admits to being an intravenous drug user. What is the most likely diagnosis in this case?

(A) Chronic mucocutaneous candidiasis
(B) Severe combined immunodeficiency disease
(C) DiGeorge's syndrome
(D) Chronic granulomatous disease

22 Which of the following clinical and laboratory features is characteristic of acute myeloblastic leukemia (AML)?

(A) Patients present with thrombocytosis
(B) Patients often develop hypernatremia and hyperkalemia
(C) Presence of Auer rods in the cytoplasm of leukemic cells
(D) Leukemic cells are negative for myeloperoxidase
(E) Leukemic cells are negative for terminal deoxynucleotidyl transferase (TdT)
(F) Leukemic cells are negative for Sudan black stain

23 The primary thyroid malignancy depicted in Figure 22 from the color plate section is best classified as

(A) papillary carcinoma
(B) follicular carcinoma
(C) medullary carcinoma
(D) insular carcinoma

24 Chronic lymphocytic leukemia (CLL) is the most common form of chronic leukemia in the United States. Which of the following statements about CLL is true?

(A) It is usually seen in patients younger than 50 years of age
(B) It is more frequent in women than in men
(C) It most commonly represents a clonal expansion of neoplastic T lymphocytes
(D) The cells commonly have trisomy 12 chromosomal abnormality
(E) Most patients develop hypergammaglobulinemia

25 After osmotic equilibrium, infusion of several liters of a hypertonic saline solution will

(A) decrease intracellular osmolality
(B) not affect intracellular volume
(C) increase extracellular fluid volume
(D) decrease the plasma osmolarity

26 The U.S. Food and Drug Administration (FDA) has announced that it will test the vaccines against human immunodeficiency virus (HIV) with the least potential for causing the disease and the best chance of inducing protective immunity. Which of the vaccination reagents listed is most likely to be tested?

(A) An attenuated virus that does not cause disease in monkeys
(B) A recombinant HIV DNA in a vaccinia virus to induce host cells to produce only the HIV p24 protein and then antibodies to p24 protein
(C) A denatured, purified CD4 (T4) protein to cause the host to mount an immune response to the HIV-infected CD4+ cells
(D) A human monoclonal antibody that reacts with the intact CD4 (T4) receptor

27 The most important allosteric activator of glycolysis in the liver is which one of the following compounds?

(A) Fructose 2,6-bisphosphate
(B) Acetyl coenzyme A (acetyl CoA)
(C) Adenosine triphosphate (ATP)
(D) Citrate
(E) Glucose 6-phosphate

28 Ingestion of 150 mEq Na+/day is usually balanced by excretion of a similar amount in urine. Because the glomerular filtrate normally contains 26,000 mEq Na+/day, several important Na+-reabsorbing mechanisms have evolved, including which of the following?

(A) Passive transport of Na+ from inside proximal epithelial cells to interstitial spaces
(B) Active transport of Na+ by the Na-K-dependent adenosine triphosphatase (ATPase) basolateral membrane in the proximal tubular epithelium
(C) Passive transport in the thick segment of the loop of Henle
(D) Hormone-independent passive reabsorption in the distal tubular epithelium

29 Which of the following statements concerning immunogenicity is most correct?

(A) Compounds with a molecular weight less than 6,000 daltons are generally immunogenic
(B) Haptens become immunogenic only when combined with low-molecular-weight carriers
(C) A polymer of lysine, methionine, and glutamate with a molecular weight of 10,000 daltons would not be immunogenic
(D) A homopolymer of lysine with a molecular weight of 30,000 daltons would not be immunogenic

30 The thyroid tumor pictured here was removed from a 60-year-old woman whose medical history likely includes

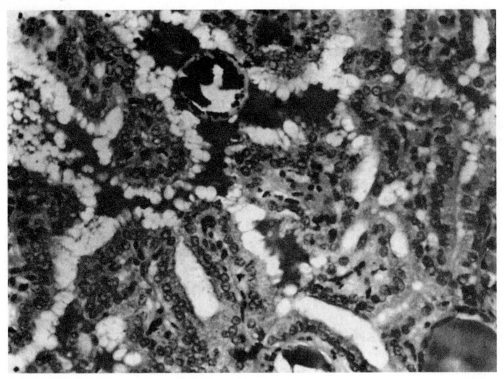

(A) hyperthyroidism
(B) hypothyroidism
(C) irradiation to the head and neck
(D) a pituitary adenoma

31 When comparing pertussis and diphtheria, true statements include which one of the following?

(A) Both pertussis and diphtheria are caused by bacteria that must adhere to respiratory tract cells

(B) Diphtheria symptoms are caused by an exotoxin, but no symptoms of pertussis result from an exotoxin

(C) The bacteria responsible for diphtheria and pertussis both produce endotoxin

(D) Pertussis is caused by an intracellular pathogen, but diphtheria is caused by an extracellular pathogen

(E) The neurologic problems observed with the current diphtheria–tetanus–pertussis (DTP) vaccine are caused by the diphtheria component of this vaccine

32 A 68-year-old widower complains of headaches, forgetfulness, decreased appetite, weight loss, insomnia, constipation, and anhedonia. An electrocardiogram shows first-degree heart block; he also has prostatic hypertrophy. Considering side effects profiles, the best choice of medication would be

(A) imipramine
(B) phenelzine
(C) lithium carbonate
(D) clonazepam
(E) chlorpromazine

33 Which of the following serological profiles are consistent with a patient that has had a self-limited hepatitis B infection? (HbsAg, hepatitis B antigen; HbcAg, hepatitis B core antigen; anti-HBs, anti-hepatitis surface antigen antibody)

(A) HBsAg negative, HBcAg positive, anti-HBs negative

(B) HBsAg negative, HBcAg negative, anti-HBs positive

(C) HBsAg negative, HBcAg positive, anti-HBs positive

(D) HBsAg positive, HBcAg positive, anti-HBs negative

(E) HBsAg positive, HBcAg negative, anti-HBs positive

34 Which of the following neurological diseases are properly matched with frontline therapies for the treatment of that disease?

(A) Myasthenia gravis—mannitol

(B) Parkinson's disease—serotonin reuptake inhibitors

(C) Multiple sclerosis—beta interferon

(D) Alzheimer's disease—lithium

(E) Bipolar disorders (type I and II)—dopamine prodrugs

35 The bone tumor depicted in Figure 23 from the color plate section is probably associated with which one of the following conditions?

(A) von Willebrand's disease

(B) von Hippel–Lindau disease

(C) Multiple myeloma

(D) Multiple osteochondromatosis

36 Which of the following statements concerning the maturation of T cells is true?

(A) It occurs earliest in the thymic medulla

(B) It is independent of thymic epithelial cells

(C) It is independent of antigen

(D) It results in functionally mature cells that are both CD4- and CD8-positive

37 Which of the following conditions is most diagnostic for Zellweger's syndrome?

(A) Increased abundance of peroxisomes

(B) Presence of catalase in the vacuoles of hepatocytes

(C) Elevated plasma C26:0/C22:0 ratio

(D) Increased serum levels of platelet-activating factor

(E) Decreased circulating levels of very long chain fatty acids

38 Which of the following components of sleep architecture is most closely associated with night terrors?

(A) Sleep spindles

(B) Sleep-onset rapid eye movement (REM)

(C) Delta waves

(D) Increased percentage of REM

(E) Normal REM sleep

39 Medications can often affect sexual responses via altering neurotransmitter levels. Which of the following effects on neurotransmitter levels is correctly paired with effect on sexual function?

(A) Increased serotonin—hindered ejaculation and orgasm

(B) Increased dopamine—hindered erection capacity

(C) Decreased norepinephrine—enhanced erection capacity

(D) Decreased dopamine—enhanced libido

(E) Increased norepinephrine—hindered erection capacity

40 A 24-year-old man presented to his family practitioner with a purulent penile discharge. The diagnosis of gonorrhea was based on the finding of intracellular gram-negative cocci in his discharge. He was given amoxicillin and probenecid. The infection improved, but 1 week later the patient still complained of a persistent urethral discharge and pain on urination. On a visit to a local clinic for sexually transmitted diseases, a diagnosis of postgonococcal urethritis was made. What is the most likely cause of his latest syndrome?

(A) A common side effect of probenecid administered during the initial treatment

(B) A lingering gonococcal infection caused by a penicillin-resistant strain of *Neisseria gonorrhoeae*

(C) An improper therapy regimen, which did not treat a coinciding chlamydial infection

(D) A side effect of the correct therapy regimen, which suppressed the patient's normal flora and allowed the establishment of a secondary infection

41 A 38-year-old man with AIDS develops meningitis. Microscopic examination of his spinal fluid shows yeast cells. India ink staining of these yeasts shows a visible, clear halo surrounding each cell. Which one of the following pathogens is responsible for the man's meningitis?

(A) A virus

(B) *Cryptococcus neoformans*

(C) *Haemophilus influenzae*

(D) *Neisseria meningitidis*

(E) *Candida albicans*

42 Which of the following statements describes a property of acetaminophen?

(A) It inhibits lipoxygenase activity
(B) It is an anti-inflammatory agent
(C) It irreversibly acetylates platelets
(D) Gastric irritation is a common side effect
(E) Hepatotoxicity can develop as a result of overdose

43 Which of the following statements about allosteric enzymes is true?

(A) Positive cooperativity desensitizes the enzyme to small changes in substrate concentration
(B) Allosteric regulation requires a quaternary level of protein structure
(C) The allosteric site must be on a different subunit from the catalytic site
(D) The binding of a ligand to the allosteric site induces a conformational change in the active site
(E) They have substrate saturation curves that frequently show first-order kinetics

44 The kidney tumor depicted in Figure 24 from the color plate section is best classified as

(A) Wilms' tumor
(B) teratoma
(C) neuroblastoma
(D) hamartoma

45 A patient presents with a torn medial collateral ligament of the left knee. Which of the following signs may be elicited on physical examination?

(A) Posterior displacement of the tibia
(B) Abnormal lateral rotation during extension
(C) Abnormal passive abduction of the extended leg
(D) Inability to lock the knee on full extension

46 The section of heart and valve depicted in Figure 25 from the color plate section demonstrates which of the following histologic changes?

(A) Mallory bodies
(B) Lewy bodies
(C) Aschoff bodies
(D) Weibel–Palade bodies

47 The female reproductive viscera are best characterized by which of the following statements?

(A) The mesosalpinx contains the tubal branches of the uterine vessels
(B) The ovarian veins drain directly into the inferior vena cava
(C) Lymph from the cervix drains into the inguinal nodes
(D) Visceral afferent nerves from the body of the uterus course along the pelvic splanchnic nerves

48 Which of the following associations between signs and disorders is most correct?

(A) Anti-liver–kidney microsomal antibody-1 (anti-LKM1), positive for hepatitis virus infection, women—autoimmune hepatitis type 3
(B) Antimitochondrial antibodies, elevated alkaline phosphatase, and γ-glutamyl transpeptidase, middle-aged women—primary sclerosing cholangitis
(C) Mallory bodies, α-fetoprotein, descarboxyprothrombin—hepatocellular carcinoma
(D) Aspartate aminotransferase (AST)/alanine aminotransferase (ALT) <2 (ALT>500)—alcoholic liver disease
(E) Ulcerative colitis, cholangiocarcinoma, men—primary biliary sclerosis

49 The primary liver tumor depicted in Figure 26 from the color plate section is which one of the following?

(A) Hepatocellular carcinoma
(B) Epithelioid hemangioendothelioma
(C) Hepatic adenoma
(D) Cholangiocarcinoma

50 Captopril is useful in the treatment of systemic hypertension because it

(A) blocks the effect of angiotensin II at its receptor in the central nervous system (CNS)
(B) directly relaxes vascular smooth muscle
(C) inhibits the movement of extracellular calcium into myocardial cells
(D) decreases the activity of angiotensin-converting enzyme (ACE)
(E) inhibits the production of renin

Answer Key

1-A	11-D	21-C	31-A	41-B
2-A	12-B	22-C	32-B	42-E
3-C	13-E	23-A	33-B	43-D
4-D	14-B	24-D	34-C	44-C
5-E	15-B	25-C	35-C	45-C
6-D	16-E	26-D	36-C	46-C
7-E	17-D	27-A	37-C	47-A
8-A	18-C	28-B	38-C	48-C
9-D	19-A	29-D	39-A	49-D
10-B	20-C	30-C	40-C	50-D

Answers and Explanations

1 The answer is A *Gastrointestinal system / Pathology / Barrett's espohagus*

Barrett's esophagus is a result of protracted reflux owing to lower esophageal sphincter incompetence, with attendant increased exposure to acid, pepsin, lysolecithin, and bile acids. Esophageal inflammation and ulceration are followed by re-epithelialization and ingrowth of immature pluripotent stem cells. Rather than squamous epithelium, the new epithelium is columnar-lined with gastric- or duodenal-type cells, which better tolerate prolonged acid exposure. Inflammation would be absent only in the case of postmortem ulceration and autolysis; such changes may be accompanied by "leopard spotting"—brown-black esophageal spots that form from acid digestion of hemoglobin. Barrett's esophagus is associated with esophageal adenocarcinoma in a few cases.

2 The answer is A *General principles / Pharmacology / Plasma protein binding of drugs*

Many drugs bind to plasma proteins, which limits glomerular filtration in the kidneys because the drugs are not freely diffusible. Drug–protein interactions generally occur between a wide variety of drugs and albumin or α_1-acid glycoprotein, but not immunoglobulins. Covalent interactions are rare, but when they occur it is generally with reactive, antineoplastic drugs. Renal tubular secretion is generally not limited by plasma protein binding of drugs because secretion reduces free plasma drug concentration, which is quickly followed by dissociation of the drug from plasma proteins.

3 The answer is C *General principles / Pharmacology / Suicide management*

Safely removing any pill fragments from the stomach by nasogastric tube is the first step in the management of the patient described in the question because amitriptyline is an anticholinergic that retards gastrointestinal absorption, increasing the likelihood that pill fragments remain. The patient may ultimately need psychiatric hospitalization; because she is unresponsive, there is no urgency in pursuing this. An electroencephalogram would not add any useful information at this time, and seizures, if they occurred, would most likely be related to the toxicity of amitriptyline and a lowering of the seizure threshold.

Tricyclic antidepressants, like quinidine, have an arrhythmic effect. The changes on electrocardiogram, especially with increased or toxic serum levels, include a prolonged PR interval, prolonged QRS duration, and a prolonged QT interval. In therapeutic dose ranges, tricyclics may suppress premature ventricular contraction.

4 The answer is D *General principles / Pathology / Inflammatory processes*

Secondary amyloidosis is associated with diseases that often result in chronic inflammation and include renal cell carcinoma, chronic heroin abuse, Hodgkin's disease, and rheumatoid arthritis, all conditions that are associated with large amounts of inflammation and cell death.

5 The answer is E *General principles / Pharmacology / Nonsteroidal anti-inflammatory drugs*

Aspirin will cause gastric bleeding and damage to the gastrointestinal tract of virtually all patients. The acidic nature of aspirin and the loss of cytoprotective eicosanoid (due to inhibition of cylco-oxygenase 1) contribute to this common effect. Indeed, this has led to the use of concomitant therapy of aspirin and stable analogues of prostaglandin E2 for patients requiring long-term therapy with nonsteroidal anti-inflammatory drugs (NSAIDs). It is important to note that aspirin will lower body temperature in febrile states only. Unlike narcotic analgesics, aspirin will alleviate mild to moderate pain only (and thus will not affect visceral pain), but will not produce tolerance or physical dependence. Although useful for affecting the pathophysiology associated with inflammation (redness, pain, edema, loss of function), aspirin will not stay the course of the disease by affecting the underlying cellular contributions.

6 **The answer is D** *Central and peripheral nervous system / Neuroscience / Neurotoxicity*

Nitrous oxide toxicity causes presentation of patients with symptoms very similar to long-term vitamin B_{12} (cobalamin) deficiency. The neuropathologic description of this phenomenon is termed subacute combined degeneration (SACD) and comprises the following findings: (1) spongy vacuolization and degeneration of myelin sheaths starting in the thoracic spinal cord region; (2) axonal degradation; and (3) macrophage infiltration and astrocytic gliosis. Chronic cyanide exposure causes optic atrophy and deafness. Symptoms of prolonged carbon monoxide exposure include headache, dizziness, and confusion, with some patients developing a persistent tremor and a wide range of psychiatric disorders. Hexachorophene ingestion causes irritability, nausea, and vomiting, while amphotericin B ingestion may lead to symptoms similar to Parkinson's disease, encephalopathy, or various myelopathies or radiculopathies.

7 **The answer is E** *General principles / Histology / Membrane structure and function*

The plasma membrane consists of amphipathic lipids (predominantly phospholipids and cholesterol) and amphipathic proteins. The hydrophilic portions of these molecules face the external and internal aqueous environments. The hydrophobic portions are in the internal portion of the bilayer. Phospholipids, which have charged head groups, prevent free diffusion of ions and water-soluble molecules, thus imparting selective permeability properties to the lipid bilayer. Proteins may be restricted to the external portion of the bilayer or span it entirely. In addition, the membrane is fluid, allowing lateral diffusion of even large proteins.

8 **The answer is A** *General principles / Biochemistry / Polymerase chain reaction*

A polymerase chain reaction is used to amplify sequences of DNA from a single copy to more than 1 million copies in a logarithmic fashion. The template DNA is initially denatured in the presence of excess primers, which are short (15 to 25 base pairs) oligonucleotides homologous to sequences on the template DNA. Because the DNA is denatured and renatured many times by multiple heating and cooling cycles, limiting amounts of primers prevents large-scale amplification of the parent strand. The temperatures at which a polymerase chain reaction is carried out are generally in the range of 55°C to 95°C. Heat-resistant DNA polymerase, such as the Taq polymerase, is resistant to heat denaturation.

9 **The answer is D** *General principles / Biochemistry / RNA structure and function*

The primary transcript for mRNA is formed in the nucleus, where the elongation proceeds from the 5′ to the 3′ end. Most eukaryotic mRNAs are distinctive in that the 5′ ends are capped by the addition of a methylated guanylic acid residue and the 3′ ends have a polyadenylate tail of 100 to 200 adenosine nucleotides. Most precursor forms of mRNA contain intervening sequences that are removed by a process known as splicing. The binding of steroid hormones with their receptors to specific genes results in the increased synthesis of the mRNA encoded in those genes.

10 **The answer is B** *Skin and related connective tissue / Pathology / Gastric carcinoma*

The development of seborrheic keratosis plus acanthosis nigricans may signify the presence of an internal malignancy, including gastric carcinoma. The Leser–Trélat sign is the development of seborrheic keratosis, acanthosis nigricans, or amyloidosis in a patient with gastrointestinal malignancy.

11 **The answer is D** *Gastrointestinal system / Pathology / Adenocarcinoma of the stomach*

The gross appearance of a leather-bottle stomach is caused by a diffuse infiltration of the wall of the stomach by a poorly differentiated adenocarcinoma, usually a signet ring adenocarcinoma. This accounts for the gray, plaque-like thickening of the stomach wall apparent in this photograph. The adjacent prepyloric stomach appears to have a glistening serosal surface. Signet ring adenocarcinomas diffusely infiltrate through the wall of the stomach, invade the serosal adipose tissue and omentum, and have a very poor prognosis.

12 **The answer is B** *Skin and related connective tissue / Anatomy / Epidermis*

The order of epidermal maturation is stratum basale, stratum spinosum, stratum granulosum, stratum lucidum, and stratum corneum. The stratum basale is the germinal layer of the epidermis. Cells migrate and differentiate from this layer at a rate equal to desquamation of keratin from the outermost layer. The stratum spinosum is superficial to the stratum basale, and its cells are in the process of growth and early keratin synthesis. The stratum granulosum is characterized by intracellular granules, which contribute to the keratinization process. The stratum lucidum is a homogeneous layer between the stratum granulosum and the stratum corneum that occurs only in thick skin. The stratum corneum is the most superficial layer of the epidermis and is mainly composed of keratin.

13 **The answer is E** *Renal/urinary system / Microbiology / Recurrent urinary tract infections*

Longitudinal studies have shown that bacteriuria in women susceptible to urinary tract infections is preceded by colonization of the vaginal introitus with the responsible organism from the rectal flora.

14 **The answer is B** *Gastrointestinal system / Pathology / Gaucher's disease*

Type II Gaucher's disease is the infantile acute cerebral pattern and is characterized by a virtual absence of glucocerebrosidase, with an accumulation of large quantities of β-glucosylceramide in macrophages and hepatocytes. Type I, or the classic form, is the adult type, in which storage of glucocerebrosides is limited to the mononuclear phagocytes. Patients with type I have reduced but detectable levels of glucocerebrosidase. Both type I and type II are autosomal recessive. Niemann–Pick disease is characterized by the accumulation of sphingomyelin, which is due to a deficiency in sphingomyelinase. Tay–Sachs disease, in which ganglioside accumulates, results from lack of N-acetyl hexosaminidase. The defective enzyme in Krabbe's disease is galactosyl ceramidase.

15 **The answer is B** *Reproductive system / Histology / Epididymis*

The micrograph shows the epididymis, a highly convoluted tubular organ that conveys sperm and fluid from the testis to the ductus (vas) deferens.

16 **The answer is E** *Central and peripheral nervous system / Neuroscience / Parkinson's disease*

Resting tremor and bradykinesia represent the most common presentation for Parkinson's disease. Most patients develop changes in personality or the development of depression, but these changes are normally overlooked due to the physical manifestations of the disease. Men develop Parkinson's disease more often than women (3:2 ratio) and the average age of onset is 55 years of age. Symptoms do not become manifest until over 80% of neurons of the substantia nigra are lost. Lewy bodies (eosinophilic cytoplasmic inclusions formed by collections of filaments) are found in neurons of patients with types of several neurological diseases. Their presence has not been linked to any particular variation in Parkinson's disease but they are normally found in the venterolateral regions of the substantia nigra in association with marked dopaminergic neuron loss.

17 **The answer is D** *Central and peripheral nervous system / Neuroscience / Myasthenia gravis*

The presentation of this patient is very suggestive for myasthenia gravis (MG). Patients with MG present with diplopia, ptosis, and weakness in commonly used muscles. Symptoms of MG are caused by autoantibodies that bind to the acetylcholine receptor, although some cellular immunity against the receptor may also be present. This limits the number of available acetylcholine receptors and leads to a limited ability to stimulate muscle contraction, especially when the muscle is repeatedly used. Edrophonium is a short-acting acetylcholinesterase inhibitor that is used in the diagnosis of MG. After administration of edrophonium the patient regains full muscle strength for up to 5 minutes. MG is sometimes found in association with thymoma, rheumatoid arthritis, systemic lupus erythematosis, or thyrotoxicosis. Treatment with neostigmine or pyridostigmine can temporarily reverse weakness. Additionally, thymectomy may reduce symptoms and lead to remission and thus should be considered for all patients under the age of 60.

18 **The answer is C** *General principles / Pathology; physiology / Anthrax*

A malignant pustule is a clinical manifestation of cutaneous anthrax. It occurs at the site of inoculation and is characterized by a black eschar at its base surrounded by an inflamed ring. Enteritis necroticans, caused by *Clostridium perfringens*, and pseudomembranous colitis, caused by *Clostridium difficile*, are diseases of the gastrointestinal tract that may be characterized by ulcerative lesions in the intestinal mucosa. Lockjaw is a lay name for tetanus; it refers to the muscle and neural spasms caused by the neurotoxin tetanospasmin. Woolsorter's disease is pulmonary anthrax, a progressive, diffuse, lethal pneumonia caused by the inhalation of spores of *Bacillus anthracis*.

19 **The answer is A** *Reproductive system / Histology; pathology / Seminomas*

Seminomas constitute 30% to 40% of testicular tumors and are divided into classic and spermatocytic forms. Classic seminomas, as in this case, are composed of nests of tumor cells with abundant clear cytoplasm with vesicular nuclei and angulated nucleoli (*left*). The nests are separated by fibrous strands that contain inflammatory cells, usually lymphocytes and plasma cells (*right*). Mumps orchitis involves large numbers of giant cells; it is an inflammatory reaction, not a neoplasm, and it is seen in the young. Teratomas contain aberrant ectopic tissues (e.g., brain, cartilage, and epithelial-lined cysts), whereas choriocarcinomas have syncytiotrophoblastic giant cells and cytotrophoblasts in close apposition.

20 **The answer is C** *Hematopoietic and lymphoreticular system / Hematology / Platelet homeostasis*

Examination of the peripheral blood smear is essential to evaluation of a patient for thrombocytopenia. Unreported abnormalities of the red cells may offer a clue to the etiology, or occasionally one may find a discrepancy between the number of platelets seen on the smear and that found by the automated count. This occurs in pseudothrombocytopenia, in which clumping of platelets in a specific anticoagulant, usually ethylenediaminetetraacetic acid (EDTA), results in marked underestimation of the count.

21 **The answer is C** *General principles / Immunology / DiGeorge's syndrome*

Patients with diseases that cause a deficiency in T cells are extremely prone to viral, fungal, and protozoal infections. The patient described in the question has severe oral thrush, which is caused by a *Candida* species, and hypocalcemia. These findings are consistent with a diagnosis of DiGeorge's syndrome, which results from a defect in the embryonic development of the third and fourth pharyngeal pouches. Both the thymus and parathyroid glands fail to develop, resulting in hypocalcemia. The white blood cell count can be within normal limits, but virtually all of the circulating leukocytes are B cells and plasma cells.

22 **The answer is C** *Hematopoietic and lymphoreticular system / Pathology / T cell acute myeloblastic leukemia*

Patients with acute leukemia often develop metabolic abnormalities. Hyponatremia and hypokalemia are common in patients with acute leukemia, because renal tubule abnormalities can be induced by lysozyme or other products of the leukemic cells. Patients with acute lymphocytic leukemia (ALL) and AML also present with pancytopenia. Detection of TdT, a nuclear protein, is seen in more than 95% of patients with ALL and 15% of patients with AML. AML is positive for Sudan black stain and myeloperoxidase, whereas ALL is negative for both. The presence of Auer rods (i.e., abnormal primary granules) in the cytoplasm of leukemic cells is diagnostic of AML.

23 **The answer is A** *Endocrine system / Pathology / Papillary carcinoma*

This portion of thyroid demonstrates multiple cysts containing a papillary proliferation of cellular elements. This papillary architecture is characteristic of a form of adenocarcinoma of the thyroid gland termed papillary carcinoma. In this neoplastic proliferation, cuboidal cells line fibrovascular cores and are associated with psammomatous calcifications. These tumors are usually cystic and exude an oily hemorrhagic fluid.

24 The answer is D *Hematopoietic and lymphoreticular system / Pathology / Chronic lymphocytic leukemia*

Chronic lymphocytic leukemia (CLL) is uncommon in persons younger than 40 years of age and is usually seen in patients older than 50 years of age. It is found more frequently in men than in women. CLL is a clonal expansion of neoplastic B lymphocytes in more than 95% of cases. These cells commonly have trisomy 12 alone or have additional chromosomal abnormalities. Most patients with CLL develop some degree of hypogammaglobulinemia.

25 The answer is C *General principles / Physiology / Fluid balance*

Infusion of a hypertonic solution instantaneously adds both volume and milliosmoles to the extracellular (and total body) water space. Because the solution is hypertonic, the osmolality increases in the extracellular space (but remains unchanged in the intracellular space), thereby causing osmosis of water out of the cells and into the extracellular compartment. At equilibrium, the extracellular volume is expanded, and its osmolality is increased. In contrast, the intracellular volume is decreased, resulting in an increase in intracellular osmolality.

26 The answer is D *General principles / Immunology / Vaccines as applied to AIDS*

Of the vaccination procedures listed, the FDA is most likely to test the procedure that uses a human monoclonal antibody that reacts with the intact CD4 (T4) receptor. Antibodies that react with CD4 should look like the portion of HIV that reacts with the CD4 receptor. Therefore, the vaccinated person should make an antibody to the human monoclonal antibody, which may protect against HIV.

27 The answer is A *General principles / Biochemistry / Glycolysis*

The primary step in the regulation of glycolysis is the conversion of fructose 6-phosphate to fructose 1,6-bisphosphate. The enzyme, 1-phosphofructokinase, is an allosteric enzyme that is inhibited by ATP and citrate and is activated by fructose 2,6-bisphosphate. The concentration of fructose 2,6-bisphosphate in turn is regulated by glucagon. Acetyl CoA is not an allosteric effector of any of the glycolytic enzymes. Glucose 6-phosphate is an inhibitor of hexokinase.

28 The answer is B *Renal/urinary system / Physiology / Renal sodium transport*

Almost 75% of Na + is reabsorbed in the proximal tubular epithelium by several processes, including active transport at the basolateral surface and cotransport of Na + at the luminal surface with glucose or amino acids. An additional 22% is reabsorbed by the active transport process in the ascending thick limb of the loop of Henle. The remaining small percentage of Na + that reaches the distal tubular epithelium is reabsorbed by a highly regulated, aldosterone-sensitive process involving exchange with K + .

29 The answer is D *General principles / Immunology / Immunologic response*

The necessary characteristics that a given compound must possess to be immunogenic include a high molecular weight, chemical complexity, and recognition as being foreign. Compounds with a molecular weight greater than 6,000 daltons are generally immunogenic, and those with a molecular weight less than 1,000 daltons generally are not. Compounds between 1,000 and 6,000 daltons may or may not be immunogenic, depending on the degree of foreignness or chemical complexity. Haptens are small, low-molecular-weight compounds that become immunogenic when combined with a high-molecular-weight carrier, such as a conjugate of dinitrophenol and albumin. Whereas a large homopolymer of lysine would not be immunogenic because of a lack of chemical complexity, a smaller polymer containing different molecules would be immunogenic.

30 **The answer is C** *Endocrine system / Pathology / Papillary carcinoma*

The photomicrograph is of a papillary carcinoma of the thyroid gland, and there is a demonstrated association of this type of tumor with previous radiation therapy to the neck. The tumor cells grow on thin, fibrovascular stalks and form papillae. The cells have large, overlapping nuclei; the nucleoplasm has marked chromatin, which gives the nuclei a clear "Orphan Annie eye" appearance. Papillary carcinomas also may have stromal calcification, forming concentric laminated concretions called psammoma bodies (*top center*). These carcinomas metastasize through the lymphatics to cervical lymph nodes, but in general they are indolent tumors.

31 **The answer is A** *Respiratory system / Pathology / Pathogenic mechanisms of respiratory pathogens*

Pertussis and diphtheria are caused by *Bordetella pertussis* and *Corynebacterium diphtheriae*, respectively. Both of these pathogens are extracellular bacteria that adhere to the respiratory tract and produce exotoxins contributing to pathogenesis. Because *B. pertussis* is gram-negative, it produces endotoxin, unlike gram-positive *C. diphtheriae*. The neurologic problems associated with the DTP vaccine are caused by the pertussis component of the vaccine that uses whole killed cells.

32 **The answer is B** *Central and peripheral nervous system / Pharmacology / Geriatric depression*

The patient has depression. Monoamine oxidase inhibitor antidepressants (e.g., phenelzine) have a safe cardiac profile (except for some initial orthostatic hypotension) and essentially no anticholinergic activity, making them a good choice for the elderly who are vulnerable to constipation, memory impairment, and urinary retention. Lithium carbonate has a prophylactic role for recurrent depression but not acute depression. The neuroleptic chlorpromazine is not indicated because the patient is exhibiting no psychotic symptoms. Benzodiazepines (e.g., clonazepam) help with anxiety, which this patient does not have, and can sedate, increase cognitive deficits, and increase depression in the elderly.

33 **The answer is B** *General principles / Virology / Hepatitis B serologies*

Self-limited hepatitis B viral infection is associated with immune clearance of the virus and a lack of hepatitis B viral replication. In the absence of viral replication, serologies should be negative for surface and core antigens. Immunity against hepatitis B virus is demonstrated by anti-hepatitis B surface antigen antibody. Thus, the answer is (B) and this should also be the serology found for individuals vaccinated against hepatitis B infection.

34 **The answer is C** *Central and peripheral nervous system / Neuroscience / Neurologic pharmacology*

The proper treatments for the above diseases are: myasthenia gravis—pyridostigmine or neostigmine; Parkinson's disease—levodopa-carbidopa (dopamine prodrugs); multiple sclerosis—beta interferon; Alzheimer's disease—various acetylcholine inhibitors have shown small amounts of efficacy; bipolar disorders—lithium compounds.

35 **The answer is C** *Musculoskeletal system / Pathology / Bone tumor*

This bone tumor is characterized by a proliferation of cells with a cartwheel-like arrangement of chromatin and abundant eccentric cytoplasm. Adjacent to the nucleus is a clear space, called a hof, that corresponds to the Golgi apparatus. This histologic appearance is characteristic of a plasma cell tumor of bone. Plasmacytomas of bone are frequently associated with systemic plasma cell disorders, such as multiple myeloma. Systemic involvement can be confirmed by demonstrating a monoclonal spike in serum protein electrophoresis or by identifying multiple lytic bone lesions by radiographic study.

36 The answer is C *General principles / Histology / T cell maturation*

Maturation of a stem cell to a resting T cell occurs earliest in the cortex. The medullary region is where the variable (V), diverse (D), and joining (J) regions of the T cell receptor undergo rearrangement. Maturation is independent of antigen and dependent on contact with thymic epithelial cells for purposes of proliferation and differentiation. Upon reaching functional maturity, T cells become positive for either CD4 or CD8, but not both.

37 The answer is C *General principles / Pathology / Zellweger's syndrome*

In Zellweger's syndrome, the amount of cytosolic catalase is elevated; phytanic acid accumulates in CNS tissues; the plasma ratio of C26:0/C22:0 fatty acids is elevated; and there is a deficiency of platelet-activating factor. Zellweger's syndrome results from the absence of or a grossly reduced number of peroxisomes. Peroxisomes are cellular microbodies where oxidation of a very long chain of fatty acids (C26 to C40) is initiated, phytanic acid is oxidized, and plasmalogens (e.g., platelet-activating factor) are synthesized.

38 The answer is C *Central and peripheral nervous system / Behavioral science / Sleep architecture*

Night terrors are characterized by partial awakening in terror from stages III and IV (when delta waves occur) of slow-wave sleep. In narcolepsy, sleep attacks are sleep-onset REM periods that intrude into wakefulness. The motor paralysis component of sleep-onset REM periods that is associated with narcolepsy is called cataplexy. REM sleep normally occurs about 90 minutes after the onset of sleep, but in major depression, it occurs after only 45 minutes. There are also increased amounts of REM throughout the night in depressed individuals.

39 The answer is A *Reproductive system / Behavioral science / Sexual function*

Increasing the levels of serotonin can decrease the ability to ejaculate and achieve orgasm. As dopamine levels increase, a patient may have enhanced libido and ability to have an erection. When dopamine levels are decreased, the erection capacity is diminished. Drugs modifying norepinephrine levels modulate erection capacity; increased levels enhance and decreased levels inhibit erection capacity.

40 The answer is C *Reproductive system / Pharmacology / Gonorrheal and chlamydial coinfections*

Of all cases presenting clinically as gonorrhea, 45% have coexisting chlamydial infections. Therefore, the correct treatment for gonorrhea is the administration of both penicillin for *Neisseria gonorrhoeae* and tetracycline for *Chlamydia trachomatis*. Amoxicillin is an oral penicillin; probenecid increases its blood level by blocking its excretion.

41 The answer is B *Central and peripheral nervous system / Microbiology / Meningitis*

Cryptococcus neoformans is responsible for meningitis in this case. The India ink microscopic staining technique demonstrated the presence of yeast cells producing a capsule (the capsule appears as a clear halo), and the only encapsulated yeast among the options is *C. neoformans*. This organism is an important fungal cause of meningitis, and it often infects AIDS patients.

42 The answer is E *Musculoskeletal system / Pharmacology / Action of aspirin and acetaminophen*

Acetaminophen, like aspirin and NSAIDs, inhibits the cyclo-oxygenase, not the lipoxygenase, pathway. The lack of anti-inflammatory effects of acetaminophen remains perplexing but may relate to selectivity toward inhibition of newly described members of the cyclo-oxygenase family. Also, unlike aspirin, it does not interfere with platelet function and rarely causes gastric side effects. When consumed in very high doses, acetaminophen can cause hepatotoxicity due to the production of reactive metabolites in the liver that eventually overwhelm the protection afforded by glutathione.

43 **The answer is D** *General principles / Physiology / Allosteric enzymes*

Allosteric enzymes have sites distinct from the active site where regulatory ligands bind and alter either the V_{max} or the K_m for the substrate. The substrate saturation curves do not obey Michaelis–Menten kinetics and often show sigmoidicity, which indicates positive cooperation between active sites. Enzymes that obey Michaelis–Menten kinetics require an 81-fold increase in substrate concentration to achieve an increase from 10% to 90% of V_{max}. Allosteric enzymes that display positive cooperation require a smaller increase in substrate concentration to achieve the same increase in V_{max}. The allosteric sites may be either on the same subunit as the catalytic site or on a separate regulatory subunit. Thus, the quaternary level of protein structure (i.e., the presence of multiple peptides in a protein) is not an absolute requirement for allosteric regulation.

44 **The answer is C** *Central and peripheral nervous system / Pathology / Neuroblastoma*

Neuroblastomas are among the most frequent tumors of early childhood. They are derived from neural crest cells, and neoplastic cells may produce epinephrine or norepinephrine. The neoplastic cells have a salt-and-pepper chromatin and frequently form rosettes, with the background matrix having a fibrillary or a reticular appearance. This appearance derives from the tendency of these cells to produce abortive neurites or dendritic connections.

45 **The answer is C** *Musculoskeletal system / Anatomy / Knee*

The medial collateral ligament prevents abduction of the leg at the knee. It extends from the medial femoral epicondyle to the shaft of the tibia. The oblique popliteal ligament resists lateral rotation during the final degrees of extension. The posterior cruciate ligament prevents posterior displacement of the tibia. The anterior cruciate ligament helps lock the knee joint on full extension.

46 **The answer is C** *Cardiovascular system / Pathology / Rheumatic carditis*

This section of heart shows the characteristic Aschoff bodies of rheumatic carditis. These bodies have a central region of degenerated collagen surrounded by histiocytes. Many of these histiocytes are multinucleated or have central stripes of chromatin within their nucleus (hence, the term caterpillar cells). Rheumatic endocarditis is typically associated with pancarditis, chorea, erythema marginatum, and migratory polyarthritis. Weibel–Palade bodies are rod-shaped, cytoplasmic organelles seen by electron microscopy in endothelial cells. Mallory bodies are eosinophilic intracytoplasmic inclusions seen in liver cells. Lewy bodies are eosinophilic round to elongated inclusions found in cholinergic cells of the basal nucleus of Meynert.

47 **The answer is A** *Reproductive system / Anatomy / Female reproductive system*

Blood flows to the fallopian tubes through branches of the uterine vessels carried in the surrounding mesentery, which is called the mesosalpinx. The ovarian veins drain blood from the ovaries. The right ovarian vein drains into the inferior vena cava; the left ovarian vein drains into the left renal vein. Lymph from the cervix eventually drains into the internal and external iliac and obturator nodes. Visceral afferent nerves from the uterus follow two pathways: fibers from the cervix follow the splanchnic nerves (nervi erigentes); however, the body of the uterus and uterine tubes send fibers in parallel to the sympathetic nerves.

48 **The answer is C** *Gastrointestinal system / Physiology / Interpretation of laboratory tests in liver disease*

In hepatocellular carcinoma, Mallory bodies and α-fetoprotein demonstrate that the tumor is of hepatocellular origin. Descarboxyprothrombin is an abnormal form of prothrombin that is often produced by hepatocellular carcinoma tumor cells. Autoimmune hepatitis (AIH) type 3 is associated with antisoluble liver antigen antibodies, not anti-LKM1. Anti-LKM1 is seen in AIH type 2. Type 3 is the only type of AIH that is not associated with hepatitis C infection. Primary biliary cirrhosis results in destruction of intrahepatic bile ducts. It is associated with antimitochondrial antibodies, increased alkaline phosphatase, and λ-glutamyl transpeptidase. Approximately 90% of patients with primary biliary cirrhosis are middle-aged women. Aspartate aminotransferase (AST) and ALT are the most accurate markers of hepatocellular necrosis. In patients with alcoholic liver disease, the AST:ALT ratio is above 2, because ALT is more sensitive to vitamin B_6 deficiency and does not increase to greater than 500 because of this disease. If the AST:ALT ratio is above 2 but the ALT is greater than 500, another diagnosis should be considered. Primary sclerosing cholangitis is a cholestatic liver disease characterized by inflammation and sclerosis of the intrahepatic and extrahepatic bile ducts. Approximately 70% of patients have concomitant inflammatory bowel disease, in particular ulcerative colitis. The incidence of cholangiocarcinoma in these patients is as high as 10% to 15%. Unlike the other immune-mediated liver diseases, 75% of patients with primary sclerosing cholangitis are men.

49 **The answer is D** *Gastrointestinal system / Pathology / Hepatic neoplasm*

This primary liver tumor is characterized by multiple white nodules involving the right lobe of the liver. Cholangiocarcinomas, which are adenocarcinomas derived from the bile ducts, tend to track along the normal biliary system of the liver, forming multiple nodules along the arborizing biliary network. The white nodules visible in this slide reflect this propensity. These tumors are extremely aggressive neoplasms and frequently cause obstructive jaundice.

50 **The answer is D** *Cardiovascular system / Pharmacology / Angiotensin-converting enzyme inhibitors*

Captopril is the prototype of a group of ACE inhibitors. These agents lower blood pressure in poorly understood ways, but a critical role for inhibition of ACE (with loss of production of angiotensin II) seems apparent. ACE inhibitors do not affect renin per se, nor do they have any activity toward angiotensin II receptors.

test **5**

Questions

Directions: Single best answer questions consist of numbered items or incomplete statements followed by answers or by completions of the statement. Select the ONE lettered answer or completion that is BEST in each case.

1 Which of the following statements concerning insulin-dependent diabetes mellitus (IDDM) type I is correct?

(A) It responds to sulfonylurea therapy

(B) Patients usually have low plasma glucagon levels

(C) Continuous subcutaneous insulin infusion therapy minimizes the danger of hypoglycemia

(D) Posthypoglycemic hyperglycemia is treated by decreasing insulin dosage during a critical period

(E) Hemoglobin A_{1C} levels are not a good indicator of diabetic control over the preceding 3 months

2 The uterine cervical tissue shown in the accompanying photomicrograph shows features of which one of the following infections?

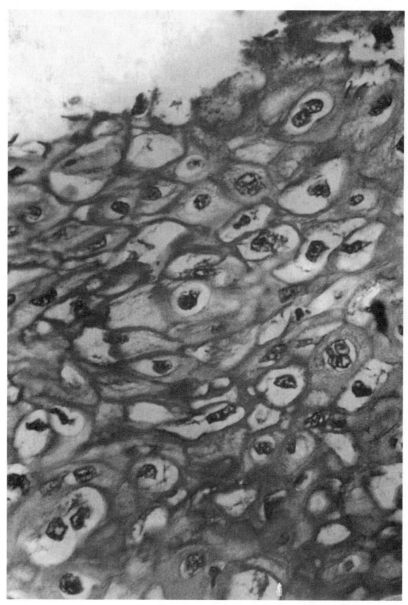

(A)   Papillomavirus
(B)   Herpes genitalis
(C)   Gonorrheal cervicitis
(D)   Carcinoma in situ

3 Which of the following vaccines for viral diseases does not require the use of live or inactivated viral compounds?

(A)   Hepatitis B
(B)   Vaccinia
(C)   Measles
(D)   Mumps
(E)   Rubella

4 Hepatic gluconeogenesis from alanine requires the participation of

(A)   glucose 6-phosphatase and pyruvate kinase
(B)   phosphofructokinase and pyruvate carboxylase
(C)   pyruvate carboxylase and phosphoenolpyruvate carboxykinase
(D)   fructose 1,6-diphosphatase and pyruvate kinase
(E)   transaminase and phosphofructokinase

5 Which of the following statements about hairy cell leukemia is true?

(A) It represents an expansion of neoplastic T lymphocytes

(B) Patients usually have symptoms caused by splenomegaly

(C) Cells are negative for tartrate-resistant acid phosphatase

(D) It occurs more frequently among females than among males

(E) It is usually seen in patients younger than 40 years of age

6 Glycine is a diprotic amino acid containing two ionizing groups available for titration. If the pK_a values for these groups are $pK_1 = 2.4$ and $pK_2 = 9.60$, what is the isoelectric point (pI) for glycine?

(A) 1.5

(B) 6.0

(C) 7.0

(D) 9.0

(E) 12.9

7 Which of the following statements concerning primitive aortic arches and their derivatives is true?

(A) The left fourth aortic arch forms the arch of the aorta

(B) The right sixth aortic arch forms the right subclavian artery

(C) The left fifth aortic arch forms the ductus arteriosus

(D) The first aortic arch forms the common carotid artery

8 If forbidden clones are not deleted during T cell development, a person may develop

(A) hypogammaglobulinemia

(B) a type I hypersensitivity reaction to exogenous antigens

(C) an autoimmune disease

(D) tolerance to autoantigens

9 A 60-year-old woman is brought to the hospital because of fever and confusion. A week earlier, she received chemotherapy for lymphoma. In the emergency department, she is noted to have rapid breathing; cool, clammy skin; and blood pressure of 70/40. Complete blood count shows a white blood cell count of $200/\mu L$. Gram stains of urine and sputum are negative. Which of the following empiric therapies would be most appropriate for this patient?

(A) Gentamicin

(B) Amikacin

(C) Chloramphenicol–gentamicin

(D) Piperacillin–gentamicin

10 The lung depicted in Figure 27 from the color plate section is filled with eosinophilic granular material. This lung is most likely affected by which one of the following conditions?

(A) Pulmonary edema

(B) Bronchioloalveolar adenocarcinoma

(C) Alveolar proteinosis

(D) Aspirated food

11 A physician who has recommended urography for her competent 68-year-old male patient is trying to decide whether or not to disclose the remote risk (1 in 10,000) of a fatal reaction. If the physician favors nondisclosure, reasoning that it would not be in the patient's best interest to worry him with such remote risks, the physician is guided by

(A) beneficence but not nonmaleficence

(B) nonmaleficence but not beneficence

(C) both beneficence and nonmaleficence

(D) justice

(E) gratitude

12 A physician who has recommended a procedure to his patient is trying to decide whether or not to disclose the remote risk of a fatal reaction associated with this procedure. The physician who believes the decision should be determined by what other physicians would do in similar circumstances is guided by

(A) both beneficence and nonmaleficence

(B) strong paternalism

(C) weak paternalism

(D) respect for autonomy

(E) the professional practice standard

13 Which of the following viruses belongs to a family of viruses characterized by life-long latency and the possibility of reactivation?

(A) Hepatitis A virus

(B) Adenovirus serotypes 1–35

(C) Influenza

(D) Respiratory syncytial virus

(E) Epstein–Barr virus

14 A scientist in the year 2350 is advising the NASA genetic engineering department concerning its attempts to engineer humans who can better survive the harsh climate of a planet that has high levels of ultraviolet (UV) light. The NASA engineers want to incorporate a group of genes that will allow epidermal cells to produce a light-absorbing pigment. Of the following genetic manipulations, which would be most advantageous in cells in a UV-rich environment?

(A) Removing intron DNA from the engineered genes

(B) Introducing the engineered genes in an overlapping fashion into the human genome

(C) Altering a theoretical human equivalent of the bacterial RecA protein in the cells to decrease RecA activity

(D) Producing genes with a low thymidine content

15 The accompanying photomicrograph shows an adrenal mass that was resected from a 2-year-old child. This lesion most likely is

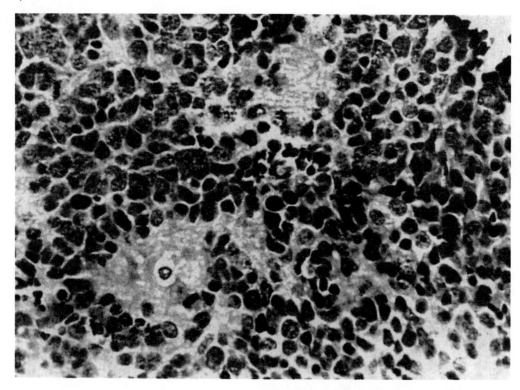

(A) Wilms' tumor

(B) a neuroblastoma

(C) a ganglioneuroma

(D) a pheochromocytoma

16 Based on the Michaelis–Menten equation, V_0, the initial velocity, equals V_{max} when

(A) $[S] \gg K_m$

(B) $K_m = [S]$

(C) $K_m \gg [S]$

(D) $[S] = 0$

17 A resident has been assigned to the operating room for a 2-month rotation. The staff surgeon under whom he will work is a stickler for theory, and on the first day of the new rotation, he asked the resident the following question. With regard to anesthetics, MAC refers to

(A) maximum allowable concentration
(B) minimum alveolar concentration
(C) maximum alveolar concentration
(D) minimum arterial concentration
(E) maximum arterial concentration

18 If an anesthetic has a high blood:gas partition coefficient, it means that

(A) recovery will likely be prolonged
(B) lean patients should receive a lower dose than heavy patients
(C) the anesthetic should be delivered at a low concentration initially
(D) the anesthetic should be mixed with an inert gas or oxygen

19 Nitrous oxide cannot be used alone to produce surgical anesthesia but is often used in conjunction with a more powerful agent, such as halothane, because nitrous oxide is

(A) explosive
(B) slow in onset of action due to a low blood:gas partition coefficient
(C) not very potent (i.e., has relatively low lipid solubility)
(D) rapidly metabolized

20 Which of the following statements about chronic myelogenous leukemia (CML) is true?

(A) Chromosomal abnormalities are uncommon
(B) Bone marrow findings reveal 50% cells and 50% fat
(C) A prominent laboratory finding is leukocytosis
(D) There is a marked decrease of serum vitamin B_{12} levels
(E) The disease occurs equally in both sexes

21 Of the following amino acids, which one is released from skeletal muscle in amounts that exceed its relative abundance in muscle protein?

(A) Aspartate
(B) Alanine
(C) Glutamate
(D) Leucine
(E) Tyrosine

22 Rapid diagnosis and determination of the causal species are essential because of the immediately life-threatening nature of which one of the following parasitic infections?

(A) Malaria
(B) Chronic Chagas disease
(C) Amebic dysentery
(D) Mucocutaneous leishmaniasis
(E) Giardiasis

23 Which one of the following classifications describes the annular lesion affecting the rectum that is depicted in Figure 28 from the color plate section?

(A) Signet ring adenocarcinoma
(B) Mucinous adenocarcinoma
(C) Leiomyoma
(D) Solitary rectal ulcer syndrome with cystic change

24 Cystic fibrosis is an autosomal recessive disease with an incidence of 1/1,600 in the white population. What is the frequency of the cystic fibrosis gene?

(A) 1/4
(B) 1/20
(C) 1/40
(D) 1/200
(E) 1/400

25 Which of the following viral gene products are needed for the replication of RNA genome viruses but are not needed for the replication of DNA genome viruses?

(A) Topoisomerase
(B) DNA polymerase (large subunit)
(C) DNA ligase
(D) Reverse transcriptase
(E) Single-strand DNA-binding protein

26 A 50-year-old woman with diabetes has an almost complete loss of renal function within 3 hours of a seemingly successful kidney transplant. Which of the following statements is most correct concerning this type of rejection?

(A) Administration of an immunosuppressive agent will restore kidney function
(B) The rejection occurs without complement activation
(C) Massive T cell infiltration leads to the destruction of the tissue
(D) The patient had preformed antibodies to the graft

27 A 23-year-old woman with borderline personality disorder is hospitalized on a surgery ward to recover from fractures sustained in a motor vehicle accident. The patient states that her resident physician is wonderful and caring, but her primary nurse is cold and cruel. The psychologic mechanism being displayed is best termed

(A) denial
(B) projection
(C) manipulation
(D) displacement
(E) splitting

28 Baroreceptors are highly branched nerve endings that generate receptor potentials proportional to the rate of change in arterial blood pressure; they can also adapt to changes in arterial blood pressure over hours to days. Which of the following statements concerning the specific properties of baroreceptors is most accurate?

(A) Baroreceptors are important for long-term regulation of blood pressure
(B) Clamping both carotid arteries after cutting both vagus nerves results in a decrease in arterial blood pressure
(C) Massaging the carotid sinus area leads to bradycardia and a decrease in arterial blood pressure
(D) A decrease in blood pressure activates baroreceptors, which in turn directly activate the vasomotor center

29 The thyroid neoplasm depicted in Figure 29 from the color plate section is most likely associated with which one of the following conditions?

(A) Giant cell tumors of bone
(B) Wernicke's encephalopathy
(C) Pheochromocytoma
(D) Renal cysts

30 Lidocaine is the prototype of an amide local anesthetic and, as such, is

(A) free of potential CNS side effects
(B) free of potential cardiac adverse effects
(C) rapidly metabolized by plasma cholinesterases
(D) a Na + channel blocker, especially in small myelinated nerve fibers
(E) inappropriate for use in spinal anesthesia

31 A 25-year-old medical student is buried by an avalanche of snow while skiing. Upon rescue, it is necessary to revive him from cardiopulmonary arrest. Although resuscitated, he remains in a coma for several hours before regaining consciousness. It is known that the patient has suffered global hypoxia. The function most likely to have been lost under this condition is the ability to

(A) move facial muscles
(B) walk
(C) move arms
(D) move eyes

32 Which of the following viruses contains a single-stranded DNA genome?

(A) Herpes simplex virus type 1
(B) Hepatitis B
(C) Poliovirus
(D) Adenovirus
(E) Parvovirus B19

33 A 28-year-old woman presents to the emergency department of her local hospital with a complaint of bladder dysfunction. She reports that several months ago she had a transient, severe worsening of her vision that resolved over several weeks. Which of the following statements concerning her disease is correct?

(A) Visual-evoked potentials would show no change in propagation speed
(B) Cerebrospinal fluid analysis would show increased immunoglobulin levels
(C) T2-weighted MRI analysis would be normal
(D) Her symptoms would be resolved by use of a short-acting acetylcholinesterase inhibitor
(E) Her symptoms would be resolved by treatment with a levodopa–carbidopa combination medicine

34 A pregnant woman who is primigravida with blood type O negative comes to the obstetrician's office for a routine visit. The patient states that her husband is AB positive, and she is concerned about the incompatibility of the Rh factors. Her isohemagglutinin titers are normal. What would the most appropriate treatment be?

(A) Administer human anti-D globulin (RhoGAM) to the mother after the birth of the child
(B) Administer RhoGAM to the child immediately after birth
(C) Administer RhoGAM to the child if the blood is Rh-positive
(D) Do nothing at this time

35 In the accompanying figure, the oxyhemoglobin dissociation curve is shown for a normal patient and for an anemic patient. A true statement concerning these patients is which one of the following?

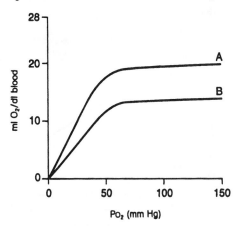

(A) Patient A is anemic
(B) Arterial Po_2 is likely to be similar for both subjects
(C) Venous Po_2 of the anemic subject will be greater than that of the normal subject at rest or during exercise
(D) If cardiac output is identical, oxygen delivery will be identical in subjects A and B

36 A 45-year-old woman has eaten some home-canned vegetables. Two days later she has blurred vision and difficulty swallowing. This is followed by respiratory distress and flaccid paralysis. The symptoms of her illness result from an intoxication caused by a bacterial toxin whose action involves which one of the following effects?

(A) Adenosine diphosphate (ADP) ribosylation of elongation factor 2
(B) Blockage of release of inhibitory neurotransmitters
(C) Blockage of release of acetylcholine (ACh)
(D) Stimulation of adenylate cyclase to elevate intracellular cyclic adenosine monophosphate (cAMP) levels
(E) Hemolysis resulting from sequestration of cholesterol in membranes

37 A 22-year-old woman reports gradual onset and relentless progression of severe pain in the lower left quadrant of her abdomen. She also reported nausea with vomiting and fever. A pelvic examination determined that there was marked tenderness both upon direct palpation and on manipulation of the cervix. A greenish-yellow discharge from the cervix also was noted, but a direct Gram stain of the discharge revealed no etiologic agents. Despite this finding, the patient began antibiotic therapy. A day later, laboratory culture of the discharge yielded growth of oxidase-positive, gram-negative diplococci on Thayer–Martin medium. A diagnosis of gonococcal salpingitis was made. A week posttherapy, the patient's symptoms were relieved and laboratory culture of her cervix revealed no pathogenic organisms. What is the patient's prognosis?

(A) The patient may not be cured and will require constant monitoring of her cervical flora for the next 6 months
(B) The patient may not be cured and is therefore encouraged to abstain from sexual intercourse or observe safe sex practices for the next 6 months
(C) The patient is cured and requires no further monitoring
(D) The patient is cured but faces an increased risk of subsequent episodes of pelvic inflammatory disease, infertility, and ectopic pregnancy

38 Which of the following structures contains Hassall's corpuscles?
(A) Thyroid gland
(B) Parathyroid gland
(C) Pineal gland
(D) Thymus
(E) Spleen

39 The hereditary lung disease depicted in Figure 30 from the color plate section is best classified as
(A) diffuse interstitial fibrosis, familial type
(B) cystic adenomatoid malformation
(C) cystic fibrosis
(D) congenital emphysema (α_1-antitrypsin deficiency)

40 Synthesis of glycogen from fructose in a person with essential fructosuria requires the activity of which one of the following enzymes?
(A) Transketolase
(B) Aldolase B
(C) Hexokinase
(D) Fructokinase
(E) Glucokinase

41 The renal tumor shown in Figure 31 from the color plate section is associated with

(A) hypotension
(B) polycythemia
(C) cerebellar glioblastomas
(D) chromosome 12 abnormalities
(E) chromosome 17 abnormalities

42 A mildly obese 20-year-old man presents to the emergency room at 5:00 A.M. He ingested several six-packs of beer the evening before and awakened at home with a sharp pain in his wrist at the radial–carpal articulation. The wrist is swollen and tender. The patient is slightly disoriented and ataxic but does not remember falling. Radiographs of the wrist are negative. A slight fever is present. For long-term therapy, the patient should be treated with

(A) acyclovir
(B) allopurinol
(C) amantadine
(D) acetazolamide
(E) ampicillin

43 A 52-year-old middle-school teacher has chronic peptic ulcer disease that has been treated for several years with ranitidine (Zantac) and metoclopramide (Reglan). On examination, the physician notes that the patient has involuntary, irregular chewing movements and repetitive tongue protrusion. The most likely cause of these movements is

(A) dystonic reaction
(B) Wilson's disease
(C) Huntington's disease
(D) cerebellar degeneration
(E) tardive dyskinesia

44 A 15-year-old girl presents for evaluation of short stature. She has not yet begun to menstruate. Examination reveals an intellectually normal child with short stature, webbing of the neck, a broad chest, and cubitus valgus. Which of the following tests will provide the best evaluation of this patient?

(A) Amino acid analysis of urine
(B) Organic acid analysis of urine
(C) Serum long-chain fatty acids
(D) Chromosome analysis
(E) Tissue glycogen content

45 A patient who weights 50 kg is given a 20-mg/kg dose of a new drug. The plasma concentrations determined over time are illustrated in the graph below. The drug's volume if distribution (V_d) is approximately

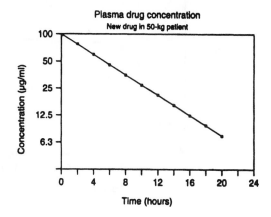

Plasma drug concentration
New drug in 50-kg patient

(A) 200 mL
(B) 1 L
(C) 2 L
(D) 10 L
(E) insufficient information to answer

46 Which of the following correctly pairs a neuronal injury with a symptom of this injury?

(A) Upper motor neuron injury—spasticity
(B) Upper motor neuron injury—muscle atrophy
(C) Upper motor neuron injury—hyporeflexia
(D) Lower motor neuron injury—Babinski reflex possible
(E) Lower motor neuron injury—muscle fasciculations not present

47 The renal disease shown in Figure 32 from the color plate section is associated with which one of the following conditions?

(A) Angiomyolipomas of the kidney
(B) Transitional cell carcinoma of the urinary bladder
(C) Glioblastomas
(D) Intracranial berry aneurysms

48 N-glycosylation of proteins occurs on which of the following amino acids?

(A) Asparagine
(B) Aspartate
(C) Lysine
(D) Serine
(E) Threonine

49 Actin is a microfilament that is involved with which of the following activities?

(A) Ciliary beating

(B) Mitochondrial division

(C) Cell locomotion

(D) Mitotic spindle formation

(E) Vesicle transport in the neuronal axon

50 The chronic inflammatory bowel disease shown in Figure 33 from the color plate section is best classified as

(A) ulcerative colitis

(B) collagenous colitis

(C) Crohn's disease

(D) ischemic colitis

Answer Key

1-D	11-C	21-B	31-C	41-B
2-A	12-E	22-A	32-E	42-B
3-A	13-E	23-B	33-B	43-E
4-C	14-D	24-C	34-D	44-D
5-B	15-B	25-D	35-B	45-D
6-B	16-A	26-D	36-C	46-A
7-A	17-B	27-E	37-D	47-D
8-C	18-A	28-C	38-D	48-A
9-D	19-C	29-C	39-C	49-C
10-C	20-C	30-D	40-C	50-A

Answers and Explanations

1 **The answer is D** *Endocrine system / Pharmacology / Insulin-dependent diabetes mellitus type I*

Sulfonylureas and other oral hypoglycemics are contraindicated in IDDM. The underlying problem is insufficient levels of insulin production. A subsequent lack of glucose uptake into the cells mimics starvation. Consequently, glucagon levels are usually elevated in type I IDDM. Insulin therapy to maintain blood glucose levels within a physiologic range is a symptomatic approach to the treatment of IDDM. Blood glucose levels are monitored routinely, and insulin is adjusted to maintain the blood glucose level. Continuous subcutaneous insulin infusion (CSII) therapy affords the best control of blood glucose level. Even under the strictest monitoring conditions, however, frequent episodes of hypoglycemia complicate CSII therapy. Rebound or posthypoglycemic hyperglycemia, also known as the Somagyi's phenomenon, is treated by reducing the dosage of insulin to avoid the causal drop in blood glucose. Levels of irreversibly glycosylated hemoglobin A_{1C} provide a good indication of diabetic control during the past several months.

2 **The answer is A** *Reproductive system / Histology; pathology / Papillomavirus*

This cervical tissue shows the squamous epithelial changes seen with human papillomavirus (HPV) infection, an epidemic affecting primarily young women. The viral infection causes crenation of nuclei and hyperconvolution, which is accompanied by perinuclear clearing of the cytoplasm. This change has been called condylomatous or koilocytic change and is caused by HPV infection. Some subtypes of HPV predispose the cervical squamous epithelium to dysplasia, and therefore, these patients are sometimes treated with ablative surgery.

3 **The answer is A** *General principles / Virology / Vaccination*

Vaccines for measles, mumps, and rubella are produced from inactivated viral particles and are given as a series of injections as part of pediatric vaccination. Vaccinia vaccine is an attenuated strain of vaccinia that is available for vaccination of toddlers. Hepatitis B vaccine is a purified viral protein of the Hepatitis B viral coat that is produced by recombinant DNA technology.

4 **The answer is C** *General principles / Physiology / Gluconeogenesis*

Gluconeogenesis uses the enzymes in glycolysis that catalyze reversible reactions. The enzymes that catalyze irreversible steps in glycolysis are hexokinase, 1-phosphofructokinase, and pyruvate kinase. To circumvent the three irreversible reactions, the de novo synthesis of glucose requires four enzymes that are unique to gluconeogenesis: pyruvate carboxylase, phosphoenolpyruvate carboxykinase, fructose 2,6-bisphosphatase, and glucose 6-phosphatase.

5 **The answer is B** *Hematopoietic and lymphoreticular system / Pathology / Hairy cell leukemia*

Hairy cell leukemia is caused by expansion of neoplastic B lymphocytes. It is usually seen in patients older than 40 years of age, and there is a definite male preponderance. Patients commonly present with splenomegaly and cytopenia. Abnormal B cells with characteristic cytoplasmic (hairy) projections can be seen on a blood smear by phase microscopy. These cells also stain positively for tartrate-resistant acid phosphatase.

6 **The answer is B** *General principles / Biochemistry / Titration of glycine, isoelectric point, pK$_a$*

Titration of the diprotic form of glycine involves the net removal of one proton from one molecule of glycine. When observing a titration curve for glycine, the addition of base results in two stages on the curve with two pK$_a$ values (pK$_a$ is the negative logarithm of the acid ionization constant). At very low pH values, the fully protonated form of glycine predominates ($+H_3NCCH_2CCOOH$). The midpoint of the first stage of the curve, the pH = pK$_1$ of the ionizing group (COOH), is equal to 2.4. At very high pH values, a proton is removed from the ionizable group $+NH_3$ so that the predominant form of glycine is H_2NCCH_2CCOO-. The midpoint of this section of the curve is 9.6 where the pH = pK$_2$. The pI is the midpoint between the two stages in the titration curve and represents the fully ionized, dipolar form of glycine with no net electric charge. Because glycine has no ionizable group in its side chain, pI is determined by the equation pI = 1/2(pK$_1$ + pK$_2$).

7 **The answer is A** *Cardiovascular system / Embryology / Cardiovascular system*

Both branches of the fourth aortic arch remain intact during fetal development. In adults, the left fourth aortic arch forms the aortic arch, and the right fourth aortic arch forms the proximal segment of the right subclavian artery. During development, the first and second aortic arches all but disappear. In adults, they form the maxillary, hyoid, and stapedial arteries. The third aortic arch forms the common carotid artery. The fifth aortic arch disappears. The sixth aortic arch forms the proximal segment of the right pulmonary artery and the ductus arteriosus.

8 **The answer is C** *General principles / Immunology / Etiology of autoimmune disease*

Forbidden clones provide a supply of cells that can recognize self-antigens and stimulate both humoral and cell-mediated immune responses, leading to autoimmunity. B cell deficiency—primarily a lack of circulating B cells—is a major cause of hypogammaglobulinemia. Type I hypersensitivity (anaphylactic hypersensitivity) is mediated by humoral antibodies, which result from a normal immune response to exogenous antigens. The deletion of forbidden clones leads to tolerance to autoantigens—the opposite of autoimmunity.

9 **The answer is D** *General principles / Pharmacology / Empiric antibacterial therapy in an immuno-compromised host*

The most likely diagnosis of this patient's condition is septic shock secondary to bacteremia. Chemotherapy for cancer is a common cause of neutropenia with fever and infection. The risk is high when the white blood cell count is less than 500/μL. In addition, cold, clammy skin indicates peripheral vascular shutdown. Lactic acid buildup will lead to metabolic acidosis and compensatory rapid breathing. Patients with neutropenic fever must be treated with double broad-spectrum antibacterial agents for gram-negative rods, including Pseudomonas. The combination of piperacillin, a broad-spectrum β-lactam, and gentamicin, an aminoglycoside that has broad gram-negative activity, is a good choice. In addition, penicillin–aminoglycoside combinations may be synergistic because of the different mechanisms of action of these agents: Penicillins are cell wall synthesis inhibitors, and aminoglycosides inhibit protein synthesis. Single-agent therapy with gentamicin or amikacin would not be as effective for resistant organisms. Both chloramphenicol and gentamicin are protein synthesis inhibitors and would not be expected to work synergistically.

10 **The answer is C** *Respiratory system / Pathology / Pulmonary alveolar proteinosis*

Pulmonary alveolar proteinosis is a condition associated with an inherited or acquired defect in macrophage function. The failure of alveolar macrophages to phagocytose surfactant produced by alveolar pneumocytes results in accumulation of eosinophilic granular material within the lung parenchyma. This material stains strongly with periodic acid–Schiff (PAS) stains and contains fat and lipoprotein. Treatment of patients with idiopathic alveolar proteinosis includes whole-lung lavage.

11 **The answer is C** *General principles / Behavioral science / Medical ethics*

If the physician's sole concern is not to harm the patient with unnecessary worry, the guiding principle is nonmaleficence. If the sole concern is to be able to benefit the patient with urography (which is impossible if the patient refuses because of concerns about the risks), the guiding principle is beneficence. Both are possible. Justice is irrelevant, and gratitude (e.g., for the patient's patronage) is, at most, marginally relevant.

12 **The answer is E** *General principles / Behavioral science / Medical ethics*

The physician who decides to do what others do in like circumstances is acting without appeal to the independent ethical principles of beneficence and nonmaleficence. Depending on what the professional practice standard dictates, the disclosure decision might prove to be respectful of autonomy or strongly paternalistic, but the decision would still be guided by professional practice. Weak paternalism is entirely irrelevant because the patient is competent.

13 **The answer is E** *General principles / Virology / Epstein–Barr virus*

Epstein–Barr virus belongs to the Herpesviridae family of viruses that includes herpes simplex virus types 1 and 2, human cytomegalovirus, Varicella zoster, and human herpes virus 6 (HHV-6). All of these viruses can attain a latent state in stable human tissues and reactivate (having a replicative cycle) under certain conditions.

14 **The answer is D** *General principles / Genetics / Ultraviolet damage to DNA*

UV light causes cross-linking of thymidine base pairs in DNA and cross-links thymidine to cytosine (forming pyrimidine–pyrimidine dimers). In bacteria such as *Escherichia coli*, these lesions are repaired by a system of proteins called the SOS system, which includes the RecA protein. RecA is involved in the recombination of normal DNA and the repair of damaged DNA, and thus it would not be advantageous to decrease its activity. Also, it would be foolish to overlap the genes, because one pyrimidine base pair has the potential to impair all of the genes involved. Removal of introns would also be disadvantageous, because introns are thought to act as buffers of inactive DNA so that a mutation can occur without disrupting the gene. However, genes with low thymidine content may be less susceptible to damage by UV radiation because fewer pyrimidine base pairs would be involved.

15 **The answer is B** *Central and peripheral nervous system / Histology; pathology / Neuroblastoma*

Neuroblastomas arise from neural crest cells of the adrenal medulla. The tumors are usually large and soft, with a red-gray cut surface. They may be calcified, with areas of hemorrhage and necrosis. The tumor cells have hyperchromatic nuclei and indistinct eosinophilic cytoplasm. The nuclei are arranged in a spoke-like pattern around a characteristic central mass of neuritic cell processes, called Homer–Wright pseudorosettes, as seen in the illustration. Like pheochromocytomas, neuroblastomas produce catecholamines, but unlike pheochromocytomas, they do not cause systemic hypertension.

16 **The answer is A** *Biochemistry / Michaelis–Menten equation*

The Michaelis–Menten equation defines the rate equation for a one-substrate, enzyme-catalyzed reaction. The equation is

$$V_0 = \frac{V_{max} [S]}{K_m + [S]}$$

where V_0 = initial velocity, V_{max} = maximum initial velocity, $[S]$ = initial substrate concentration, and K_m = Michaelis–Menten. This equation was derived to explain the rate of a reaction catalyzed by an enzyme that is affected by a continuously changing substrate concentration as substrate is converted to product. Based on this equation, at low levels of $[S]$, $K_m \gg [S]$ so that $[S]$ in the denominator of the equation is insignificant. This changes the equation to $V_0 = V_{max} [S]/K_m$, so that V_0 is linearly dependent on $[S]$. When $[S] \gg K_m$, the equation is $V_0 = V_{max}$ because K_m becomes insignificant and the term $[S]$ cancels out. When V_0 is exactly half of V_{max}, $K_m = [S]$. $V_0 = 0$ when the equation is now $V_0 = 0$ and not V_{max}.

17 **The answer is B** *Respiratory system / Pharmacology / Properties of anesthetic gases*

Minimum alveolar concentration (MAC) is the concentration of anesthetic at 1 atm that produces immobility in 50% of patients exposed to a noxious stimulus.

18 **The answer is A** *General principles / Pharmacology / Properties of anesthetic gases*

If an anesthetic has a high blood:gas partition coefficient, it is very soluble in blood and is eliminated from the bloodstream into the alveolar air relatively slowly. This tends to prolong recovery time.

19 **The answer is C** *General principles / Pharmacology / Properties of anesthetic gases*

Relative potency of anesthetics is directly proportional to their lipid solubility. Among the commonly used agents, nitrous oxide has a very low oil:gas partition coefficient. In contrast, nitrous oxide has a rapid onset of action because of a low blood:gas partition coefficient. Nitrous oxide is neither explosive nor highly metabolized.

20 **The answer is C** *Hematopoietic and lymphoreticular system / Pathology / Chronic myelogenous leukemia*

CML is diagnosed by identifying a clonal expansion of a hematopoietic stem line with a distinctive molecular abnormality–translocation that positions the BCR gene on chromosome 9 next to the ABL gene on chromosome 22. In more than 95% of cases, the balanced t(9;22)(q34;q11) translocation results in a characteristic Philadelphia (Ph) chromosome. Leukocytosis is the most prominent laboratory finding in patients with CML. The bone marrow biopsy usually reveals almost 100% cells. Accompanying the leukocytosis of CML is a marked elevation of serum vitamin B_{12} levels and an increased serum vitamin B_{12}-binding capacity. Elevated levels in the serum of patients with CML are caused by the turnover of the increased granulocytic mass. The age-adjusted incidence of CML is higher among men than among women.

21 **The answer is B** *Musculoskeletal system / Biochemistry / Amino acid catabolism*

The amount of alanine released from skeletal muscle is greater than the amount that can be accounted for in muscle protein. The catabolism of many amino acids in muscle involves the transamination of α-amino groups from amino acids to pyruvate, producing alanine. Thus, the carbon skeleton of much of the alanine released from muscle is derived from glucose via the glycolytic pathway.

22 **The answer is A** *General principles / Microbiology / Malaria*

Of the major diseases with geographic relevance, malaria is one of the few that can be rapidly life-threatening. Chronic Chagas disease, amebic dysentery, mucocutaneous leishmaniasis, and giardiasis are either chronically debilitating or subpatent. Amebic dysentery and giardiasis are not life-threatening conditions, and it is not necessary to determine the causative species for treatment of either. No effective treatment exists for chronic Chagas disease, so rapid diagnosis is not essential. Although determination of the species of Leishmania is useful in distinguishing cutaneous and mucocutaneous leishmaniasis in terms of treatment, both are long-term infections and are not life-threatening.

23 **The answer is B** *Gastrointestinal system / Pathology / Adenocarcinoma of the large intestine*

This section of the large intestine shows an infiltrating adenocarcinoma, with neoplastic cells arranged in cords and glands. They are free-floating within large pools of mucin, which is produced by the neoplastic cells. By definition, adenocarcinomas either form glandular structures or produce neutral mucin. They are the most common form of carcinoma affecting the large intestine. Tumors that produce abundant amounts of mucin (colloid carcinomas) have an especially poor prognosis. The cord-like and tube-like arrangement of the neoplastic cells in this mucinous adenocarcinoma contrasts with the vacuoles and displaced nucleus typical of signet ring adenocarcinoma.

24 **The answer is C** *General principles / Genetics / Cystic fibrosis*

The frequency of the cystic fibrosis gene is 1/40, the square root of the incidence. Remembering the Hardy–Weinberg law, the gene frequency is equal to the square root of the incidence (q^2). If the incidence $= q^2 = 1/1,600$, the square root of the incidence, the gene frequency (q) $= 1/40$.

25 **The answer is D** *General principles / Virology / Reverse transcriptase*

Reverse transcriptases convert RNA into DNA and allow for the production of new RNA genomic strands for incorporation into newly formed viral particles and thus are necessary for the replication of RNA viruses, but are not necessary for the replication of DNA genome viruses. Thus, inhibitors of reverse transcriptases have become important drugs in the arsenal of infectious disease specialists to treat RNA genome viruses and are most commonly used for the treatment of HIV infections.

26 **The answer is D** *General principles / Immunology / Transplants*

Rejection that occurs a few minutes to a few hours after transplantation is called hyperacute rejection. It is the result of preformed circulating antibodies to the graft that were made as a result of previous transplantations, blood transfusions, or pregnancies. It usually transpires minutes after the donor kidney is anastomosed, although it can proceed over a few days. The antibodies activate the complement sytem, with ensuing swelling, interstitial hemorrhage, and thrombotic occlusion followed by outright infarction of the kidney. The only therapy is removal of the transplanted tissue.

27 **The answer is E** *Central and peripheral nervous system / Behavioral science / Defense mechanisms*

Borderline patients tend to view things as extremes of black and white, with little ability to perceive the gray zones. In splitting, negative feelings are split off and attributed to one person (or thing), while positive feelings are attributed to another, without the realization that people have both good and bad features. Borderline patients may also project, deny, displace, and manipulate, but the example in the question is of splitting.

28 **The answer is C** *Central and peripheral nervous system / Physiology / Regulation of arterial blood pressure*

A rise in arterial blood pressure within the carotid sinus or an increase in pressure secondary to mechanical massage leads to activation of baroreceptors, which subsequently causes inhibition of the central vasoconstrictor center with activation of the central vagal center. The net short-term effect is a decrease in blood pressure, heart rate, and cardiac output. Ultimately, baroreceptors adapt to the stimulus and are unimportant in the long-term regulation of blood pressure. Clamping of the carotid arteries (in a vagotomized animal) will decrease baroreceptor firing and remove inhibitory pathways from the central nervous system (CNS), leading to increases in pressure and heart rate.

29 **The answer is C** *Endocrine system / Pathology / Multiple endocrine neoplasia*

This thyroid proliferation consists of nests of cells with abundant eosinophilic cytoplasm and round to uniform nuclei with salt-and-pepper chromatin. This morphology is characteristic of a medullary carcinoma of the thyroid gland, which is a neuroendocrine carcinoma derived from the thyroid C cells. Medullary carcinoma is often a component of the multiple endocrine neoplasia (MEN) syndromes, in particular MEN 2 (Sipple's syndrome) or MEN 3 (mucosal neuroma syndrome). These syndromes frequently have associated parathyroid hyperplasia and may or may not be associated with adenomas of the pancreas and pituitary glands. Recent research has identified an association of MEN syndromes with the RET proto-oncogene on chromosome 10.

30 **The answer is D** *General principles / Pharmacology / Properties of lidocaine*

Local anesthetics block Na+ channels and decrease conductance of Na+, thereby inhibiting depolarization and normal conduction of action potentials. Small myelinated nerve fibers are most sensitive, and differential sensitivity explains preferential blockade for pain sensation as opposed to other sensory modalities. Lidocaine is highly lipid soluble and may cause convulsions in the CNS if sufficient amounts are delivered to the brain. Because Na+ channels in cardiovascular tissue are affected, dysrhythmia and decreased contractility may ensue. The ester anesthetics, such as procaine, are substrates for plasma cholinesterases, whereas lidocaine is more slowly metabolized in the liver. Local anesthetics, such as lidocaine, are often used in spinal anesthesia to produce widespread blockage of neurotransmission.

31 **The answer is C** *Central and peripheral nervous system / Physiology; neuroanatomy / Hypoxic injury*

The first of the motor functions to become deficient during hypoxic injury to the brain is the ability to move the arms. This is because the most distal ends of the anterior and middle cerebral arteries anastomose in the cerebral hemispheres over the location on the motor gyrus controlling the arms. The neurons in this anastomosing zone are very sensitive to hypoxic injury.

32 **The answer is E** *General principles / Virology / Parvovirus*

Parvovirus B19 contains a single-stranded DNA viral genome. Parvovirus B19 has been shown to cause hydrops fetalis in infants, and an association with pure red cell aplasia and an inflammatory articular inflammation. Hepatitis B contains a mixed, partial, double-stranded DNA genome. All members of the Herpesviridae family and Adenoviruses have a double-stranded DNA genome, while poliovirus contains a single-stranded RNA genome.

33 **The answer is B** *Central and peripheral nervous system / Neuroscience / Multiple sclerosis*

This woman is presenting with symptoms highly suggestive of early-stage multiple sclerosis (MS). MS develops more commonly in women than men at a 3:2 ratio. The average age for symptoms to occur is 30 year of age. The disease is characterized by bouts of demyelinization in the CNS, termed relapses. The ultimate trend of relapses varies from patient to patient but it is not uncommon for one of the first symptoms to be associated with optic neuritis. In this case, visual-evoked potentials would be expected to show significant slowing, and by the time a patient has endured multiple relapses white matter changes are present on T2-weighted MRI analyses. These changes are due to collection of scar-like tissue or plaques within the myelinated areas of the brain. Over 90% of MS patients show increases in CSF immunoglobulin levels versus about 13% for the normal population. Short-acting acetylcholinesterase inhibitors would resolve disease symptoms in patients with myasthenia gravis but not MS. Levodopa–carbidopa medications would result in improvement of Parkinson's disease but not MS.

34 **The answer is D** *General principles / Immunology / Hypersensitivity reactions*

ABO or Rh incompatibility, the cause of erythroblastosis fetalis, is the result of blood group differences between the mother and the child. Normally, in cases of Rh-incompatible mating, RhoGAM, an anti-Rh antibody, is given to the mother shortly after the birth of her first Rh-positive child. This clears the child's Rh-positive red cells from the mother's circulation before she can be immunized. In the case described in the question, the mother has blood type O negative with normal isohemagglutinin titers, so the preexisting ABO compatibility should clear her system of any leaked fetal blood cells. Administration of RhoGAM to an Rh-positive child will cause hemolytic anemia in that child.

35 **The answer is B** *General principles / Physiology / Gas exchange*

Anemia reduces the oxygen-carrying capacity of the blood but does not affect arterial oxygen tension. Thus, oxygen delivery is decreased and venous oxygen has a lower partial pressure at rest and during exercise in the anemic subject. The anemic subject is patient B because his oxygen content is reduced for every level of Po_2.

36 The answer is C *Central and peripheral nervous system / Physiology / Toxins; neurotransmission*

The woman has botulism, which is caused by the neurotoxin botulin. The action of botulin involves inhibition of ACh release from peripheral nerve endings at the neuromuscular junction. Other bacterial toxins have actions described in (A), (B), (D), and (E): diphtheria toxin, tetanus toxin, cholera toxin, and streptolysin O, respectively.

37 The answer is D *Reproductive system / Pathology / Gonococcal salpingitis*

For all practical purposes, the patient is cured. However, women who have had gonorrhea are at risk for future complications, such as subsequent episodes of pelvic inflammatory disease, infertility, and ectopic pregnancy.

38 The answer is D *Hematopoietic and lymphoreticular system / Histology / Hassall's corpuscles*

Hassall's (thymic) corpuscles are found in the thymus. They are concentrically laminated structures of unknown function that appear during fetal development and increase in number with age. Thought to be degenerated medullary epithelial cells, they display varying degrees of keratinization or calcification.

39 The answer is C *Respiratory system / Pathology / Cystic fibrosis*

Cystic fibrosis is characterized by production of abnormal mucin. This mucin tends to accumulate within the pulmonary tracheobronchial tree, causing extreme dilation of the airways. This gross picture shows dilated airways with hyperplastic smooth muscle in their walls, resulting in a trabeculated appearance. This is a classic example of bronchiectasis, which causes pulmonary insufficiency in cystic fibrosis patients.

40 The answer is C *General principles / Biochemistry / Fructosuria; glycogen synthesis*

Essential fructosuria results from a deficiency in fructokinase, which is found only in the liver and which catalyzes the first step in the assimilation of fructose by the liver. Under normal conditions, almost all of the fructose is converted to fructose 1-phosphate and is metabolized in the liver. Hexokinase, which is present in all extrahepatic tissues, can convert fructose to fructose 6-phosphate; however, the K_m of hexokinase for fructose is sufficiently high that this reaction does not occur to any significant extent. When, as a consequence of a deficiency in fructokinase, the accumulation of fructose is high enough, it is converted to fructose 6-phosphate in extrahepatic tissues and metabolized by the glycolytic pathway. Glucokinase, which is found in the liver, is specific for glucose and cannot catalyze the phosphorylation of fructose. Aldolase B is specific for fructose 1-phosphate. Transketolase is a part of the nonoxidative phase of the pentose phosphate pathway.

41 The answer is B *Renal/urinary system / Pathology / Renal neoplasia*

This renal tumor is a classic renal cell carcinoma reflected in its parenchymal location and deep golden appearance (due to abundant cytoplasmic fat). Patients with renal cell carcinomas often present with costovertebral pain, hematuria, and a palpable abdominal mass; polycythemia, hypercalcemia, and Cushing's syndrome (among other endocrinopathies) also may be associated. Polycythemia results from abnormal production of erythropoietin-like hormones by the tumor. These tumors arise from proximal tubular epithelium and may appear in patients with von Hippel–Lindau syndrome, which is associated with chromosome 3 abnormalities. These individuals also have a risk for cerebellar hemangioblastomas.

42 The answer is B *General principles / Pharmacology / Gout*

Colchicine is the anti-inflammatory drug of choice for gout. Allopurinol inhibits xanthine oxidase, the enzyme that converts hypoxanthine to xanthine and xanthine to uric acid. Thus, allopurinol decreases urate production and is efficacious for the treatment of gout.

43 **The answer is E** *General principles / Pharmacology / Dopamine receptor antagonism; tardive dyskinesia*

Metoclopramide is a potent dopamine receptor antagonist that can cause tardive dyskinesia in nonpsychiatric patients. Tardive dyskinesia frequently involves the orobuccal area. Dystonia is a sustained muscle spasm that occurs as an early complication of treatment with an antidopaminergic drug. Wilson's and Huntington's diseases cause chorea, but there is no history to suggest these diseases.

44 **The answer is D** *General principles / Genetics / Turner syndrome*

The patient presented in the question is a classic example of a child with Turner syndrome (i.e., short stature, webbed neck, cubitus valgus), which is best diagnosed through chromosome analysis. The genotype of this patient is most likely to be 45,X. None of the other tests listed in the question would contribute to the diagnosis of Turner syndrome.

45 **The answer is D** *General principles / Pharmacology / Volume of distribution; half-life of elimination*

The volume of distribution (V_d) is approximately 10 L. V_d is defined as V_d = dose/Cp, where Cp is the plasma concentration at zero time. In this case, the Cp can be estimated easily because the log plasma concentration versus time plot is linear; it is approximately 100 µg/mL. Thus,

$$V_d = (20 \text{ mg/kg}) (50 \text{ kg})/0.1 \text{ mg/mL}$$
$$= 10,000 \text{ mL}$$
$$= 10 \text{ L}$$

46 **The answer is A** *Central and peripheral nervous system / Anatomy / Motor neuron injury*

Upper motor or lower motor neuron injuries are linked to certain constellations of symptoms that may be very helpful in diagnosis. Upper motor neuron injuries result in spasticity and hyperreflexia without muscle fasciculations or significant muscle atrophy. Lower motor neuron injuries result in flaccid paralysis, hyporeflexia, muscle atrophy, and muscle fasciculations. An easy way to remember these symptoms is to understand the actions of muscles in the absence of neuronal input. No input from lower motor neuron equals no muscle action and thus the muscle atrophies and is hyporeflexic.

47 **The answer is D** *Renal/urinary system / Pathology / Renal disease*

This resection specimen shows a kidney affected by multiple cysts of varying size, some with recent hemorrhage. This diffuse process is diagnostic of adult polycystic kidney disease, an autosomal dominant disease with high penetrance that usually manifests in adulthood. The disease is bilateral and progressive, and ultimately it requires dialysis or transplantation. Often, cystic disease affects other organs, including liver, spleen, pancreas, and lungs. Berry aneurysms are present in 10% to 30% of patients and may cause subarachnoid hemorrhage. A slight risk of renal cell carcinoma accompanies this condition.

48 **The answer is A** *General principles / Biochemistry / Protein posttranslational modifications*

After proteins are synthesized (translated), many are glycosylated in the lumen of the endoplasmic reticulum and the Golgi complex. Oligosaccharides are attached to proteins by N-glycosylation of asparagine side chains or by O-glycosylation of serine and threonine side chains. The transfer of oligosaccharides is mediated by an activated lipid carrier, dolichol phosphate.

49 **The answer is C** *General principles / Histology / Cytoskeleton*

In muscle cells, actin and myosin filaments cause muscle contraction by a process known as the sliding filament hypothesis. In nonmuscle cells, actin is involved with endocytosis, exocytosis, cell locomotion, and cytokinesis. The mitotic spindle consists of the microtubule protein tubulin; actin is not present. Likewise, ciliary beating and axonal transport depend on microtubules and do not depend on actin filaments. Mitochondrial division is not known to involve either microtubules or actin.

50 The answer is A *Gastrointestinal system / Pathology / Inflammation of bowel*

This diffuse, nonsegmental process is characterized by dramatic, needle-like polyps projecting from the mucosal surface. Such pseudopolyps are features of chronic ulcerative colitis, in which zones of hyperplasia alternate with areas of mucosal flattening and atrophy. Crohn's disease is a segmental process, as is ischemic colitis, and it is not associated with such pronounced pseudopolyps. Collagenous colitis, a microscopic disease with thickening of the basement membrane of the colonic mucosa, shows a grossly normal mucosa.

test **6**

Questions

Directions: Single best answer questions consist of numbered items or incomplete statements followed by answers or by completions of the statement. Select the ONE lettered answer or completion that is BEST in each case.

1 Tricyclic antidepressants (e.g., imipramine and amitriptyline) are useful agents for the management of endogenous depression because they
- (A) reverse symptoms within days of initial administration
- (B) have little effect on cardiovascular function
- (C) affect dopamine receptors within the central nervous system (CNS)
- (D) affect neuronal amine uptake mechanisms
- (E) deplete brain serotonin levels

2 Mitochondria are important to the cells of eukaryotes for generating the adenosine triphosphate (ATP) necessary to carry out all energy-requiring processes. Which of the following statements concerning mitochondria are true?
- (A) They contain a linear DNA molecule
- (B) Mitochondrial proteins come solely from the nucleus
- (C) The codons used by mitochondrial transfer RNA (tRNA) are identical to those used in other mammalian genes
- (D) Mitochondrial proteins are encoded by gene sequences that overlap one another

3 A very painful, spreading, cutaneous edematous erythema is clinically descriptive of
- (A) erysipeloid
- (B) diphtheria
- (C) Pontiac fever
- (D) listeriosis
- (E) nocardiosis

4 Which of the following statements concerning gene duplication is most correct?
- (A) Gene duplications are necessary to meet the cell's requirements for some RNA transcripts
- (B) Pseudogenes are translated into proteins but lack function
- (C) β-Tubulins and β-like globins are examples of genes that arose independently yet carry out similar functions
- (D) Gene duplication involves unequal crossover between homologous repetitive DNA sequences during mitosis

5 Tay–Sachs disease occurs almost exclusively among Ashkenazi Jews, with an incidence of 1/3,600. The frequency of carriers of the Tay–Sachs gene, which can be calculated by using the Hardy–Weinberg law $(p^2 + 2pq + q^2 = 1)$, is which of the following?
- (A) 1/4
- (B) 1/30
- (C) 1/60
- (D) 1/600

6 Which of the endogenous substances listed is derived from the cyclo-oxygenase pathway of arachidonic acid metabolism?
- (A) Platelet activating factor (PAF)
- (B) Leukotriene D_4
- (C) Eosinophil chemotactic factor (ECF)
- (D) Thromboxane (TXA_2)

7 Which of the following statements about the protein kinase C (PKC) signal transduction pathway is true?
- (A) After activation, PKC is degraded to protein kinase A
- (B) PKC phosphorylates tyrosines on proteins
- (C) PKC requires Mg^2+ for full activation
- (D) PKC requires lipids for full activation
- (E) PKC is normally found in the nucleus

8 Renal osteodystrophy is a condition that may follow chronic renal failure. Features of this condition include osteitis fibrosa cystica admixed with osteomalacia. The pathogenesis of this condition is characterized by which of the following?
- (A) Hypophosphatemia
- (B) High levels of 1,25-dihydroxyvitamin D_3 (calcitriol)
- (C) Enhanced calcemic response to parathyroid hormone
- (D) Hyperparathyroidism
- (E) Hypercalcemia

9 A 65-year-old woman is seen before cataract surgery. She has had no previous surgery except for a dental extraction, after which she bled for 10 days and required a 2-unit blood transfusion. One sibling died of postoperative hemorrhage during childhood, and there is a history of bleeding in a number of relatives, both male and female. Her partial thromboplastin time (PTT) is markedly prolonged, and the bleeding time is within normal limits. The most likely diagnosis is

(A) factor VIII deficiency
(B) factor XI deficiency
(C) factor XII deficiency
(D) Fletcher factor deficiency
(E) von Willebrand's disease

10 Enteric pathogens vary with respect to their ability to invade the intestinal mucosa. After infection, which one of the following enteric pathogens is most likely to invade the intestinal submucosa and then disseminate throughout the body?

(A) *Vibrio cholerae*
(B) *Salmonella typhi*
(C) *Shigella dysenteriae*
(D) Nontyphoid *Salmonella*
(E) *Campylobacter jejun*

11 A 45-year-old woman is admitted to the hospital with an unremitting sore throat. She has undergone radical mastectomy for breast carcinoma and recently underwent adjuvant chemotherapy. Two weeks before, she received a 7-day course of amoxicilin-clavulanic acid (Augmentin) for a recurrent urinary tract infection. Examination of her palate reveals several patches of white, creamy, curd-like friable lesions on the tongue and other mucosal surfaces. This patient most likely has which type of fungal infection?

(A) Sporotrichosis
(B) Dermatomycosis
(C) Candidiasis
(D) Cryptococcosis

12 Which of the following therapies would be most appropriate for treating a patient with oropharyngeal candidiasis?

(A) Topical undecylenic acid
(B) Topical tolnaftate
(C) Oral nystatin
(D) Topical clotrimazole
(E) Oral griseofulvin

13 An elderly woman had a synovial biopsy and total knee replacement for degenerative joint disease. Sections of the synovium revealed the findings shown in the accompanying photomicrograph, indicating a history of which one of the following conditions?

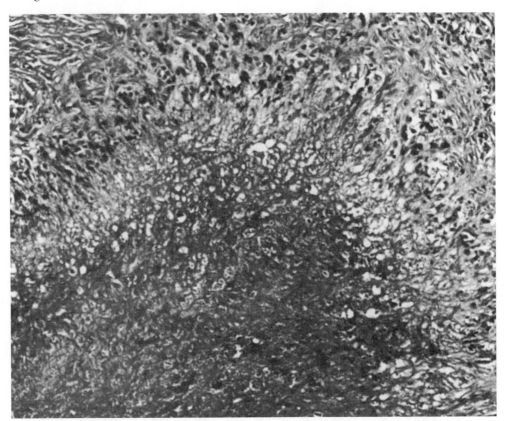

(A) Colchicine therapy for gout
(B) Repeated fractures
(C) Rheumatoid arthritis
(D) Trauma and foreign body within the joint space

14 The accompanying figure shows a portion of large bowel resected from a middle-aged woman who had repeated bouts of crampy abdominal pain. It would be concluded from the histology that the gross appearance of the bowel would show which one of the following features?

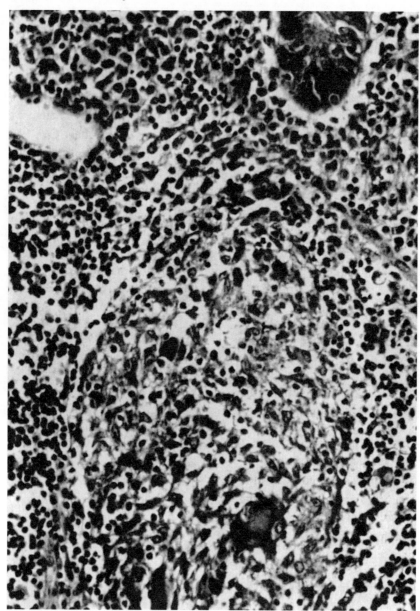

(A) Uniform inflammation extending from the rectum
(B) Creeping fat
(C) A thinned bowel wall
(D) Pseudopolyps
(E) Inflammation confined primarily to the mucosa

15 Which of the following statements about RNA is true?

(A) RNA occurs only in a single-stranded form
(B) RNA can act to catalyze certain reactions, much like an enzyme
(C) RNA cannot act as primary genetic material
(D) A molecule of RNA differs from DNA in the number of carbon atoms in the sugar moieties
(E) Thymidine is one of the pyrimidine bases used by RNA

16 Cimetidine is the prototype of a histamine receptor antagonist that

(A) causes sedation
(B) is useful for motion sickness
(C) enhances hepatic drug-metabolizing enzymes
(D) reduces gastric acid secretion
(E) is useful in the treatment of certain allergies

17 Which of the following statements about the peptide bond is true?

(A) A peptide bond is tetrahedral
(B) A peptide bond has restricted rotation
(C) α-Carbon atoms are in a *cis* configuration
(D) Peptide bond atoms do not participate in the secondary structure of proteins
(E) A peptide bond has a charge associated with it

18 Ca^{2+} is required for various processes, such as neurotransmission and muscle contraction. However, an elevated level of Ca^{2+} can be cytotoxic to cells. Which of the following mechanisms is used by cells to regulate intracellular Ca^{2+} concentration?

(A) Chelation of Ca^{2+} by ethylenediaminetetraacetic acid (EDTA)
(B) ATP-dependent $H+$ pumping
(C) ATP-dependent Ca^{2+} pumping
(D) Sequestration of Ca^{2+} in the nucleus
(E) Sequestration of Ca^{2+} in the Golgi apparatus

19 The resected mitral valve in Figure 34 from the color plate section shows which one of the following?

(A) Calcific deposits
(B) Vegetations
(C) Mural thrombi
(D) Perforation

20 Which of the following statements about fenestrated capillaries is true?

(A) Fenestrations are 150 to 200 nm in diameter
(B) Their basal lamina is discontinuous
(C) They may be partially surrounded by pericytes
(D) They are present in exocrine glands
(E) In the renal glomerulus, they have a slit diaphragm that forms a filtration barrier

21 Pathogenic bacteria enter the body by various routes, and entry mechanisms are critical for understanding the pathogenesis and transmissibility of each agent. Which one of the following is a correct association between a pathogen and its common entry mechanism?

(A) *Neisseria meningitidis*—sexually transmitted entry
(B) *Corynebacterium diphtheriae*—foodborne entry
(C) *Rickettsia rickettsii*—entry by contamination of wound with soil
(D) *Clostridium tetani*—inhalation entry
(E) *Borrelia burgdorferi*—arthropod vectorborne entry

22 A 70-year-old man is brought to the hospital, and a neurologist is called for a consultation. The residents caring for the patient tell the physician that he has spastic paralysis on one side of his body but has no sensory deficit. On examination, the physician finds that the patient can move neither the right side of his face nor his left extremities. He has right-sided ptosis of the eyelid, and the right eye deviates laterally. The right eye also does not respond to light or exhibit accommodation. What is the most likely site of the patient's lesion?

(A) The midbrain
(B) The pons
(C) The medulla
(D) The upper cortex

23 A transient blockage of the right middle cerebral artery would cause which constellation of symptoms?

(A) Right-sided muscular weakness, leg more than arm, face unaffected
(B) Left-sided muscular weakness, leg more than arm, face unaffected
(C) Right-sided muscular weakness, arm more than leg, face unaffected
(D) Left-sided muscular weakness, arm more than leg, face affected
(E) Right-sided muscular weakness affecting arm, leg, and face

24 Huntington's disease is an inherited, neurodegenerative disease that usually presents in the fifth or sixth decade of life. What is the type of genetic mutation that is case of this disease?

(A)   Single nucleotide deletion
(B)   Single nucleotide mutation
(C)   Promoter sequence mutation
(D)   Unbalanced translocation
(E)   Trinucleotide repeat expansion

25 Which of the following statements concerning cyclic adenosine monophosphate (cAMP) is true?

(A)   Intracellular cAMP levels are not under hormonal control
(B)   It is the second messenger for the action of parathyroid hormone (PTH) on the kidney
(C)   It activates PKC by binding to the regulatory subunit and causing dissociation of the catalytic subunit
(D)   It is degraded intracellularly by a family of adenylate cyclases
(E)   It is synthesized from adenosine diphosphate (ADP)

26 Which of the following is most characteristic of Tay–Sachs disease?

(A)   It is characterized by an absence of α-galactosidase
(B)   It results in widespread subcutaneous deposition of lipids
(C)   It is characterized by an abnormal accumulation of hexosaminidase A
(D)   It is characterized by a deficiency of GM_2 gangliosides
(E)   It is more prevalent among Ashkenazi Jews than among other population groups

27 In a family with a disease that has an autosomal dominant inheritance pattern, seven children have been born, four of whom have the disease and three of whom do not. One parent is affected and one is not. What is the probability of the next child born having the disease?

(A)   100%
(B)   50%
(C)   25%
(D)   Zero
(E)   Cannot be determined

28 The lesion affecting the large intestine in Figure 35 from the color plate section is most likely a

(A)   hyperplastic polyp
(B)   tubular adenoma
(C)   villous adenoma
(D)   polypoid adenocarcinoma

29 The inhibition observed in the Lineweaver–Burk plot below is subject to which one of the following actions?

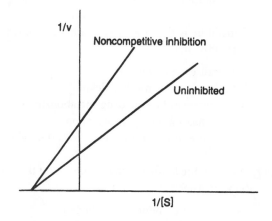

(A)   It can be reversed by a high concentration of substrate
(B)   It results from compounds that are transition state analogs
(C)   It occurs through the interaction of the inhibitor at the active site
(D)   It results in a decrease in the V_{max} of the reaction
(E)   It is characterized by an increase in the K_m for the substrate

30 An action potential recorded from a microelectrode in a nerve fiber is shown in the accompanying figure. Which of the following statements accurately describes the changes that occur during the action potential recorded by this electrode?

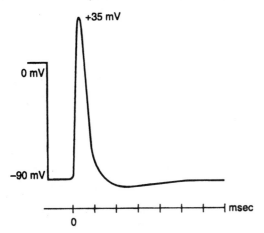

(A) At the peak of the action potential, the number of open K+ channels greatly exceeds the number of open Na+ channels

(B) Depolarization is caused by an abrupt increase in K+ conductance

(C) Repolarization is caused primarily by an increase in Na+ conductance

(D) Repolarization is caused by activation of the $Ca^2+ -Na+$ channel

(E) Chloride channel permeability does not change during an action potential

31 A 35-year-old man presents with loss of pain sensation in the skin of the forearm and lateral border of the leg. He also exhibits loss of tendon reflexes and complains of severe stabbing pains of the legs. This condition could have been prevented by

(A) avoiding the bullet that damaged his cingulate gyrus 13 years ago

(B) early penicillin treatment

(C) avoiding exposure to varicella zoster virus infection

(D) early administration of acyclovir

32 Which one of the following conditions is represented in Figure 36 from the color plate section, a photomicrograph of the lung?

(A) Asthma

(B) Klebsiella infection

(C) Cystic fibrosis

(D) Thermophilic actinomyces

(E) Pulmonary neoplasia

33 Which of the following are proteins that regulate transcription initiation?

(A) Origins of replication

(B) Promoters

(C) Enhancers

(D) Repressors

34 Which of the following factors decreases glomerular filtration rate (GFR)?

(A) Constriction of the afferent arteriole

(B) An increase in renal blood flow (RBF)

(C) An increase in systemic arterial pressure from 100 to 150 mm

(D) Constriction of the efferent arteriole

35 At which of these blood neutrophil levels do patients acquire a significant risk of opportunistic infection?

(A) $<1,000/\mu L$

(B) 1,000 to $1,500/\mu L$

(C) 1,500 to $2,000/\mu L$

(D) 2,000 to $2,500/\mu L$

(E) 2,500 to $3,000/\mu L$

36 A physician interested in evaluating the effects of a drug on the synthesis of RNA has decided to measure RNA production in cells after treatment with the drug by radiolabeling RNA. Which of the following radiolabeled bases should this physician use?

(A) Tritiated thymine ($[^3H]$-thymine]

(B) Tritiated (^3H) guanine

(C) ^3H-adenine

(D) ^3H-uracil

(E) ^3H-cytosine

37 For a patient trying to prevent intercourse-related urinary tract infections, which of the following antibiotics would be the most effective and economical when administered only once after coitus?

(A) Cephalexin

(B) Nitrofurantoin

(C) Trimethoprim–sulfamethoxazole

(D) Ciprofloxacin

(E) Penicillin G

38 The best diagnosis for the process shown in Figure 37 from the color plate section, which occurs approximately 30 cm from the ileocecal valve, is

(A) Meckel's diverticulum

(B) mucocele

(C) intestinal reduplication

(D) false diverticulum

39 For which one of the following organisms do opsonic antibodies play a major role in acquired immunity to infection?

(A) *Neisseria meningitidis*, group A
(B) *Vibrio cholerae*
(C) *Clostridium botulinum*
(D) *Shigella flexneri*

40 If end diastolic volume is approximately 115 mL in the volume–pressure curve of the left ventricle in the accompanying figure, which of the following statements is most accurate?

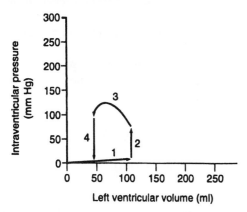

(A) The ejection fraction is approximately 30%
(B) Aortic diastolic pressure is approximately 80 mm Hg
(C) Isovolumic contraction is during the section labeled 3
(D) Stroke volume is approximately 45 mL
(E) Left ventricular end diastolic pressure is approximately 100 mm Hg

41 The change shown in the cross section of the heart (Figure 38 from the color plate section) is

(A) artifactual
(B) 2 days old
(C) 6 days old
(D) 14 days old
(E) 48 days old

42 A 45-year-old man has complained of increasing abdominal girth, fever, and malaise for the previous 4 months; he denies having a cough. Physical examination shows a greatly enlarged spleen but no lymphadenopathy. Laboratory evaluation shows a normal chest radiograph, a hemoglobin concentration of 15 g/dL, a white blood count of 45,000 cells/μL. The most likely diagnosis is

(A) malignant lymphoma
(B) acute leukemia
(C) chronic myeloproliferative disorder
(D) pulmonary tuberculosis
(E) myelodysplastic disorder

43 Which of the following descriptions concerning the autonomic nervous system is correct?

(A) The parasympathetic ganglion are located near the spinal cord
(B) The first synapse in the chain of autonomic control is cholinergic for the parasympathetic nerves and adrenergic for the sympathetic nerves
(C) The parasympathetic nervous system cell bodies exit the spinal cord at levels T1–L2
(D) The primary cell bodies of the sympathetic nervous system are located in the intermediolateral columns of the spinal cord
(E) The final synapse for secondary neurons of the parasympathetic and sympathetic nervous system is largely cholinergic

44 Chronic Chagas disease should be considered in patients from Central and South America presenting with which set of the following signs and symptoms?

(A) Periodic fever and chills
(B) Cardiac conduction defects
(C) Multiple mucocutaneous lesions
(D) Persistent diarrhea
(E) Pneumonia

45 The patient with the transversely transected heart at autopsy shown in Figure 39 from the color plate section most likely presented with which one of the following conditions?

(A) Pulmonary emboli
(B) Metastatic carcinoma
(C) Cerebral infarct
(D) Cardiac tamponade

46 Which of the following is the most likely cause of the abnormalities in the spleen shown in Figure 40 from the color plate section?

(A) Histoplasmosis
(B) Infarct
(C) Lymphoma
(D) Chronic congestion

47 A patient is on a ventilator. The patient's anatomic dead space is 150 mL, and the ventilator's dead space is 250 mL. The ventilatory rate is set at 20 per minute. How should the output (tidal volume) of the ventilator be adjusted so that alveolar minute ventilation is 4 L/min?

(A) 150 mL
(B) 250 mL
(C) 400 mL
(D) 600 mL
(E) 1,000 mL

48 Lidocaine has a half-life of approximately 2 hours and a relatively low therapeutic index. It is useful in the treatment of life-threatening arrhythmias during myocardial infarction. In an emergency situation, lidocaine might be administered by which of the following methods?

(A) Orally, despite extensive first-pass elimination in the liver
(B) Intravenously (3 to 4 mg/kg) over a short period (20 to 30 minutes) followed by a continuous maintenance dose (1 to 4 mg/min)
(C) As a slow intravenous infusion for 4 to 6 half-lifes
(D) As rapidly as possible, as a single, large bolus

49 Which of the following components is found in chromatin?

(A) Tubulin
(B) Histone
(C) Inositol triphosphate
(D) Connexin

50 A hospitalized patient is found to have a urinary tract infection owing to Serratia. A course of antimicrobial therapy with an aminoglycoside is planned. However, the patient has mild renal impairment. The best means to determine the appropriate drug dosage is

(A) body surface area
(B) serum creatinine
(C) serum blood urea nitrogen
(D) creatinine clearance
(E) peak and trough drug levels

Answer Key

1-D	11-C	21-E	31-B	41-B
2-D	12-D	22-A	32-A	42-C
3-A	13-C	23-B	33-D	43-D
4-A	14-B	24-E	34-A	44-B
5-B	15-B	25-B	35-A	45-C
6-D	16-D	26-E	36-D	46-C
7-D	17-B	27-B	37-E	47-D
8-D	18-C	28-B	38-A	48-B
9-B	19-B	29-D	39-A	49-B
10-B	20-C	30-E	40-B	50-E

Answers and Explanations

1 **The answer is D** *General principles / Pharmacology / Properties of tricyclic antidepressants*

Tricyclic antidepressants, such as imipramine, inhibit neuronal uptake of norepinephrine, serotonin, and other CNS amines. Potentiation of local concentrations of these amines may underlie the ability of these agents to reverse symptoms of depression after chronic administration over several weeks. The parent and metabolite compounds of many of these drugs can directly or indirectly affect cardiac function (including α-adrenergic receptor blockade) and thus may cause orthostatic hypotension and cardiac dysrhythmias. Indeed, suicide with these agents is quite common, and the cause of death is related to cardiac toxicity. The drugs do not appear to affect dopamine receptors significantly in the concentrations used clinically. Some agents (e.g., fluoxetine, which is not a tricyclic antidepressant) are more selective for serotonin uptake than for norepinephrine uptake. By contrast, desipramine, which is a tricyclic antidepressant, is more selective for norepinephrine uptake than for serotonin uptake.

2 **The answer is D** *General principles / Histology / Mitochondria*

Mitochondria are organelles unlike the others within the cell. They contain a ring of DNA that codes for some of the proteins they require; the other proteins are encoded by nuclear genes. Mitochondria also use a genetic code that is slightly different from that used by other mammalian genes: Mitochondria have only 22 tRNA molecules (as opposed to 32 in the nucleus), so that 1 tRNA must cover more codons. Some codons are also different (e.g., UGA, a termination codon normally, is a tryptophan codon to mitochondrial tRNA). Finally, genes encoding the proteins overlap one another, perhaps reflecting the fact that the genome is so small (16,500 base pairs).

3 **The answer is A** *Skin and related connective tissue / Microbiology / Presentation of cutaneous erythema*

The etiologic agent of erysipeloid is *Erysipelothrix rhusiopathiae*, a bacterium widely distributed in the environment. Human erysipeloid is clinically described as slowly spreading cutaneous erythema. Cutaneous edema is characteristic, and erysipeloid is very painful. Cutaneous diphtheria is characterized by a necrotic lesion sometimes associated with insect bites; the bite apparently provides the break in the skin through which toxigenic *Corynebacterium diphtheriae* enters the tissue. Cutaneous nocardiosis is characterized by draining sinus tracts discharging purulent exudate-containing granules. Pontiac fever and listeriosis do not have cutaneous manifestations.

4 **The answer is A** *General principles / Genetics / Gene duplications*

As many as 100 to 1,000 gene families contain similar sequences; β-tubulins and β-like globins are perfect examples of duplicated gene families. At least two nonfunctional regions in the human β-like globin gene cluster have sequences similar to functional β-like genes. Analysis of their DNA sequences shows that they retain their intron–exon structure, but some sequence drift has resulted in sequences that block transcription or terminate protein translation. Some gene duplications, such as those for ribosomal RNA (rRNA) and tRNA, along with genes coding for histones, are necessary to meet the demands of the cell for messenger RNA (mRNA) transcripts. Although there is no accepted model for duplication, it is thought to involve unequal crossover during meiosis.

5 **The answer is B** *General principles / Genetics / Hardy–Weinberg law*

The frequency of carriers of Tay–Sachs disease can be calculated from the Hardy–Weinberg law, in which the carrier frequency is equal to 2 pq: q is calculated by taking the square root of the incidence, which gives the frequency of the gene, 1 in 60, and p is equal to $1 - q$, or $60/60 - 1/60$, which gives 59/60. As can be seen here, in most cases of rare diseases, p becomes equal to 1, and the carrier frequency then becomes 2q, or $2 \times 1/60$, which gives a carrier frequency of 1/30.

6 **The answer is D** *General principles / Biochemistry / Lipids and arachidonic metabolism*

Leukotrienes are compounds formed as the result of the action of lipoxygenase on arachidonic acid. PAF is an ether phospholipid. ECF is a set of peptides that produces a chemotactic gradient to attract eosinophils. TXA_2, like prostaglandins, are synthesized through the action of cyclo-oxygenase, a reaction that is inhibited by acetylsalicylic acid.

7 **The answer is D** *General principles / Biochemistry / Serine and theonine kinases*

PKC is a member of a class of kinases that phosphorylates serine and threonine but does not phosphorylate tyrosine. PKC is activated by a lipid known as diacylglycerol, and its activation requires Ca^{2+} (Mg^{2+} is not required for activation). PKC is normally a cytoplasmic protein. When activated, it moves from the cytoplasm to the plasma membrane via translocation. PKC is degraded by a calcium-activated protease to form the lipid- and Ca^{2+}-independent protein kinase M. Protein kinase A is a cyclic adenosine monophosphate-dependent protein kinase and is unrelated to PKC.

8 **The answer is D** *Renal/urinary system / Physiology / Pathogenesis of renal osteodystrophy*

Normally, approximately 90% of serum phosphate is not protein-bound and thus it is filterable at the glomerulus. Of the filtered phosphate, approximately 75% is actively reabsorbed, mainly by cotransport with sodium in the proximal tubule. In chronic renal failure, hyperphosphatemia occurs as the glomerular filtration rate declines. Hyperphosphatemia produces a secondary hyperparathyroidism as excess phosphate ties up the free serum calcium, in essence leading to hypocalcemia. A reduced calcemic response to parathyroid hormone, often seen, is another cause of hypocalcemia. 1,25-Dihydroxyvitamin D_3 levels are reduced directly by the inability of the damaged kidney to convert the 25-hydroxyvitamin D_3 produced by the liver from inactive vitamin D_3 to 1,25-dihydroxyvitamin D_3 and indirectly by the ability of high serum phosphate levels to directly inhibit renal 25-hydroxyvitamin D_3 hydroxylase activity.

9 **The answer is B** *Hematopoietic and lymphoreticular system / Hematology / Differential diagnosis of coagulation disorders*

Factor XI deficiency is autosomally transmitted and can result in serious postoperative bleeding, although it may be mild enough to cause no spontaneous symptoms. Neither factor XII nor Fletcher factor deficiencies result in a bleeding disorder, and inherited factor VIII deficiency occurs only in male subjects. Severe von Willebrand's disease could result in a positive family history and significant bleeding, but rarely is the factor VIII:C low enough to prolong the PTT, especially when the bleeding time is normal.

10 **The answer is B** *General principles / Microbiology / Enteric infections*

Salmonella typhi is a highly invasive pathogen that is readily disseminated throughout the body. In typhoid fever, this organism invades through the intestinal mucosa and spreads through the body via the lymphatic system. In nontyphoid *Salmonella* infections, the bacteria invade the intestinal submucosa but usually do not spread into other regions of the body. *Campylobacter jejuni* and *Shigella dysenteriae* invade the intestinal mucosa but usually do not penetrate the submucosa or spread throughout the body. *Vibrio cholerae* is noninvasive.

11 **The answer is C** *General principles / Microbiology / Etiology of fungal infections*

The clinical signs and history are consistent with oropharyngeal candidiasis (thrush). This patient is most likely immunocompromised because of her adjuvant chemotherapy. In addition, antibacterial therapy for urinary tract infection predisposes her to develop a fungal infection because of depletion of floral bacteria. Opportunistic, endogenous *Candida* infections in the mouth are common under these conditions. Sporotrichosis is an endogenous systemic infection. Cryptococcosis is also a systemic infection. Dermatophytes usually appear on the hair, nails, and skin.

12 **The answer is D** *General principles / Microbiology / Antifungal therapy*

Griseofulvin is effective for dermatophyte infections of the nails and hair; it concentrates in the stratum corneum and outer epidermis and stops fungal growth in these tissues. Ketoconazole, fluconazole, and clotrimazole are ergosterol synthesis inhibitors, which are fungistatic or fungicidal (at high concentrations) for *Candidia*. Nystatin, a polyene, binds to membrane ergosterol and affects membrane permeability and integrity. Nystatin, like the more commonly used polyene amphotericin B, is fungicidal. Nystatin is effective only in topical preparations for candidiasis, whereas amphotericin B is commonly used systemically. Clotrimazole is effective topically against candidiasis. Tolnaftate and undecylenic acid are employed against ringworm, but both are ineffective in treating candidiasis.

13 **The answer is C** *General principles / Histology / Histopathology of rheumatoid arthritis*

The synovium in the photomicrograph shows the classic features of a rheumatoid nodule in a patient with rheumatoid arthritis, a disease that affects primarily women. Rheumatoid arthritis initially affects the small joints of the hands and feet and then the larger joints of the knees and elbows. The synovium becomes infiltrated by lymphocytes and plasma cells with lymphoid follicle formation. In some cases, central fibrinoid necrosis occurs, with an intense palisade of histiocytes and giant cells forming around the necrotic material, as in this case. Rheumatoid nodules occur in the skin and subcutis, particularly on extensor surfaces, but may also occur in unusual sites such as the lungs, heart, and spleen.

14 **The answer is B** *Gastrointestinal system / Pathology / Macroscopic features of Crohn's disease*

The photomicrograph shows chronic inflammation of the bowel, which is typical of Crohn's disease, or terminal ileitis. The presence of a small granuloma at the base of the colonic gland is helpful in confirming the diagnosis. Grossly, the bowel demonstrates involved areas interrupted by apparently normal skip areas. In Crohn's disease, inflammation extends through all layers of the bowel wall and leads to a thickened, leathery-appearing bowel. If the process extends into pericolic fat, thick, edematous creeping fat and fistulas are seen. Pseudopolyps, uniform involvement of the colon, and inflammation that does not extend beneath the submucosa occur in ulcerative colitis and provide a means of differentiating ulcerative colitis from Crohn's disease.

15 **The answer is B** *General principles / Cell biology / Functions of nucleic acids*

RNA differs from DNA by the number of hydroxyl groups on the sugar moieties and in the kind of pyrimidine bases used; RNA has uracil substituted for thymidine. Because these differences are fairly minor, RNA can take on the same configurations as DNA; that is, it can be linear, circular, double-stranded, or single-stranded. Molecules of tRNA are a perfect example of RNA that has base-paired with itself to form double strands. RNA acts as a catalyst in certain mRNA splicing reactions and is the primary genetic material for a number of viruses.

16 **The answer is D** *General principles / Pharmacology / Histamine receptor antagonists*

Cimetidine and ranitidine are H_2-receptor blockers whose main clinical use is in the treatment of ulcers and other peptic disorders. They block the effects of histamine on gastric acid secretion. H_2 antagonists inhibit, not enhance, cytochrome P450 enzymes of the liver. H_1 antagonists (e.g., diphenhydramine, chlorpheniramine) are useful in treating allergies. They also have central effects that are useful in preventing motion sickness; however, they can also cause unwanted sedation.

17 **The answer is B** *General principles / Biochemistry / Peptide bonds*

The chemistry of the peptide bond imposes restrictions on higher orders of protein structure. The secondary structure of proteins is stabilized by hydrogen bonds that are formed between the amide hydrogen and carbonyl oxygen of the peptide bond. Because the atoms of the peptide bond lie in a plane, the only permissible rotations are around the Cα-C and the N-Cα bonds. There is no formal charge associated with the peptide bond; the electrons of the carbonyl oxygen and the lone pair of electrons on the nitrogen atom are delocalized. The α-carbon atoms are in a *trans* configuration.

18 **The answer is C** *General principles / Physiology / Calcium homeostasis*

EDTA is a chelator of Ca^{2+} but is not normally found within cells and thus is not a mechanism by which cells regulate Ca^{2+} concentration. Two important transmembrane proteins in Ca^{2+} homeostasis are the Ca^{2+} adenosine triphosphate (ATPase) pump and the $Na+/Ca^{2+}$ transport chain; an ATP-dependent $H+$ pump is not known to be important. Ca^{2+} binds to a number of intracellular proteins, such as calsequestrin, and these proteins are found in high concentration in the endoplasmic reticulum. Ca^{2+} can move between the nucleus and the cytoplasm freely, and thus there is no nucleus sequestration, nor is there significant sequestration in the Golgi apparatus.

19 **The answer is B** *Cardiovascular system / Pathology / Microbiology*

The polypoid hemorrhage tissue adherent to this white fibrotic and stenotic valve is characteristic of bacterial vegetations associated with endocarditis. These vegetations derive from bacterial seeding of defective or congenitally abnormal valves. In this case, the white fibrosis thickening of the valve cusps was associated with stenosis. Vegetations may be associated with bacteria of low virulence (e.g., *streptococcus*) or those that are highly aggressive and destructive (e.g., *staphylococcus*). They may cause valve perforation and insufficiency, or they may embolize, causing infarction and secondary infection.

20 **The answer is C** *Cardiovascular system / Anatomy / Microcirculation*

Fenestrated capillaries have circular pores (fenestrae) 60 to 100 nm in diameter that may be partially surrounded by pericytes. Like nonfenestrated capillaries, their basal lamina is continuous; only sinusoid capillaries (located in the spleen, liver, and bone marrow) have discontinuous basal lamina. Fenestrated capillaries are present where there is a great deal of molecular exchange with blood (e.g., kidneys, small intestine, endocrine glands, choroid plexus). Exocrine glands contain nonfenestrated capillaries. The fenestrae are often spanned by a slit diaphragm, which is filamentous and thus does not possess a unit membrane structure. Although glomerular capillaries are fenestrated, they lack the slit diaphragm; rather, a thick basement membrane forms the filtration barrier.

21 **The answer is E** *General principles / Microbiology / Pathogenesis of infectious microorganisms*

Borrelia burgdorferi is spread by ticks and is the cause of Lyme disease. *Rickettsia rickettsii* also is usually spread by ticks. *Clostridium tetani* enters the body through wounds. *Neisseria meningitidis* and *Corynebacterium diphtheriae* both enter via the respiratory tract.

22 **The answer is A** *Central and peripheral nervous system / Neuroanatomy / Neurologic lesions and syndromes*

The deficits described in the question indicate destruction of cranial nerve (CN) III motor function and total autonomic function of the eye, combined with spastic paralysis of the contralateral body, indicating upper motor neuron destruction (as opposed to flaccid paralysis, indicating lower motor neuron disease). CN III fibers leave the brain at the level of the midbrain to continue to the ipsilateral eye. CN III is responsible for moving the eye nasally and vertically in both directions; therefore, loss of CN III function results in lateral deviation of the eye. CN III also carries autonomic fibers that originate in the Edinger–Westphal nucleus and are responsible for constriction of the pupil to light and for accommodation. Riding with the oculomotor nerve are sympathetic fibers responsible for dilation of the pupil. The destruction of all of these functions together indicates a lesion of the midbrain where it intersects with the corticospinal tract.

23 **The answer is B** *Central and peripheral nervous system / Anatomy / Circulation*

The internal carotid artery is responsible for blood flow above the midbrain, including the cerebral hemispheres. The internal carotid artery divides into the anterior cerebral artery that provides blood flow to anterior and midline areas of the cerebral hemispheres, while the middle cerebral artery provides blood flow to the more lateral areas of the cerebral hemispheres, including the areas of the motor cortex controlling the head and arm (remember the homunculus with the face most lateral; then the hand, arm, and leg as you go more medial; then in between the two hemispheres). The right side of the brain controls left-sided muscular control, so the correct answer would include involvement of the left side of the body with the face affected and the arm more compromised than the leg.

24 **The answer is E** *General principles / Genetics / Huntington's disease*

Huntington's disease is an inherited, neurodegenerative disease that often occurs in the fourth or fifth generation of life. The cause of the disease is an increased number of CAG repeats that build gradually over several generations. When that number of repeats becomes too large, it results in the synthesis of a protein that has an abnormal shape because a section of it is expanded. As a result, the abnormal protein causes the deterioration in neurological function that is associated with Huntington's disease. As the size of the repeat section increases over generations, the age of onset of the disease becomes earlier.

25 **The answer is B** *General principles / Physiology / Signal transduction; protein kinase*

Hormonal regulation of intracellular cAMP levels is widespread in mammalian organ systems. For example, cAMP is the second messenger for the effect of PTH on the kidney. Although cAMP may affect several signal transduction pathways, it does not regulate PKC by binding to its regulatory subunit and causing dissociation of the catalytic subunit; this is the activation mechanism for cAMP-dependent protein kinase A. cAMP is synthesized from ATP in a reaction that is catalyzed by adenylate cyclase. The degradation of cAMP is mediated by a family of phosphodiesterases, which catalyze the hydrolysis to 5'-AMP.

26 **The answer is E** *Central and peripheral nervous system / Biochemistry / Tay–Sachs disease*

Tay–Sachs disease has a reported 1/30 carrier rate among Ashkenazi Jews, which is about 10 times the rate in other population groups. It is a lysosomal storage disease caused by mutations in the gene coding for hexosaminidase A, leading to a virtual absence of this enzyme. Deficiency of hexosaminidase A results in an accumulation of GM_2 gangliosides, which normally make up 1% to 3% of total brain gangliosides but comprise over 90% in individuals with Tay–Sachs disease. Lack of the enzyme β-galactosidase is an autosomal recessive disorder; however, unlike Tay–Sachs disease, it results in lysosomal storage of GM_1 gangliosides.

27 **The answer is B** *General principles / Genetics / Autosomal dominant inheritance*

Every child has a 50% chance of inheriting a condition with an autosomal dominant mode of inheritance. This does not necessarily mean that in a family with eight children, four will be affected and four unaffected, although this is statistically the most likely possibility. It is also possible that all children will be affected or all will be unaffected, although these possibilities are unlikely.

28 **The answer is B** *Gastrointestinal system / Pathology / Gastrointestinal tract*

This gross picture shows a pedunculated polyp with a cauliflower-like neoplasm attached to the colonic mucosa by a thin stalk. These neoplastic polyps contain dysplastic colonic glands and may be precursors to colonic adenocarcinomas. Malignant transformation is related to the size, severity of dysplasia, and amount of villous architecture on histologic examination. Hyperplastic polyps are small, sessile proliferations of hyperplastic epithelium. They lack stalks and are smooth, hemispheric mucosal protrusions. Villous adenomas are sessile-based tumors with a finger-like, brushy surface resembling a sea anemone.

29 **The answer is D** *General principles / Biochemistry / Emzyme inhibition*

The data in the Lineweaver–Burk plot are diagnostic of noncompetitive inhibition. The intercept on the $1/[S]$ axis indicates that the inhibitor has no effect on the K_m for the substrate. The increase in the $1/v$ intercept observed in the presence of the inhibitor indicates a decrease in the V_{max} of the reaction. Noncompetitive inhibitors interact at a site other than the active site. They usually bear no structural resemblance to either the substrate or the transition-state analogs, and their effects cannot be reversed by high concentrations of substrates. Competitive inhibitors, however, interact at the active site, are structurally related to transition state analogs, and can be reversed by high concentrations of substrate.

30 **The answer is E** *General principles / Physiology / Membrane physiology and excitation*

The resting membrane potential is -90 mV, which is primarily due to diffusion potentials caused by $K+$ (and $Na+$) and the electrogenic $Na+/K+$ pump. Stimulation at time zero (e.g., as occurs with ACh) activates a $Na+$ channel, thus greatly increasing $Na+$ conductance and leading to depolarization. At the peak of the action potential, the number of open $Na+$ channels is 10 times the number of open $K+$ channels. Within a short time, voltage-gated $Na+$ is inactivated, and a $K+$ channel opens, greatly increasing the conductance to $K+$ and hence repolarization. The $Ca^{2+}/Na+$ channel (if present) is slow to be activated and would normally depolarize the membrane. Chloride channel permeability does not change during an action potential and thus functions passively in this process.

31 **The answer is B** *General principles / Pathology / Neurologic disease*

The patient described in the question most likely has tabes dorsalis, a disease that results from an untreated syphilis infection. The causative agent is *Treponema pallidum*, and the antibiotic of choice is penicillin. This disease results in the selective destruction of neurons in the spinal cord near the dorsal root of the spinal nerves, which causes the symptoms described in the question. Varicella zoster virus (VZV) causes shingles, a disease resulting from the activation of the virus in dorsal root ganglia of the spinal nerves, and chickenpox, a vesicular disease that usually affects children. Acyclovir is an antiviral agent that interferes with VZV as well as herpes simplex virus replication and therefore is not useful here.

32 **The answer is A** *Respiratory system / Pathology / Pulmonary disease*

The photomicrograph shows consolidation of air spaces by bilobed leukocytes—eosinophils. This pattern is diagnostic of eosinophilic pneumonia, an allergic reaction mediated by immunoglobulin E. This condition occurs in asthmatic patients and is accompanied by peripheral air space consolidation and peripheral blood eosinophilia. Known causes include drug reactions, filarial infections, and some fungal diseases (e.g., Coccidioides, Aspergillus). Klebsiella infections are bacterial pneumonias with multilobate neutrophils, not eosinophils. Thermophilic actinomyces cause a type IV immune reaction mediated by lymphocytes and histiocytes that results in the histopathology associated with hypersensitivity pneumonitis.

33 **The answer is D** *General principles / Biochemistry / Transcription*

Transcription begins when RNA polymerase recognizes and binds to specific promoter sequences on the DNA molecule found very close to the RNA synthesis start site. Therefore, to regulate transcription initiation, the interaction between an RNA polymerase protein and its promoter DNA sequence must be controlled. Enhancers are regions of DNA that increase the transcriptional activity of a gene. Three types of proteins regulate transcription initiation, including specificity factors, repressors, and activators. Specificity factors regulate the specificity of an RNA polymerase for a given promoter or set of promoters. A repressor binds to a specific DNA region and induces negative regulation by blocking RNA polymerase binding or movement along DNA strands. An activator offers positive regulation by binding to sites adjacent to the promoter region on DNA and enhancing RNA polymerase binding and activity. Origins of replication are regions of DNA that are the start sites for copying DNA during DNA replication.

34 **The answer is A** *Physiology / Glomerular filtration rate*

Blood enters the glomerulus via an afferent arteriole and leaves via an efferent arteriole. A decrease in RBF or a decrease in glomerular hydrostatic pressure tends to decrease the GFR. Accordingly, constriction of the afferent arteriole generally has this effect. An increase in RBF that increases hydrostatic pressure increases the GFR. This effect of the RBF persists even without an increase in hydrostatic pressure because of a subtle oncotic effect. Although a rise in systemic pressure would theoretically increase hydrostatic pressure and the GFR, the effect is greatly minimized by normal autoregulation in the kidney. Thus, the RBF and hydrostatic pressure are maintained by afferent arteriolar constriction in the presence of this increase over normal systemic pressures. Constriction of the efferent arteriole increases hydrostatic pressure and the GFR, but this effect is also offset by the aforementioned decrease in RBF; thus, only a modest increase in GFR is normally observed.

35 **The answer is A** *General principles / Hematology / Neutropenia and infection*

Neutropenia is defined as an absolute neutrophil count of less than 1,500/μL. Although there is a modest risk of acquired infection beginning at this level, patients with neutrophil counts of less than 1,000/μL for any length of time are at significant risk for acquiring infection, and patients with counts below 500/μL are at extreme risk. The percentages of formed elements determined by peripheral blood count have limited value; they must be multiplied by the total white cell count to arrive at absolute numbers of circulating granulocytes, monocytes, and lymphocytes. Leukocyte percentages determined by a 100-cell manual differential count have extremely broad 95% confidence intervals that may yield broad apparent shifts in absolute numbers. New cell counters with machine analysis of percentages of neutrophils, monocytes, and lymphocytes (even eosinophils and basophils) offer a better estimate of absolute number.

36 **The answer is D** *General principles / Biochemistry / DNA and RNA composition*

DNA is composed of the purines adenine and guanine and the pyrimidines thymine and cytosine. RNA is composed of the same bases with the exception that thymine is replaced by uracil. Therefore, DNA or RNA can be selectively labeled by using ^{3}H-thymine or ^{3}H-uracil, respectively.

37 **The answer is E** *Reproductive system / Pharmacology / Urinary tract infection therapy*

Penicillin G is the treatment of choice. It is inexpensive, and it is a broad-spectrum antibiotic effective in the treatment of urinary tract infections. The serum levels are so low that it is unlikely to alter the natural bacterial flora of the host.

38 **The answer is A** *Gastrointestinal system / Pathology / Gastrointestinal tract*

A small sac or outpouching occurring at this site (30 to 70 cm from the ileocecal valve) is most likely Meckel's diverticulum. These true diverticula are vestiges of the vitelline duct, and they are usually less than 6 cm long. Meckel's diverticula are present in 2% of the population. Interestingly, the intestinal mucosa of the Meckel's diverticulum may show heterotopic rests of gastric mucosa in 50% of cases. The production of acid by this mucosa may lead to peptic ulceration distal to the diverticulum and possibly perforation.

39 **The answer is A** *General principles / Immunology / Opsonic antibodies*

Opsonic antibodies are important for acquiring immunity to infection by group A *Neisseria meningitidis* because they permit recognition and destruction of *N. meningitidis* at the onset of infection. *V. cholerae*, *C. botulinum*, and *S. flexneri* exert their pathogenic effects via toxins. Opsonic antibodies are not known to protect against the action of *V. cholerae*, *C. botulinum*, or *S. flexneri*.

40 **The answer is B** *Cardiovascular system / Physiology / Mechanics of the heart*

At the end of the period of isovolumic contraction (2), the pressure inside the ventricle has risen to equal the pressure in the aorta at end diastole (80 mm Hg). At this point, ventricular pressures push the aortic valve open, and blood begins to pour out of the left ventricle (3) while it continues to contract. The fraction of end diastolic volume (115 mL) that was ejected was 60% because stroke volume was $115 - 45 = 70$ mL. After isovolumic relaxation, left ventricular end diastolic pressure was near atmospheric pressure.

41 **The answer is B** *Cardiovascular system / Pathology / Myocardial infarct*

This gross specimen shows the classic appearance of a recent (2 to 4 days old) subendocardial infarct. Early after vascular occlusion, the most distal myocardium (the subendocardial zone) undergoes coagulative necrosis. This is accompanied by vasospasm and extravasation of red blood cells. The gross appearance is of subendocardial hemorrhage and edema. Over time, red cells lyse, macrophages phagocytose debris, and myocardial fibers degenerate; this later stage (6 to 14 days) has a pale gray appearance. In time, white fibrosis scar tissue replaces necrotic muscle fibers.

42 **The answer is C** *Cardiovascular system / Pathology / Chronic myeloproliferative disorder*

An elevated platelet count and a low white blood cell count suggest chronic myeloproliferative disorder. Malignant lymphoma can be eliminated because of the lack of lymphadenopathy, and acute leukemia can be eliminated because of the lack of blasts on the blood smear. The absence of a cough and the normal chest radiograph eliminate pulmonary tuberculosis, which is often associated with myeloproliferative disorders.

43 **The answer is D** *Central and peripheral nervous system / Anatomy / Neurotransmitters*

The actions of parasympathetic and sympathetic nervous systems are largely antagonistic. The sympathetic nervous system is primarily a catabolic system associated with "fight or flight" responses and increased heart rate and blood flow to muscles and the heart. The parasympathetic nervous system is largely in control of anabolic processes and one function is to shunt blood flow to the digestive tract for use in the efficient digestion of food and collection of nutrients. The cell bodies of the parasympathetic and sympathetic nervous system found in the spinal cord are located in the intermediolateral columns of the spinal cord with the sympathetic nerves leaving from levels T1–L2 and the parasympathetic nerves leaving the spinal cord at levels S2–S4. Both of these systems use two neurons to convey their signals. The secondary neurons of the sympathetic nervous system are located in a string of paravertebral ganglion, while parasympathetic secondary neurons come from ganglion located much closer to target tissue. The primary nerve signaling for both pathways is cholinergic while the secondary signaling of the parasympathetic pathway is cholinergic and the sympathetic signaling is adrenergic.

44 **The answer is B** *General principles / Pathology / Chagas disease*

Patients with chronic Chagas disease present with cardiac conduction defects. The other signs and symptoms listed are classic for several diseases that are endemic in Central and South America, including malaria, visceral and cutaneous leishmaniasis, and amebiasis. Chronic Chagas disease (chronic trypanosomiasis) results from gradual tissue destruction of the heart, most likely caused by damage to myofibrils and the autonomic innervation of the heart. This results in the conduction defects and megacardia that are hallmarks of the disease. Parasitemia at this point is subpatent; parasites are difficult to detect in either the blood or tissues. Periodic fever and chills indicate malaria. Cutaneous and mucocutaneous lesions are seen in leishmaniasis. Persistent diarrhea and pneumonia can be the result of a number of infectious agents endemic in this region, although these symptoms are not seen in either acute or chronic Chagas disease.

45 **The answer is C** *Cardiovascular system / Pathology / Cardiology*

The heart shows extensive replacement of myocardium by dense white fibrous scars, the consequence of previous infarcts. Adherent to the endocardium is a white mural thrombus. Portions of the thrombus ejected from the left ventricle can cause distal infarcts, including those in the brain. Cerebral infarcts are a common cause of such thromboembolic events. No tumor nodules are seen in this case, and no evidence of rupture is seen, although this may be noted in patients with large infarcts.

46 **The answer is C** *Hematopoietic and lymphoreticular system / Pathology / Neoplasia*

The spleen is affected by large, white nodules having a fleshy appearance and central hemorrhage and necrosis. The most common cause of large nodular masses in the spleen is malignant lymphoma. Nodules larger than 5 mm are usually attributed to large cell lymphoma or Hodgkin's disease, whereas small nodules usually result from low-grade, non-Hodgkin's lymphomas (i.e., small lymphocytic, follicular center cell). Infarcts of the spleen are wedge-shaped and capsule-based. Histoplasmosis can cause a granulomatous splenitis, but the granulomas are usually small (size of millet seed) and calcified. Chronic congestion of the spleen causes a diffuse, brownish discoloration because of hemosiderin-laden macrophages with white fibrous plaques along the capsular surface.

47 **The answer is D** *Respiratory system / Physiology / Alveolar ventilation*

Alveolar ventilation is the product of respiratory rate × (tidal volume − dead space). In this situation, total dead space (400 mL) is the sum of the patient's anatomic dead space (150 mL) and the ventilator's dead space (250 mL). Thus, if the total output of the ventilator is adjusted to 600 mL, 200 mL of the alveolar volume will be delivered 20 times per minute, and total minute alveolar ventilation will be 4 L/min.

48 **The answer is B** *Cardiovascular system / Pharmacology / Antiarrhythmic agents; pharmacokinetics*

Lidocaine is a local anesthetic that can be used for the treatment of ventricular arrhythmias, especially those associated with acute myocardial infarction. Lidocaine can depress membrane responsiveness and, at therapeutic concentrations, appears to have minimal effects on normal myocardial cells (neither ventricular nor conducting tissue), but will favorably affect damaged or depolarized myocardial cells. Lidocaine is quantitatively removed by the liver and thus is only administered intravenously. Because of its narrow margin of safety (e.g., significant adverse effects in the CNS), lidocaine is never given as a single, large bolus but, rather, is infused slowly over a short period of time (loading dose) followed by a slow, continuous infusion (maintenance dose).

49 **The answer is B** *General principles / Biochemistry / Chromatin*

Chromatin contains the chromosomal material in nondividing eukaryotic cells. Upon cell division, chromatin condenses into a specific number of chromosomes. Chromatin is made up of equal portions of protein and DNA plus a small amount of RNA. The protein portions consist of histone proteins, which are tightly associated with DNA, and nonhistone proteins, which regulate gene expression. The DNA in chromatin is wrapped tightly around five classes of histones to form distinct structural units called nucleosomes. This forms an arrangement known as beads on a string. These nucleosome structures are compacted further into 30-nm fibers before arrangements into one loop (50 × 106 base pairs), one rosette (6 loops), one coil (30 rosettes), and two chromatids (2 × 10 coils). Inositol triphosphate functions in signal transduction cascades, whereas connexins act to stabilize gap junctions.

50 **The answer is E** *General principles / Pharmacology / Pharmacokinetics of drugs*

Nomograms (e.g., body surface area, creatinine clearance) are reliable indicators of appropriate drug dosages in only approximately 50% of patients with renal insufficiency. Actual peak and trough levels are the only way to guarantee a therapeutic level of antimicrobial agents and avoid toxicity.

test **7**

Questions

Directions: Single best answer questions consist of numbered items or incomplete statements followed by answers or by completions of the statement. Select the ONE lettered answer or completion that is BEST in each case.

1 Which one of the following statements about glycogen storage disease type Ia is true?

(A) Liver glycogen is decreased
(B) Renal glycogen is increased
(C) Phosphorylase A is deficient
(D) Debranching enzyme is deficient

2 Which of the following statements regarding coronary artery blood flow in a healthy person is true?

(A) During systole, coronary artery blood flow is uniform from subendocardial to epicardial regions of the left ventricle
(B) Myocardial oxygen extraction, not coronary artery blood flow, increases during exercise
(C) Coronary artery blood flow is directly proportional to arterial blood pressure over a range of pressures within 20 to 30 mm Hg of normal
(D) Coronary artery blood flow is proportional to myocardial oxygen demands
(E) Coronary artery blood flow is maximal during systole

3 Which of the following facts about oxidized nicotinamide adenine dinucleotide (NAD+), oxidized nicotinamide adenine dinucleotide phosphate (NADP+), flavin mononucleotide (FMN), and flavin adenine dinucleotide (FAD) nucleotide cofactors in metabolism is true?

(A) They are lipid-soluble
(B) They are very tightly bound to flavoproteins
(C) They undergo irreversible oxidation
(D) They are used by many dehydrogenase enzymes

4 Ascorbic acid is a six-carbon ketolactone that is

(A) commonly known as vitamin D
(B) required for conversion of proline and lysine residues in procollagen to hydroxyproline and hydroxylysine
(C) synthesized from glucose via conversion of L-gulonolactone in humans
(D) the cause of beriberi
(E) adequately obtained from a diet with liver, meat, fish, or poultry

5 A 27-year-old woman presents with muscle weakness, including eyelid ptosis, slurred speech, and difficulty swallowing. She is being treated with gentamicin for a gram-negative infection. The following tests have been ordered: thyroid function studies, serum creatine kinase, electromyogram, and muscle biopsy. The attending physician chides the resident on the case for not ordering edrophonium, which produces a dramatic improvement in the patient's muscle strength when administered intravenously. All of the other tests that were ordered returned with normal values. The attending physician's working diagnosis is

(A) Duchenne's muscular dystrophy (DMD)
(B) monoadenylate deaminase deficiency
(C) myasthenia gravis
(D) hyperthyroidism
(E) toxic drug myopathy

6 Which of the following areas of the colon would be most affected by a blockage in the inferior mesenteric artery?

(A) Lower stomach and duodenum
(B) Entire small intestine and right side of colon
(C) Right and transverse colon
(D) Descending and sigmoid colon
(E) Transverse, descending and sigmoid colon, rectum

7 Which of the following statements regarding prenatal testing is correct?

(A) Amniocentesis is the earliest form of testing that can be performed

(B) Chorionic villus testing can diagnose all of the diseases diagnosed by amniocentesis

(C) Chorionic villus sampling is considered safer than amniocentesis

(D) Amniocentesis is normally performed in the first trimester of pregnancy

(E) Amniocentesis provides more information than chorionic villus sampling

8 The distal constricting lesion at the gastroesophageal junction shown in Figure 41 from the color plate section is most likely caused by

(A) impacted foodstuffs

(B) varices

(C) Barrett's esophagus

(D) Crohn's disease

9 A research laboratory has been asked to study a new viral disease that the researchers think is caused by an arenavirus. They need a relatively simple test to determine whether this is indeed true. By pure chance they have found a cell line in which they can culture the virus. The most specific trait of Arenaviridae that would help classify the new virus as a member of this family would be

(A) an insect vector

(B) the presence of multiple genomic segments

(C) the presence of particles resembling ribosomes within the virions

(D) the presence of a viral envelope

10 In a male patient with the most common anatomic locations of arterial branch points, what is the proper order of arteries that originate from the aorta?

(A) Celiac, superior mesenteric, renal, inferior mesenteric, common iliac

(B) Celiac, renal, superior mesenteric, inferior mesenteric, common iliac

(C) Superior mesenteric, celiac, renal, inferior mesenteric, common iliac

(D) Renal, superior mesenteric, celiac, inferior mesenteric, common iliac

(E) Superior mesenteric, renal, celiac, common iliac, inferior mesenteric

11 Which one of the following is not a eukaryotic regulatory sequence element found upstream of the mRNA initiation site?

(A) α-Helix

(B) TATA box

(C) GC box

(D) CAAT box

(E) Enhancers

12 The bony abnormality seen in the femur shown in Figure 42 from the color plate section is caused by which one of the following conditions?

(A) Metastatic carcinoma

(B) Sickle cell disease

(C) Gout

(D) Fracture

(E) Asthma

13 Of the following statements, which best describes integral membrane proteins?

(A) They have at least one α-helical domain of approximately 20 amino acids, which spans the bilayer

(B) They are stabilized within the bilayer by a combination of hydrogen bonds and electrostatic interactions

(C) They may be solubilized by altering the pH or the ionic strength

(D) They are frequently glycoproteins in which the carbohydrate is on the cytosolic side of the membrane

(E) They may display transverse movement in the lipid bilayer

14 The tumor pictured in the accompanying photomicrograph arises from which one of the following types of cells?

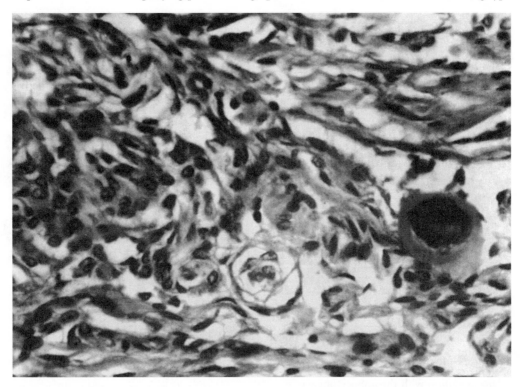

(A) Cerebellar astrocytes
(B) Leptomeningeal cells
(C) Neurons
(D) Oligodendrocytes
(E) Schwann cells

15 A 55-year-old man with a history of chronic alcoholism presents with complaints of fatigue and weakness. His laboratory values are as follows:

Hgb/Hct	11.5/34.0	
MCV	110	
MCH	38.0	
RDW	19.5	
WBC	6.0×10^9/L	
Differential:		
Polys	80%	4.8×10^9/L
Bands	7%	0.42×10^9/L
Lymphs	10%	0.6×10^9/L
Monos	5%	0.3×10^9/L

Microscopic examination of a peripheral blood smear shows poikilocytosis and hypersegmented neutrophils. This patient most likely has

(A) anemia caused by vitamin B deficiency
(B) anemia caused by iron deficiency
(C) anemia following hemorrhage
(D) sickle cell anemia
(E) β-thalassemia minor
(F) severe β-thalassemia

16 The hepatic neoplasm shown below has which one of the following characteristics?

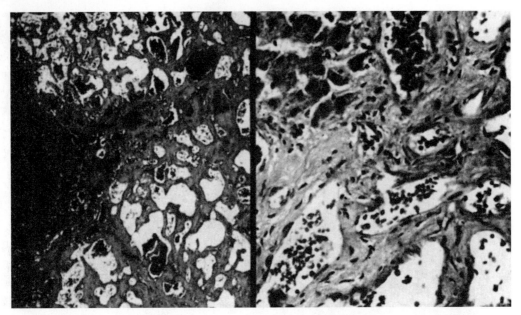

(A) An association with exposure to the carcinogen Thorotrast
(B) Highly aggressive behavior
(C) An association with thrombocytopenia
(D) Foci of hemorrhage and necrosis

17 Which of the following events occurs during receptor-mediated endocytosis for uptake of cholesterol into cells?

(A) Cholesterol binding to the low-density lipoprotein (LDL) on the plasma membrane
(B) Degradation of apoprotein B (apoB)-100
(C) Enzymatic condensation of cholesteryl esters
(D) LDL receptor degradation
(E) Endosomal/peroxisomal fusion

18 Which one of the following protein segments is characterized by its ability to bind to phosphotyrosine-containing peptides?

(A) A helix–loop–helix domain
(B) A leucine zipper
(C) An Src homology 2 (SH2) domain
(D) An Src homology 3 (SH3) domain
(E) A basic region
(F) A pleckstrin motif

19 Pain from the ovary is usually referred to which of the following regions?

(A) Inguinal and pubic regions
(B) Perineum, posterior thigh, and leg
(C) Shoulder
(D) Back

20 Cholera toxin can affect cells by blocking the guanosine triphosphatase (GTPase) activity of their G_s proteins. On a cellular level, which one of the following would be helpful in reducing the harmful effects of cholera toxin?

(A) Increasing the amount of intracellular cyclic adenosine monophosphate (cAMP)
(B) Inhibiting the activity of the adenylate cyclase in the cell
(C) Inhibiting the G_i proteins within the cell
(D) Adding ligand for the G_s protein-linked receptor
(E) Increasing the amount of protein kinase A (PKA) in the cell

21 In the following diagram of the placenta, which structure is the decidual plate and is penetrated by maternal blood vessels?

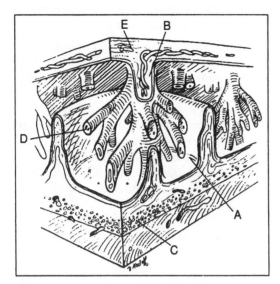

22 The spleen shown in Figure 43 from the color plate section demonstrates which one of the following abnormalities?

(A) Infarct
(B) Granuloma
(C) Angiosarcoma
(D) Hemangioma

23 A 12-year-old boy is jaundiced, and palpation reveals an enlarged liver. Laboratory values show elevated alanine aminotransferase (ALT), aspartate aminotransferase (AST), and direct bilirubin. In addition, the physician noticed Kayser–Fleischer rings on a slit-lamp examination. A diagnosis of Wilson's disease is suspected. Which of the following statements would be true?

(A) The patient is likely to have increased urinary copper with D-penicillamine challenge
(B) The primary defect is a mutation in ceruloplasmin
(C) Wilson's disease is inherited in an autosomal dominant pattern
(D) Patients can demonstrate elevated serum ceruloplasmin
(E) Patients present with increased serum free copper and decreased liver copper levels

24 Which one of the following statements about the desensitization of receptors is accurate?

(A) Homologous desensitization of nicotinic receptors requires several minutes of repeated stimuli
(B) Desensitization of adrenergic receptors can occur only if the expression of the receptor gene is reduced
(C) Desensitization does not change the affinity of a receptor for a ligand, only the activity
(D) Receptor desensitization can be affected by the phosphorylation state of the receptor
(E) Desensitization of one type of receptor cannot be mediated by the actions of another receptor pathway
(F) Desensitization occurs only for nicotinic receptors, not adrenergic receptors

25 The gross abnormality shown in the liver in Figure 44 in the color plate section most likely is caused by which one of the following conditions?

(A) Kaposi's sarcoma
(B) Massive hepatic necrosis
(C) Viral hepatitis
(D) Chronic congestion
(E) Testicular neoplasia

26 Surgical instruments are boiled for 10 minutes in a saline solution containing *Escherichia coli, Mycobacterium tuberculosis, Salmonella typhi,* and *Bacillus cereus.* Which one of the following organisms is most likely to survive this procedure?

(A) *E. coli*
(B) *M. tuberculosis*
(C) *B. cereus*
(D) *S. typhi*

27 In which of the following organs does hypoxia cause vasoconstriction?

(A) Heart
(B) Brain
(C) Lung
(D) Liver

28 In the embryo, which of the following structures is correctly paired with its adult derivative(s)?

(A) Mesonephric ducts—epididymis, ejaculatory duct, ductus deferens, seminal vesicles
(B) Urogenital folds—scrotum, scrotal raphe
(C) Gonads—vestigial appendix of testes
(D) Labioscrotal swellings—labia minora
(E) Paramesonephric ducts—ovary, follicles, rete ovarii

29 A length–tension diagram for a single sarcomere is illustrated here. Tension that develops is maximal between points *B* and *C* because

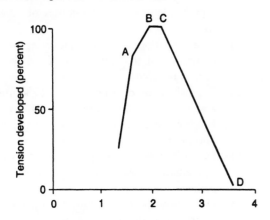

(A) there is maximal overlap between the actin filaments and the cross bridges of the myosin filaments

(B) the actin filament has pulled all the way out to the end of the myosin filament

(C) the Z disks of the sarcomere touch the ends of the myosin filament

(D) the myosin filament is at its minimal length

(E) actin filaments are overlapping for maximal interaction with myosin

30 The cortical reaction refers to which of the following processes involved in fertilization?

(A) Fusion of the female and male pronuclei

(B) Degeneration of the sperm mitochondria and tail

(C) Binding of a sperm with the oocyte zona pellucida

(D) Making the oocyte impermeable to additional sperm

(E) Fusion of the oocyte and sperm cell membranes

31 The most likely origin for the abnormality of the large intestine shown in Figure 45 in the color plate section is which one of the following conditions?

(A) Volvulus

(B) Prolapse

(C) Ulcerative colitis

(D) Colonic polyps

32 The most common cause of cystic fibrosis is the ΔF508 mutation in the cystic fibrosis transmembrane conductance regulator (CFTR) gene. Which one of the following statements concerning potential strategies to fix this defect is correct?

(A) The entire gene or protein should be replaced, because this mutation eliminates a key amino acid within the ATPase domain of the CFTR gene

(B) This mutation causes the chloride channel to be constitutively active, so it could be corrected if the regulatory region could be repaired

(C) This mutation causes the chloride channel to remain closed due to an abnormal fold of the protein, so it could be corrected if the blockage was removed

(D) This mutant protein would be able to function normally if it could be inserted in the membrane

(E) Patients with this disease could be cured if the expression of the mutated gene could be increased to normal levels

(F) This mutation causes abnormal splicing of mRNA, leading to a greatly truncated protein; therefore, correction of the splicing defect or replacement of the entire gene or protein is required

33 Which of the following enzymes may be targets of a new drug that specifically inhibits retroviral replication?

(A) DNA-dependent DNA polymerase

(B) Topoisomerase II

(C) RNA-dependent DNA polymerase

(D) RNA polymerase

(E) DNA ligase

34 The left ventricular and aortic pressure tracings shown below were recorded during cardiac catheterization of a 62-year-old patient who complains of chest pain and dizziness on exertion. The left ventricular and aortic pressure tracings indicate that this patient has

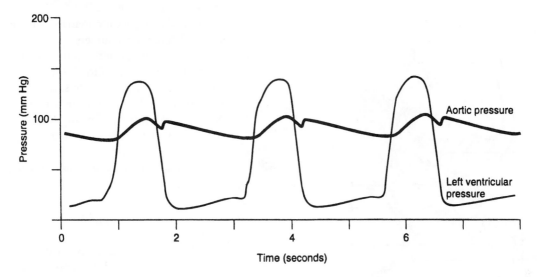

(A) pulmonary stenosis
(B) aortic stenosis
(C) mitral stenosis
(D) aortic insufficiency
(E) mitral insufficiency

35 Which of the following lists of anatomical compartments properly describes the path of sperm from within the testis to the prostatic urethra?

(A) Rete testis, seminiferous tubules, efferent ductules, epididymus, vas deferens
(B) Efferent ductules, rete testis, head of epididymus, tail of epididymus, ductus deferens
(C) Seminiferous tubules, rete testis, efferent ductules, head of epididymus, ductus deferens
(D) Tail of epididymus, seminiferous tubules, head of epididymus, ductus deferens
(E) Rete testis, ductus deferens, efferent ductules, head of epididymus

36 Which of the following signs is characteristic of an upper motor neuron injury?

(A) Flaccid paralysis
(B) Atrophy
(C) Positive Babinski sign
(D) Loss of deep tendon reflexes
(E) Fasciculations

37 A prepubertal, phenotypic girl is referred to a geneticist because a recent karyotyping that was performed for an unrelated reason showed this patient to be 46,XY. Which one of the following statements may correct?

(A) The patient may have a 17,20-lyase mutation that leads to increased production of testosterone
(B) The patient may have a deletion of the transmembrane domain of the androgen receptor, leading to androgen insensitivity
(C) The patient may have a deletion of the DNA-binding domain of the androgen receptor, leading to androgen insensitivity
(D) Because testosterone does not require a receptor, the defect must be in the synthesis pathway of testosterone
(E) The karyotype must have been performed incorrectly because it is impossible for someone to be 46,XY and phenotypically female

38 Using the following illustration of the inferior aspect of the cranium, select the lettered foramen or fissure through which the middle meningeal artery courses.

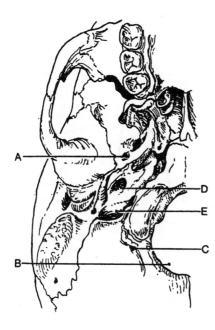

39 A 40-year-old man with short-bowel syndrome due to a resection for Crohn's disease has had large-volume diarrhea during the past few weeks. He has vesicular rash, alopecia, skin ulcers, depression, confusion with regard to time and place, and inability to discriminate tastes. He is deficient in which one of the following nutrients?

(A) Vitamin B_2 (riboflavin)
(B) Niacin
(C) Folic acid
(D) Zinc
(E) Iron
(F) Vitamin C
(G) Selenium

40 Which one of the following can be used as an antiemetic agent for patients with motion sickness?

(A) Apomorphine, a dopamine agonist
(B) Chlorpromazine, a dopamine antagonist
(C) Promethazine, an antihistamine agent
(D) Pilocarpine, a muscarinic agonist
(E) Ondansetron, a 5-HT$_3$ serotonin receptor antagonist

41 Which of the following statements concerning the informed consent of minors is true?

(A) Parental consent is required for pregnancy-related medical care
(B) Minors who are legally married still require parental consent for surgery
(C) Parental consent is not required for care related to sexually transmitted diseases
(D) Courts cannot order even life-saving treatment for a minor if it is against the parents' wishes
(E) Minors seeking treatment for alcohol dependency must have parental consent

42 Which of the following structures passes through the jugular foramen?

(A) Cranial nerve V_3
(B) Cranial nerves IX, X, and XI
(C) Cranial nerve XII
(D) Vertebral arteries and the brain stem
(E) Ophthalmic artery and the central retinal vein

43 Which of the following cranial nerves, if damaged, would leave a patient unable to shrug the shoulders?

(A) Cranial nerve V
(B) Cranial nerve XI
(C) Cranial nerve VI
(D) Cranial nerve XII
(E) Cranial nerve II
(F) Cranial nerve I

44 A 46-year-old man has symptoms of vomiting and midepigastric pain 45 minutes after having two slices of pepperoni pizza and a couple of draft beers. The pain is constant (not crampy) and radiates to the back. Vomiting does not seem to improve the patient's symptoms. His abdomen was diffusely tender with guarding but without rebound tenderness. The patient was not jaundiced. Laboratory values showed an elevated serum amylase level. Which of the following statements is most correct?

(A) Most cases of acute pancreatitis can be attributed to heredity or trauma
(B) Ranson's criteria can be useful in determining the risk of serious complications in this patient
(C) Serum amylase remains elevated longer than serum lipase in acute pancreatitis
(D) Elevated serum amylase is specific for the diagnosis of acute pancreatitis
(E) The patient may have hypercalcemia
(F) A decrease in blood urea nitrogen will be observed in this patient

45 Which of the following conditions causes unconjugated hyperbilirubinemia?

(A) Wilson's disease
(B) Crigler–Najjar syndrome type I
(C) Primary biliary cirrhosis
(D) Viral hepatitis
(E) Rotor syndrome
(F) Gallstones
(G) Alcoholic liver disease

46 A 25-year-old woman presents with a 3-week history of periumbilical pain, diarrhea, fever, and weight loss. She reports that she had these symptoms once before and that there was evidence of perianal involvement. The result of the stool culture is negative for bacteria, ova, and parasites. The radiologic barium films of the small bowel and colon demonstrate a string sign in the terminal ileum. The endoscopic evaluation, with biopsy of the affected areas, reports transmural inflammation. Which of the following statements about this disease is true?

(A) This disease does not affect the mesenteric fat
(B) This disease carries an increased risk of carcinoma
(C) Smoking is thought to be protective against this disease
(D) This disease occurs anywhere along the gastrointestinal tract but favors the terminal ileum
(E) This disease affects the bowel in a continuous fashion

47 Which of the following statements about gastric acid secretion and peptic ulcer disease (PUD) is true?

(A) Prostaglandins play an aggressive role in the development of PUD
(B) Consumption of ethanol, caffeine, tobacco, salicylates, and nonsteroidal anti-inflammatory drugs are risk factors for PUD
(C) Hereditary factors do not play a role in PUD
(D) *Helicobacter pylori* in the duodenum play a role in PUD
(E) Acetylcholine inhibits acid secretion by the parietal cells

48 A 36-year-old man complains of low-volume bloody diarrhea, crampy abdominal pain, and a fever. Microscopic examination of his stool shows fecal leukocytes. A likely cause of this man's symptoms is

(A) cholera
(B) Zollinger–Ellison syndrome
(C) laxative ingestion
(D) mannitol ingestion
(E) *shigella*

49 A lesion in which of the following anatomic structures would cause the visual defect of left anopsia?

(A) Optic chiasm
(B) Right optic nerve
(C) Left optic tract
(D) Right optic tract
(E) Left optic nerve

50 At which of the following age ranges is a child expected to develop anxiety in response to strangers?

(A) 3 to 6 months
(B) 7 to 9 months
(C) 12 to 18 months
(D) 19 to 24 months
(E) 3 to 5 years

Answer Key

1-B	11-A	21-C	31-D	41-C
2-D	12-B	22-A	32-D	42-B
3-D	13-A	23-A	33-C	43-B
4-B	14-B	24-D	34-B	44-B
5-C	15-A	25-D	35-C	45-B
6-D	16-C	26-C	36-C	46-D
7-E	17-B	27-C	37-C	47-B
8-C	18-C	28-A	38-A	48-E
9-C	19-A	29-A	39-D	49-E
10-A	20-B	30-D	40-C	50-B

Answers and Explanations

1 **The answer is B** *General principles / Physiology / Glycogen storage disease*

Glycogen storage disease type Ia, or von Gierke's disease, is caused by defective glucose-6-phosphatase activity and is characterized by hepatomegaly, renomegaly, and hypoglycemia. The liver shows intracytoplasmic accumulation of glycogen and a small amount of lipid along with some intranuclear glycogen. The kidney has intracytoplasmic accumulations of glycogen in the cortical tubular epithelial cells. The intestine also shows increased concentrations of glycogen.

2 **The answer is D** *Cardiovascular system / Physiology / Coronary artery blood flow*

Coronary blood flow closely matches myocardial work (or oxygen consumption). Myocardial oxygen extraction is near maximal at rest and does not increase appreciably, even during exercise. Coronary blood flow is maximal during diastole, in which ventricular compression of the capillaries is minimal. In addition, there is significant heterogeneity across the ventricular wall during systole, such that subendocardial blood flow is reduced and blood flow is shifted to the epicardial vessels. Autoregulation is normally observed in the myocardium, such that blood flow does not change over a large range of perfusion pressures.

3 **The answer is D** *General principles / Biochemistry / Oxidation reaction; cofactors*

In many reactions catalyzed by dehydrogenases, hydrogen atoms are transferred from a substrate to a hydrogen exceptor. This process involves the use of electron carriers, such as the following nucleotides: oxidized NAD +, oxidized NADP +, FMN, and flavin FAD. These cofactors are water-soluble and involved with several reversible oxidation–reduction reactions. NAD + and NADP + are freely diffusible in that they move from one dehydrogenase to the next. They are transformed to their reduced form after accepting one proton and two electrons. Unlike the freely diffusible NAD + and NADP +, FAD and FMN are tightly bound to flavoproteins, which catalyze oxidation–reduction reactions using these flavonucleotides as cofactors. Because they can accept either one or two electrons, flavoproteins containing FAD and FMN prosthetic groups are involved in a wide variety of reactions.

4 **The answer is B** *General principles / Biochemistry / Nutrition*

Ascorbic acid or vitamin C cannot be synthesized from precursor glucose in humans (or nonhuman primates and guinea pigs and some bats) and thus must be a critical part of the diet. It is readily obtained from citrus fruits as well as potatoes and other food sources. Ascorbic acid is a cofactor in hydroxylation (and amidation reactions) and is particularly important in collagen synthesis. A deficiency in dietary ascorbic acid leads to scurvy, a disorder typified by defect in collagen synthesis (wound healing defects, rupture of capillaries). The disorder can be treated by ingestion of citrus fruits; orange and lemon juice are particularly good sources and 60 mg per day is the daily recommended dose for adults. Beriberi is the result of vitamin B1 (thiamine) deficiency. Deficiencies in nicotinic acid cause pellagra. Nicotinic acid can be maintained by adequate ingestion of animal proteins (in which tryptophan is an important precursor).

5 **The answer is C** *Central and peripheral nervous system / Pathology / Myasthenia gravis*

Myasthenia gravis is a neuromuscular disorder with muscle weakness caused by blockade of ACh receptors by autoantibodies to the ACh receptors. The antibody–receptor complex is incapable of responding to ACh and is rapidly internalized and degraded. Edrophonium is a short-acting acetylcholinesterase inhibitor that increases synaptic ACh levels. An increase in muscle strength on administration of edrophonium is diagnostic of myasthenia gravis.

6 **The answer is D** *Gastrointestinal system / Anatomy / Circulation*

Since the duodenum is developed from the foregut and midgut, it has blood flow support from the celiac (foregut) and superior mesenteric artery (midgut). The superior mesenteric artery provides blood flow to tissues of the midgut, and that area extends from the duodenum through the jejunum, ileum, right colon, and some supply to the transverse colon. The inferior mesenteric artery provides blood flow primarily to the descending and sigmoid colon. Given these patterns of blood flow, the only possible correct answer is (D).

7 **The answer is E** *Reproductive system / Genetics / Amniocentesis*

Amniocentesis is among the most commonly performed, invasive prenatal diagnostic procedure. Amniocentesis is usually performed in the second trimester of pregnancy. The chromosome analysis is usually completed 1 to 2 weeks after the procedure is performed, and additional testing such as biochemical analyses and DNA testing usually take an additional 2 to 4 weeks. Chorionic villi sampling (CVS) is a test performed to detect specific genetic abnormalities earlier in pregnancy; it is generally done at 10 to 13 weeks. It provides genetic information earlier than CVS and can provide all of the data that amniocentesis provides except for information about neural tube defects. Chorionic villi sampling also carries a slightly higher risk of miscarriage.

8 **The answer is C** *Gastrointestinal system / Pathology / Gastrointestinal neoplasia*

This gross photomicrograph shows an annular, ulcerating, and infiltrating carcinoma arising at the gastroesophageal junction. Most distal esophageal carcinomas are gland-forming tumors, or adenocarcinomas. Their constrictive growth results in dysphagia and chest discomfort. Many adenocarcinomas occur in association with Barrett's esophagus, a metaplastic phenomenon in which glandular mucosa replaces the normal squamous epithelium of the esophagus; the most common cause of this change is reflux esophagitis. The only other consideration is Crohn's disease, which may affect the esophagus and stomach where it induces zones of stenosis. This is extremely unusual at the cardioesophageal junction, and this inflammatory process lacks the infiltrative quality of the specimen shown.

9 **The answer is C** *General principles / Microbiology / Eukaryotic and viral commonalities*

Arenaviruses are multisegmented RNA viruses with inclusion granules in the virions that contain ribosomes derived from their host cells. Although arenaviruses have envelopes, this is a trait shared by many viruses, including herpesviruses and orthomyxoviruses. Likewise, many viruses, including orthomyxoviruses and paramyxoviruses, have multiple genomic sequences. Only arenaviruses contain ribosomes; in fact, the Latin word *arena* means sand. The presence of ribosome-containing granules makes the virus look grainy under the electron microscope.

10 **The answer is A** *Gastrointestinal system / Anatomy / Circulation*

The most common anatomical order of arterial branching from the aorta is: celiac, superior mesenteric, renal, inferior mesenteric, common iliac.

11 **The answer is A** *General principles / Biochemistry / Eukaryotic transcription; regulatory sequences*

RNA transcription initiation in eukaryotic cells is highly dependent on positive regulatory elements. RNA polymerases have very little (if any) affinity on their own for their corresponding promoters. Therefore, transcription initiation depends on several activator proteins that recognize specific regulatory elements upstream of the mRNA initiation site. The TATA box is found 25 to 30 base pairs upstream of the initiation site with the sequence TATAAAA. This site is recognized by the transcription factor TFIID required for RNA polymerase binding to DNA. The GC box (GGGCGG), which is several hundred base pairs from the initiation site, regulates transcription initiation by binding the transcription factor SP1. CCAAT boxes (GCCAAT) are also several hundred base pairs upstream from the mRNA initiation site, and they are bound by the transcription activator CTF1. An additional regulatory element in eukaryotic cells, known as an enhancer, has a more complex structure and exerts its regulatory effects regardless of its position relative to the mRNA initiation site. An α-helix is a common secondary protein structure not directly associated with nucleic acids or mRNA initiation sites.

12 The answer is B *Musculoskeletal system / Pathology / Hematology*

The bone shows a wedge-shaped subcortical infarct, so-called avascular necrosis of the femoral head. Since bone is an end organ with a single vascular supply, bone infarcts tend to be pyramid-shaped, abut on the cortical surface, and be sharply defined. The causes of bone infarcts are usually related to thromboembolic events. Patients with sickle cell disease are predisposed to vaso-occlusive events and avascular necrosis of bones. Patients with metastatic carcinoma often have multiple, well-circumscribed white nodules within the medulla. Fractures tend to be hemorrhagic, irregular, jagged, not well-defined, and triangular. Gout usually affects the synovium as grainy, chalk-gray deposits. Asthma is not associated with bony abnormalities.

13 The answer is A *General principles / Biochemistry / Integral membrane proteins*

Integral membrane proteins are stabilized by hydrophobic interactions between the lipid bilayer and the amino acid side chains. Detergents are required for solubilization. Approximately 20 amino acids in an α-helical conformation are required to span the width of the bilayer. These proteins display compositional asymmetry, with the carbohydrate moieties always on the side of the membrane away from the cytoplasm. They may display lateral but not transverse movement within the membrane.

14 The answer is B *Central and peripheral nervous system / Histology / Histopathology of meningiomas*

The tumor in the photomicrograph is a meningioma, which has a marked predilection for women and arises from the pia–arachnoid cells of the leptomeninges. It is usually well-circumscribed and may be associated with a hyperostotic reaction of overlying bone. The tumor cells are arranged in whorls or nests, and they are frequently observed with concentric calcified concretions called psammoma bodies, as shown on the *right* of the photomicrograph.

15 The answer is A *Hematopoietic and lymphoreticular system / Pathology / Pathophysiology of anemia*

The result of a diet deficient in vitamin B_{12} or folate can be macrocytic, normochromic anemia with characteristic hypersegmented neutrophils. Anemia caused by folate or vitamin B_{12} deficiency often also presents with thrombocytopenia and agranulocytopenia. Microcytic hypochromic erythrocytes are observed in iron deficiency anemia and β-thalassemia minor. In addition, basophilic stippling and target cells can be seen in thalassemia minor. In sickle cell crisis, the anemia is normocytic and normochromic, as is the anemia associated with hemorrhage. Severe β-thalassemia is uniformly fatal in children.

16 The answer is C *Gastrointestinal system / Pathology / Microscopic features of hemangioma*

This hepatic neoplasm is a benign cavernous hemangioma. This is the most common mesenchymal tumor of the liver, and if it reaches an enormous size, it may be associated with a bruit over the liver and thrombocytopenia owing to venous stasis and in situ thrombosis. The neoplasm is composed of dilated vascular spaces lined by flattened, cytologically bland endothelial cells (*right*). Angiosarcomas of the liver have highly aggressive behavior and usually have foci of hemorrhage and necrosis. They are associated with particular carcinogens, one of which is Thorotrast, a radioactive medium widely used 60 years ago.

17 The answer is B *General principles / Biochemistry / Cholesterol uptake into cells*

Cholesterol is carried through the bloodstream as plasma lipoproteins. LDL is abundant in cholesterol, cholesteryl esters, and apoB-100 (the major apoprotein). LDL carries cholesterol through the blood plasma until apoB-100 is recognized by specific LDL receptors on the cell surface. Receptor binding initiates receptor-mediated endocytosis, which brings the LDL particle and the receptor into the cell via an endosome. The endosome then fuses with a lysosome, causing enzymatic hydrolysis of cholesteryl esters and degradation of apoB-100. This releases cholesterol, fatty acid, and amino acids into the cytosol. The LDL receptor escapes degradation and returns to the cell surface to begin the process again.

[18] The answer is C *General principles / Biochemistry / Motifs of DNA binding and protein–protein interaction*

Motifs are structural elements that, when combined, form the core of a domain, the functional structural unit of a polypeptide. An SH2 domain has approximately 100 amino acids, two β-pleated sheets, and two α-helices. SH2 domains are also known to bind specifically to phosphotyrosine-containing peptides. SH3 domains, helix–loop–helix domains, and leucine zippers are also involved in protein–protein interactions, but they have different binding requirements. SH3 domains bind proline-rich sequences, whereas helix–loop–helix domains and leucine zippers are involved in forming dimers, usually of transcription factors. Basic regions of a protein are often found to bind DNA. Pleckstrin motifs are known to bind phospholipids.

[19] The answer is A *Central and peripheral nervous system / Anatomy / Pelvic innervation*

Afferent nerves from the pelvic viscera travel along autonomic pathways. Afferent nerves from the ovary, testis, upper to middle ureter, uterine tubes, urinary bladder, and uterine body travel along the least splanchnic nerve to the lower thoracic segment and along the lumbar splanchnic nerves to the upper lumbar segments of the spinal cord; thus, pain is referred to the inguinal and pubic regions as well as to the lateral and anterior aspects of the thigh.

[20] The answer is B *General principles / Cell biology / G proteins*

G_s (s for stimulatory) proteins function by activating adenylate cyclase to produce more cAMP. The G_s proteins are able to activate adenylate cyclase when bound to guanosine triphosphate (GTP). Thus, the GTPase activity of the G_s proteins is a mechanism that allows the protein to turn itself off. The cholera toxin that blocks the GTPase activity leads to a constitutively active G_s protein; therefore, the levels of cAMP within the cell increase, and the cAMP acts as a second messenger. Thus, whereas increasing the amount of intracellular cAMP would make the situation worse, inhibition of adenylate cyclase would act to counteract the effects of cholera toxin. Because PKA is activated by cAMP, increasing the concentration of PKA would not be protective. cAMP can act directly on certain ion channels. Therefore, even a reduction of the amount of PKA may not eliminate the effects of the toxin. Additional ligand for the G_s protein-linked receptor would increase the activation of the G_s proteins. G_i proteins (i for inhibitory) act to reduce the activity of adenylate cyclase; therefore, inhibition of these proteins would also make the situation worse. However, activation of G_i proteins may be helpful.

[21] The answer is C *Reproductive system / Anatomy / Placenta*

The placenta consists of a decidual plate (*C*) facing the endometrium and a chorionic plate (*E*) facing the fetus. The decidual plate and chorionic plate are fused at the margins of the discoid placenta. These two plates are interconnected by cytotrophoblastic cell columns (*B*). Large numbers of chorionic villi (*D*) project away from them into the intervillous space (*A*). Maternal blood vessels end on the decidual plate and pour maternal blood into the intervillous space. Maternal blood directly bathes the chorionic villi. Thus, the human placenta is said to be a hemochorial placenta.

[22] The answer is A *Hematopoietic and lymphoreticular system / Pathology / Spleen*

The spleen in this case shows a wedge-shaped zone of hemorrhage and consolidation that abuts the capsular surface and has its apex pointing at the center of the organ. The circulation to the spleen occurs through progressive branching of the splenic artery, forming arcades that feed pyramid-shaped zones with their bases at the capsule. Occlusion of the arteries—usually through thromboembolic events or progressive atherosclerosis—results in initial hemorrhage and then, after red cell lysis and mononuclear cell infiltration, a pale, whitish infarct. Granulomas of the spleen are round, white, and have central necrosis. These granulomas do not rest adjacent to the splenic capsule. Angiosarcoma and hemangiomas form tumor nodules, with hemorrhage and necrosis. A sponge-like quality is seen with well-differentiated endothelial processes.

23 **The answer is A** *General principles / Genetics / Wilson's disease*

Although patients with Wilson's disease often have decreased serum ceruloplasmin, the primary defect is not in ceruloplasmin (chromosome 3). The genetic defect is on chromosome 13, and it is thought to be a deficiency of a P-type ATPase. This enzyme is important in the assembly of ceruloplasmin; thus, a defect in this enzyme can yield low serum ceruloplasmin. Normally, more than 90% of plasma copper is bound to ceruloplasmin. Thus, patients with Wilson's disease can have increased serum free copper and increased urinary copper (which may increase further upon challenge with D-penicillamine). Liver copper is always elevated in Wilson's disease. Wilson's disease is inherited as an autosomal recessive trait.

24 **The answer is D** *General principles / Pharmacology / Desensitization*

Desensitization can occur in a number of ways, including homologous pathways, in which only one type of receptor is involved, and heterologous pathways, in which one type of receptor is desensitized through the activity of another type of receptor. For nicotinic receptors, desensitization may take less than 1 second, whereas desensitization is slower for adrenergic receptors. However, adrenergic receptors have mechanisms to desensitize them in ways other than regulation of transcription. These methods include phosphorylation of the receptor by cAMP-dependent kinases or β-adrenergic receptor kinase. Nicotinic desensitization can also be affected by phosphorylation, because addition of a phosphate group may speed desensitization. Although desensitization may change the affinity of the receptor for its ligand (either increase or decrease), this is usually not the mechanism of desensitization. It is the decrease in receptor function, not ligand binding, that is the actual method of desensitization.

25 **The answer is D** *Gastrointestinal system / Pathology / Liver*

This gross photograph displays the classic changes of chronic congestion, resulting in the prototypic "nutmeg" liver. Regions of reddish discoloration reflect the presence of sinusoidal congestion around the central veins of the hepatic lobule. Chronic congestion is most often caused by congestive heart failure, but it may result from many conditions that cause hepatic vein congestion, including heart failure and obstruction to the inferior vena cava or hepatic veins (Budd–Chiari syndrome). Kaposi's sarcoma is a local lesion in the liver, not a diffuse process, and massive hepatic necrosis would not have this repetitive reticulated pattern. Instead, necrosis would be diffuse and uniformly brown in color.

26 **The answer is C** *General principles / Microbiology / Sterilization; disinfection*

Bacterial endospores are the life forms most resistant to heat, and they can survive boiling for several minutes. Medically important endospore formers include members of the genera *Bacillus* and *Clostridium*. Nonspore formers, such as *Escherichia coli*, *Salmonella typhi*, and *Mycobacterium tuberculosis*, are more heat-sensitive than spore formers and are usually killed after several minutes of boiling.

27 **The answer is C** *Cardiovascular system / Physiology / Vasoconstriction*

Compared with other tissue, the lung is unusual in having a vasoconstrictor response to hypoxia rather than a vasodilator response. Although the mechanism remains obscure, the rationale seems to be to divert blood flow from poorly ventilated regions of the lung, thus improving the matching of ventilation and perfusion.

28 **The answer is A** *Reproductive system / Anatomy / Embryo–adult derivatives*

The embryonic mesonephric ducts become the vestigial duct of Gartner in the woman and in the man become the epididymis, ejaculatory duct, ductus deferens, and seminal vesicles. The urogenital folds are responsible for forming the labia minora in the woman and the penile raphe, penis, and ventral portion of the penis in the man. Gonads become the ovary, follicles, and rete ovarii in the woman; in the man, the gonads develop into the testes, rete testes, and seminiferous tubules. Labioscrotal swellings in the woman become the labia majora; in the man, these swellings become the scrotum and scrotal raphe. The paramesonephric ducts form the upper part of the vagina, cervix, uterus, and uterine tubes in the woman and the vestigial appendix of the testes in the man.

29 **The answer is A** *General principles / Biochemistry / Effect of actin and myosin filament overlap on muscle contraction*

It is generally accepted that maximal contraction of muscle fiber will occur when the overlap between actin filaments and the cross bridges of the myosin filaments is optimal. At point *D*, the actin filament has pulled all the way out to the end of the myosin filament without overlap, and tension is minimal. As the muscle shortens past the optimal length, *C*, actin filaments tend to overlap each other and the myosin filaments decrease in length *A*, contributing to the decline in contraction at shorter-than-optimal lengths.

30 **The answer is D** *Reproductive system / Physiology / Fertilization*

Fertilization occurs in a series of steps beginning with the sperm binding to the oocyte's zona pellucida. This triggers the acrosome reaction, which releases enzymes used in the penetration of the oocyte by the sperm. Once penetration occurs, the cortical reaction is triggered, which prevents other sperm from fusing with the oocyte. The membranes of the sperm and oocyte fuse, followed by the degeneration of sperm mitochondria and tail. The oocyte, which was stuck in metaphase, now goes on to finish meiosis II to become an ovum. When the male and female genetic material (i.e., pronuclei) fuse, the ovum becomes a zygote.

31 **The answer is D** *Gastrointestinal system / Pathology / Intestines*

This gross photo shows an ulcerating lesion with heaped-up, rolled edges, a classic appearance of carcinomas of the large intestine. Such tumors in the proximal colon tend to present as polypoid fungating masses, whereas those in the distal colon (as in this case) form annular lesions that produce napkin-ring constrictions of the bowel. These carcinomas are thought to arise in colonic polyps in which progressive molecular perturbations result in malignant transformation. Most colonic carcinomas are adenocarcinomas, and prognosis depends on the extent of the tumor at the time of diagnosis. The most widely used classifications focus on the depth of invasion of the colonic wall and the presence of lymph node metastases (Dukes classification, Astler Coller classification).

32 **The answer is D** *Respiratory system / Genetics / Cystic fibrosis; molecular medicine; gene therapy*

Although replacing the entire gene or protein provides a cure for the disease, the ΔF508 mutation is not within an ATPase domain of the CFTR gene. This mutation is within the NBF1 domain and leads to degradation of the mutant protein within the endoplasmic reticulum because it is folded improperly and cannot travel to the plasma membrane. However, if this protein could be inserted into the membrane, it would function normally. The patency of the chloride channel is unaffected by the ΔF508 mutation except for its inability to reach the membrane. As for altering the regulation of the channel activity, increasing expression of this mutant protein would not be helpful because the CFTR would be unable to reach the membrane and perform its normal function. Splicing of the CFTR is also unaffected by this mutation.

33 **The answer is C** *General principles / Biochemistry / DNA replication; retroviruses*

RNA-dependent DNA polymerase synthesizes DNA from an RNA template and is essential for the replication of retroviruses (but not for cells), and therefore is a potential target of the new drug. Topoisomerase II relaxes supercoiled DNA. RNA polymerase synthesizes a primer fragment for DNA-dependent DNA polymerase. DNA ligase anneals the Okazaki fragments on the lagging strand of DNA synthesis.

34 **The answer is B** *Cardiovascular system / Physiology / Cardiac dynamics*

The gradient between the ventricular and aortic systolic pressures is diagnostic of aortic stenosis. The normal aortic valve provides negligible resistance, and the aortic pressure is nearly identical to the ventricular pressure during rapid ventricular ejection. A similar picture is seen if right ventricular and pulmonary pressures are measured in the presence of pulmonary valve stenosis, but the pressures are proportionately reduced because of the low resistance of the pulmonary circulation.

35 **The answer is C** *Reproductive system / Anatomy / Male reproductive tract*

Sperm are formed in the seminiferous tubules of the testes, which join together to produce the rete testis. Small, efferent ductules connect the rete testis to the head of the epididymis. The pathway from the head of the epididymis to the prostatic urethra travels from the head of epididymis to the body to the tail and then to the ducutus deferens that concludes with the ejaculatory duct that opens into the prostatic urethra.

36 **The answer is C** *Central and peripheral nervous system / Anatomy / Clinical assessment*

The Babinski sign is elicited by stroking the palmar surface of the foot along the lateral aspect from the heel to the smallest toe and then across toward the biggest toe. Normally the toes flex inward; however, in the case of upper motor neuron damage, the toes may instead fan outward, with the big toe dorsiflexing (a positive Babinski sign). Other signs of upper motor neuron damage include spastic paralysis and hyperactive deep tendon reflexes. Atrophy and fasciculations indicate lower motor neuron damage.

37 **The answer is C** *General principles / Genetics / Testosterone and its receptor*

17,20-Lyase is an enzyme involved in the production of testosterone. Deficiency of this enzyme does not affect adrenal cortex function. It can cause a 46,XY person to be phenotypically female if the deficiency is severe enough to sufficiently reduce the production of testosterone. Androgen insensitivity can also cause a 46,XY individual to be phenotypically female. This syndrome is caused by mutations in the androgen receptor. Like other steroid hormone receptors, it contains a steroid-binding domain and a DNA-binding domain; however, it does not contain a transmembrane domain, as the steroid hormones are able to diffuse through the plasma membrane to bind with the receptor intracellularly.

38 **The answer is A** *Cardiovascular system / Anatomy / Cranial vasculature*

The foramen spinosum transmits the middle meningeal artery (A), a branch of the maxillary artery. The carotid canal (D) transmits the internal carotid artery, whereas the jugular foramen (E) contains the internal jugular vein in addition to the glossopharyngeal, vagus, and spinal accessory nerves. Each posterior condylar canal (C) transmits a large emissary vein. The vertebral arteries enter the cranial cavity through the foramen magnum (B) along with the spinal accessory nerve; the spinal cord also transmits the foramen magnum.

39 **The answer is D** *General principles / Biochemistry / Vitamin/mineral deficiencies*

Zinc deficiency is characterized by facial and extremity rash, skin ulcers, alopecia, confusion, apathy, depression, dysgeusia, and poor wound healing. Riboflavin deficiency is characterized by angular stomatitis, anemia, cheilosis, geographic tongue, skin desquamation, and seborrheic dermatitis. Niacin deficiency is identified by pellagra or dermatitis, dementia, diarrhea, angular stomatitis, painful tongue, and headache. Folic acid deficiency is marked by anemia, sore tongue, mouth ulcers, nausea, diarrhea, depression, and fatigue. Iron deficiency manifests as anemia, angular stomatitis, atrophic tongue, and spoon nails (koilonychia). Vitamin C deficiency can present as scurvy with gingivitis, joint and muscle pain, and bleeding abnormalities. Selenium deficiency can result in myositis or even cardiomyopathy. Patients with short-bowel syndrome require vitamin and mineral supplements, particularly zinc and the fat-soluble vitamins.

40 **The answer is C** *General principles / Pharmacology / Antiemetic agents*

Dopamine stimulates vomiting and inhibits gut motility. Apomorphine is a dopamine (D_2) agonist that acts at the chemoreceptor trigger zone to induce vomiting. Chlorpromazine is a D_2 receptor antagonist that also blocks α-adrenergic receptors. It is a useful antiemetic agent in cancer chemotherapy, but it is ineffective against motion sickness. Antihistamines and antimuscarinic agents (e.g., promethazine and scopolamine) are effective for prevention of the vomiting caused by motion sickness because they act at the vestibular nuclei and possibly at other sites that are involved in the response of motion sickness. However, they are not effective against other causes of vomiting. Pilocarpine is a muscarinic agonist that can increase gastric secretions and can be used to treat glaucoma; therefore, it is not useful as an antiemetic. Ondansetron and other serotonin antagonists work centrally and peripherally to reduce vomiting; however, they are ineffective against motion sickness. These agents work mainly at the chemoreceptor trigger zone but also have some prokinetic activity.

41 **The answer is C** *General principles / Behavioral science / Informed consent*

People younger than 18 years of age are required to have parental consent for treatment of sexually transmitted diseases, pregnancy-related medical care, or treatment of drug and alcohol dependence. However, if a minor is declared self-sufficient or is legally married, parental consent is no longer required because that person is considered to be emancipated. If parents refuse standard medical care when the child is in life-threatening circumstances, physicians can obtain a court order allowing them to treat the child.

42 **The answer is B** *Central and peripheral nervous system / Anatomy / Cranium*

The jugular foramen contains cranial nerves IX, X, and XI, along with the jugular vein. Cranial nerve V_3 courses through the foramen ovale. The hypoglossal nerve, XII, passes through the hypoglossal canal. Vertebral arteries and the brain stem accompany the spinal roots of cranial nerve XI through the foramen magnum. The optic canal contains the ophthalmic artery, the central retinal vein, and cranial nerve II.

43 **The answer is B** *Central and peripheral nervous system / Anatomy / Cranial nerves*

The accessory nerve (XI) is responsible for the ability to shrug shoulders and turn the head. The trigeminal nerve (V) carries sensory fibers for the face and motor fibers for the muscles of mastication. The abducens nerve (VI), along with the oculomotor (III) and trochlear (IV) nerves, controls eye movement. The hypoglossal nerve (XII) controls movement of the tongue. The optic nerve (II) carries the sensory fibers that are responsible for vision. The olfactory nerve (I) carries the sensory fibers responsible for smelling.

44 **The answer is B** *Gastrointestinal system / Physiology / Acute pancreatitis*

An elevated serum amylase level is a useful test result for evaluating a patient with suspected acute pancreatitis, but it is not specific for acute pancreatitis. Serum amylase can be elevated in other conditions (e.g., acute cholecystitis, dissecting abdominal aortic aneurysms, mesenteric ischemia or infarction, and common bile duct stones). Serum lipase can also be elevated in acute pancreatitis. Serum lipase is more specific for pancreatitis, and levels remain high longer than amylase, making lipase useful for patients who present late. When determining the severity of acute pancreatitis, two classification systems can be used. Ranson's criteria include 11 clinical signs and laboratory tests that are performed during the first 48 hours after admission to assess the risks of complications. Among these criteria are higher than 10% decrease in hematocrit, higher than 5 mg/dL increase in blood urea nitrogen (BUN), serum calcium lower than 8 mg/dL, and partial pressure of oxygen in arterial blood (PaO_2) less than 60 mm Hg. Glasgow's criteria can be completed on admission. Glucose, lactate dehydrogenase (LDH), and BUN levels are included in both the Ranson and Glasgow scoring systems, so they should be tested in a patient who is thought to have pancreatitis. Approximately 80% of cases of acute pancreatitis are caused by alcohol and gallstones. Another 10% of cases are due to metabolic abnormalities (e.g., hyperlipidemia), drugs (e.g., steroids, thiazide diuretics), and trauma. Ten percent of cases are idiopathic, with a small role (~1%) for hereditary pancreatitis.

45 **The answer is B** *Gastrointestinal system / Physiology / Causes of hyperbilirubinemia*

Wilson's disease, primary biliary cirrhosis, viral hepatitis, gallstones, alcoholic liver disease, and Rotor's syndrome do not impair the liver's ability to conjugate bilirubin; however, they can lead to conjugated or direct hyperbilirubinemia. In Crigler–Najjar syndrome type I, there is no functional bilirubin uridine diphosphate-glucuronosyltransferase (the enzyme responsible for conjugation). Thus, Crigler–Najjar syndrome is associated with unconjugated (or indirect) hyperbilirubinemia.

46 The answer is D *Gastrointestinal system / Pathology / Crohn's disease*

This patient has Crohn's disease. Crohn's disease is associated with patchy involvement and skip lesions. It also frequently involves the mesentery, resulting in thickened, finger-like projections known as creeping fat. Although Crohn's disease occurs anywhere along the gastrointestinal tract, it often involves the terminal ileum. Fistulas, sinus tracts, and the string sign can be seen on radiographs. Microscopic examination may show transmural inflammation, aphthoid ulcers, and noncaseating granulomas. Endoscopy demonstrates "cobblestone" mucosa. Crohn's disease is directly associated with smoking. Smoking is thought to be protective against ulcerative colitis but not against Crohn's disease. Unlike ulcerative colitis, Crohn's disease does not increase the risk of carcinoma.

47 The answer is B *Gastrointestinal system / Pathology / Peptic ulcer disease*

Peptic ulcer disease (PUD) is thought to result from an imbalance between aggressive and protective factors. The most important aggressive factors are acid secretion and pepsin. Normally, histamine, gastrin, and ACh lead to acid secretion, with gastrin being the most potent of the three. *Helicobacter pylori* play a central role in PUD; however, they do not reside in the duodenum. *H. pylori* are found in the gastric antrum of more than 95% of patients with duodenal ulcers. Other risk factors for PUD include hereditary traits, as demonstrated by the Zollinger–Ellison syndrome, as well as consumption of ethanol, caffeine, tobacco, salicylates, and NSAIDs. Major, protective mucosal defense factors include mucus and bicarbonate secretion. Prostaglandins protect gastric mucosa from injury and stimulate the production of mucus and bicarbonate.

48 The answer is E *General principles / Pathology / Causes of diarrhea*

Shigella is an invasive bacterium that leads to inflammation, fever, and white blood cells in the stool. None of the other choices lead to tissue invasion and inflammation. Cholera causes severe secretory diarrhea without invasion or fecal leukocytes. Zollinger–Ellison syndrome of acid hypersecretion results from a non-β cell tumor of the endocrine pancreas. The tumor leads to the production of excess gastrin. Mannitol ingestion would lead to osmotic diarrhea without inflammation. Laxative use would not involve inflammation, and chemical ingredients in laxatives could be detected in the stool.

49 The answer is E *Central and peripheral nervous system / Anatomy / Visual fields*

Left anopsia is complete blindness in the left eye; it can result from damage to the left optic nerve or from damage to the left eye itself. Similarly, damage to the right optic nerve would cause right anopsia. The optic chiasm is where nerve fibers carrying visual information from the nasal half of each retina cross to the other side of the brain. Damage there or farther along the tracts causes visual defects in both eyes. A lesion of the optic chiasm alone causes loss of the temporal half of the right and left visual fields. The optic tracts carry information from the same side of the retina in both eyes. As a result, a lesion there causes homonymous hemianopsia. If the left optic tract is damaged, the patient cannot see the right half of each eye's visual field. If the right optic tract is damaged, the left halves of the visual fields are missing.

50 The answer is B *General principles / Behavioral science / Child development*

Before 7 to 9 months of age, children generally have a positive response to human faces. It is not until 7 to 9 months of age that they exhibit fear around strangers. At 10 to 18 months, they tend to exhibit anxiety when the primary caregiver is not within sight.

test **8**

Questions

Directions: *Single best answer questions consist of numbered items or incomplete statements followed by answers or by completions of the statement. Select the ONE lettered answer or completion that is BEST in each case.*

1 A 32-year-old volunteer fireman receives second-degree burns over approximately 30% of his body and third-degree burns over another 40%. Intravenous fluid and electrolyte therapy is initiated on-site, and the patient is transported to the burn ward of a large metropolitan hospital. Approximately 2 weeks after thermal injury, the patient becomes septic with *Pseudomonas aeruginosa*. The patient's sepsis possibly developed because of

(A) inability of B cells to produce opsonins
(B) inhibition of chemotactic activity of mononuclear leukocyte
(C) lack of circulating segmented neutrophils in the bloodstream
(D) inhibition of the production of immunoglobin (Ig) M
(E) induction of Bruton's agammaglobulinemia by the severe thermal injury

2 The most promising chemotherapeutic agent for treatment of a patient who has become septic with *P. aeruginosa* belongs to which of the following categories?

(A) Imidazole antibiotics
(B) Immune modulators
(C) Quinolone antibiotics
(D) Thymosin fractions
(E) Amphotericin B

3 A 52-year-old man has blood in his stools. He reports that his bowel habits have changed over the past 18 months and, recently, he has sensed that his evacuations are not complete. Proctoscopic examination reveals a large ulcerating mass in the descending colon. Biopsy results confirm the diagnosis of carcinoma of the colon, and the malignant mass is surgically removed. The patient is prescribed appropriate chemotherapy and discharged 2 weeks later to be followed in the oncology clinic. Monthly blood specimens taken during the next year reveal the following carcinoembryonic antigen (CEA) levels:

TABLE 8-1

	CEA (ng/ml)
Preoperative sample	50.0
Postoperative sample (day 1)	65.0
Month 1	15.0
Month 2	5.0
Months 3–9	<2.5
Month 10	10.0
Month 11	25.0
Month 12	40.0

The patient's serum CEA levels were assayed periodically because of the usefulness of CEA in

(A) localization of certain tumors in vivo
(B) diagnosing carcinoma of the colon
(C) diagnosing carcinoma of the pancreas
(D) diagnosing carcinoma of the prostate
(E) follow-up for the recurrence of certain malignancies

4 A 45-year-old woman presents to her primary care physician (PCP) concerns about a lump in her medial right breast. The PCP sends her to a breast cancer specialist who biopsies the mass, which is later diagnosed as ductal carcinoma of the breast. Before the mass is excised, the surgeon injects a radiolabeled dye into the tumor. Which of the following lymph node grouping would most likely drain the dye and therefore be the most likely site of cancer metastases?

(A) Axillary nodes, intraclavicular group
(B) Axillary nodes, apical group
(C) Axillary nodes, pectoral group
(D) Abdominal nodes
(E) Parasternal nodes

5 A 28-year-old white man presents with unexplained weight loss and lymphadenopathy of 2 months' duration. He admits to using intravenous drugs and states that he has shared needles with his girlfriend, whom he has been dating for 5 years. He has also shared needles and had unprotected intercourse with one other woman. The physician suspects that the man is infected with the human immunodeficiency virus (HIV). Which of the following tests is useful in evaluating this patient for HIV infection?

(A) Enzyme-linked immunosorbent assay (ELISA) for anti-HIV antibody
(B) Complete blood count with differential
(C) Restriction fragment length polymorphism (RFLP) search for viral proteins
(D) Absolute number of CD8 + lymphocytes
(E) Western blot for viral antigens

6 Myoclonic seizures, infantile spasms, and absence seizures are examples of which of the following?

(A) Status epilepticus
(B) Primary generalized seizures
(C) Complex-partial seizures
(D) Simple-partial seizures

7 A 20-year-old woman presents with ptosis and diplopia that fatigues with use and recovers with rest. The patient has high levels of antibody against ACh receptors. The best diagnosis among the following diseases is

(A) Lambert–Eaton myasthenic syndrome
(B) porphyria
(C) myasthenia gravis
(D) Guillain–Barré syndrome

8 Which one of the following statements concerning HIV-1 is correct?

(A) The gp 120 envelope protein of the virus binds specifically to the CD8 antigen on T lymphocytes
(B) HIV-1 is a member of the lentivirus group of retroviruses and causes transformation of T lymphocytes in culture
(C) Viral reverse transcriptase causes incorporation of the viral genome into the host DNA; however, the viral DNA is not copied during cell division
(D) Viral reverse transcriptase lacks a proofreading mechanism, which results in the well-documented microheterogeneity of envelope proteins
(E) HIV can be transmitted from one cell to another only by direct contact of an infected lymphocyte with a healthy cell

9 Which of the following complications is most commonly associated with late-stage HTLV type 1 (HTLV-1) infection?

(A) Burkitt's lymphoma
(B) Adult T cell leukemia or lymphoma
(C) Kaposi's sarcoma
(D) Immunoblastic lymphoma
(E) Primary central nervous system lymphoma

10 A 45-year-old man presents to the emergency department with shortness of breath. He has never traveled before and went to the doctor yesterday to prepare for his trip to central Africa. His doctor told him that his health was fine and prescribed him a course of primaquine to prevent malaria. During the physical examination, the emergency department physician notes icterus, a jaundiced appearance to the skin, and lack of color under the tongue. The patient's pulse is 102, his blood pressure is 125/85, and his respiration rate is 19. Which of the following diseases is indicated by the history and physical examination?

(A) Wilson's disease
(B) Polycythemia vera
(C) Disseminated intravascular coagulation
(D) Acute hemolytic anemia
(E) Hereditary spherocytosis

11 An 8-month-old African American girl was taken to the emergency department with shortness of breath, icterus, and pallor under the tongue. The infant measured below the 5th percentile for her age with respect to height and weight, despite her weighing above the 80th percentile at birth. Examination of the peripheral smear indicates hypochromic microcytic anemia with some target cells and some teardrop-shaped erythrocytes. Unconjugated bilirubin is markedly elevated. Hemoglobin electrophoresis reveals increased fetal hemoglobin (Hb F) and double the normal amount of hemoglobin A_2 (Hb A_2); there is very little Hb A. There are no other hemoglobin bands. What is the primary diagnosis for this patient?

(A) β-Thalassemia major
(B) Iron deficiency
(C) Sickle cell disease
(D) Hereditary spherocytosis
(E) Methemoglobinemia

12 Which one of the following statements about the retinoblastoma protein (Rb) is most likely true?

(A) Hypophosphorylated Rb binds to transcription factor E2F and causes a G_1 arrest
(B) Hyperphosphorylated Rb binds to p21 and causes a G_2 arrest
(C) Hyperphosphorylated Rb binds to E2F and causes a G_2 arrest
(D) Hyperphosphorylated Rb binds to p21 and causes a G_1 arrest
(E) Rb is phosphorylated by the cyclin B/cdc2 kinase complex

13 The accompanying diagram shows the heart in an infant with congenital heart disease. Which cyanotic congenital heart disease does this infant have?

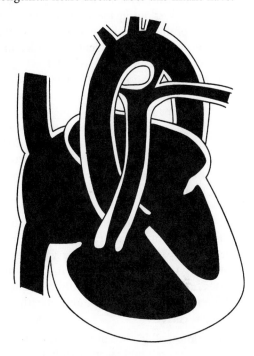

(A) Truncus arteriosus
(B) Transposition of the great arteries
(C) Patent ductus arteriosus
(D) Tetralogy of Fallot
(E) Coarctation of the aorta

14 Many congenital heart defects produce nonlaminar jet stream patterns of blood flow. These turbulent jets frequently leave infants susceptible to

(A) myocardial infarction
(B) rheumatic heart disease
(C) infective endocarditis
(D) valvular calcification
(E) mitral valve prolapse

15 Which of the following correctly describes the normal function of carnitine in fatty acid metabolism?

(A) A coenzyme that is required for the dehydrogenation of acyl coenzyme A (CoA), forming a double bond between the β- and γ-carbons
(B) A coenzyme that is added to free fatty acids on the outer mitochondrial membrane
(C) A carrier protein that holds the growing acyl chain in fatty acid synthesis
(D) A carrier protein that shuttles long-chain fatty acids into the mitochondrial matrix
(E) A carrier protein that shuttles short-chain fatty acids out of the liver to adipose tissue

16 Which of the following statements concerning the β-oxidation of fatty acids is correct?

(A) Single carboxylic acids are released in successive cycles during the metabolism of fatty acids

(B) All of the energy released is stored in the form of reduced equivalents of nicotinamide-adenine dinucleotide (NADH)

(C) Phosphorylation of fatty acid and the subsequent generation of acyl CoA are the committed steps in oxidation

(D) Fatty acids are converted into glucose by the formation of pyruvate from acetyl CoA

(E) Elevated levels of malonyl CoA activate the transfer of fatty acyl CoA into the mitochondrial matrix

17 A 2-year-old girl is taken to her pediatrician because of progressive muscular weakness and recurrent episodes of hepatic encephalopathy with nausea and vomiting. An inherited defect in metabolism is suspected, and tests reveal low serum carnitine. Which of the following characterizations of carnitine deficiency is correct?

(A) Almost all victims of this autosomal recessive disease respond to oral carnitine therapy

(B) A diet restricted to short- and medium-chain fatty acids may prove useful

(C) Pathologic deposition of iron is often seen in muscle biopsies

(D) A form of the disease confined to muscle is the most severe and may involve defective transport of carnitine into the cell

(E) A deletion mutation in the gene for carnitine palmitoyltransferase would result in an entirely different phenotype

18 Which of the following statements correctly pairs a metabolic pathway with its appropriate subcellular location?

(A) Oxidative phosphorylation occurs in the mitochondria and cytosol

(B) Fatty acid synthesis occurs in the mitochondria

(C) Glycolysis occurs in the cytosol and mitochondria

(D) Gluconeogenesis occurs in both the cytosol and the mitochondria

(E) Ganglioside degradation occurs in lysosomes and the mitochondria

19 A 30-year-old woman lawyer presents to her physician's office for an increase in fatigue over the last 2 months. She has been involved in a difficult case at work and has lost 5 pounds. During the physical examination, the physician notes delayed capillary refill in the nailbeds and a pale appearance of the inner lining of the eyelids. A peripheral smear reveals hypochromic erythrocytes. Which of the following tests would be most useful in confirming the probable diagnosis?

(A) Serum ferritin and total iron-binding capacity (TIBC)

(B) Schilling's test

(C) Glucose 6-phosphate dehydrogenase assay

(D) Hemoglobin electrophoresis

(E) Serum folate serum cobalamin (vitamin B_{12})

20 Which of the following statements about cdk is true?

(A) The cyclin B/cdc2 complex regulates the G_0/G_1 transition

(B) The cyclin D/cdk4 complex mutations dysregulate commitment to the S phase

(C) p53 is a cdk

(D) Cyclin levels are maintained constant through all stages of the cell cycle

(E) The retinoblastoma gene product Rb is not under cdk control

21 Which of the following statements regarding the control of transferrin and ferritin synthesis is correct?

(A) Hepatic synthesis of transferrin and ferritin is principally regulated at the level of mRNA transcription by the presence of iron

(B) Hepatic synthesis of transferrin and ferritin is principally regulated by the level of tissue oxygenation and the presence of sufficient heme

(C) Hepatic synthesis of transferrin and ferritin is principally regulated after mRNA transcription by an iron-binding protein that is inactive in the presence of iron

(D) The rate of transferrin turnover in the serum is a function of the presence of iron

(E) The half-life of ferritin mRNA is the site of critical regulation in ferritin synthesis

22 Which of the following statements correctly pairs a commonly prescribed ulcer medication with its mechanism of action?

(A) Atropine blocks ACh release by the vagus nerve

(B) Ranitidine and cimetidine competitively block the gastrin receptor

(C) Colloidal bismuth inhibits gastrin release

(D) Omeprazole irreversibly inhibits the hydrogen–potassium ATP

(E) Sucralfate competitively inhibits carbonic anhydrase

23 A neurologist postulates that the extent of physical disability following a cerebrovascular accident (CVA) is related to personality type. Some 500 such patients were classified according to the severity of their physical deficit (mild or severe) and assigned to one of four personality groups (1 = most prone to depression and 4 = least prone to depression), based on a personality assessment questionnaire developed by the investigator. Table 8-2 below depicts the number of subjects in each category. This study is an example of an

TABLE 8-2

Personality Type	Severity of Condition (Number of Patients)		
	Severe	Mild	Totals
1	60	40	100
2	60	40	100
3	132	68	200
4	48	52	100
Totals	300	200	500

(A) prospective cohort study

(B) case-control study

(C) cross-sectional study

(D) experimental stochastic study

(E) randomized controlled clinical trial

24 A surgeon desires to enter the lung cavity and withdraw a sample of pleural fluid. In order to perform this operation safely, he must avoid the neurovascular bundles associated with each rib. Which of the following descriptions concerning the position of neurovascular bundles with respect to each rib is correct?

(A) The neurovascular bundles are located superior to each rib with the nerve, artery, and vein from superior to inferior

(B) The neurovascular bundles are located inferior to each rib with the nerve, artery, and vein from superior to inferior

(C) The neurovascular bundles are located superior to each rib with the vein, artery, and nerve from superior to inferior

(D) The neurovascular bundles are located inferior to each rib with the vein, artery, and nerve from superior to inferior

(E) The neurovascular bundles are located equidistant between each rib with the vein, artery, and nerve from superior to inferior

25 Which of the following statements about the causes of acquired anemia is correct?

(A) Cobalamin deficiency is often secondary to chronic liver disease

(B) Methotrexate is frequently associated with hypochromic, microcytic anemias

(C) Women are more susceptible to iron deficiency anemia than men because women tend to eat less red meat

(D) Folate deficiency frequently leads to neurologic disease, which may not respond to therapy

(E) Folate deficiency can develop over months in a poorly nourished person

26 A 29-year-old man with no prior medical history is transported to the hospital after being in a serious motor vehicle accident. The bleeding has been slowed by the paramedics, but the man has lost a substantial amount of blood. His blood pressure on arrival at the hospital is 72/30. Right heart catheterization with a Swan–Ganz catheter is performed. The physician begins volume replenishment with units of packed red blood cells and plasma. Which of the following pharmacologic agents would be most useful in supporting this man's cardiovascular system?

(A) Albuterol

(B) Propranolol

(C) Furosemide

(D) Dobutamine

(E) Tubocurarine

27 A physician estimates that the systemic circulation of his 29-year-old male patient, who had lost a lot of blood in a construction accident, was compromised for a total of 4 hours. In the intensive care unit 36 hours later, his serum potassium level is 5.7, increased from 4.8 when he was admitted (normal = 3.4 to 5). Which of the following tests would be most useful in confirming the origin of this man's problem?

(A) Antinuclear antibody screen
(B) Blood urea nitrogen (BUN) and serum creatinine
(C) Antistreptolysin O (ASO) titer
(D) Complete blood count
(E) Digoxin level

28 Which of the following statements is a correct description of bias?

(A) Confounding bias is introduced by comparing groups that differ with respect to determinants of the outcome other than those under study
(B) Selection bias is introduced by selecting methods of measurement that are consistently dissimilar among groups
(C) Measurement bias is introduced when two factors are associated, and the effect of one measured factor is confused or distorted by the effect of the other
(D) Bias is random variation of the primary determinants
(E) A measurement introduces bias if it produces results that depart systematically from the true values

29 An 8-year-old girl is taken to her pediatrician's office because of blood in her urine and puffiness. Her mother indicates that the child has also been lethargic for the past 2 or 3 days. The girl has no history of cardiac or renal disease. The mother reveals that her child had a sore throat that kept her from 2 days of school about 12 days ago. The girl's blood pressure is 140/100. Which of the following diseases is suggested by the history and physical findings?

(A) Systemic lupus erythematosus
(B) Acute tubular necrosis
(C) Acute glomerulonephritis
(D) Juvenile-onset (insulin-dependent) diabetes mellitus
(E) Hyperaldosteronism

30 A 35-year-old woman goes to the emergency room with severe, stabbing abdominal pain that is constant and radiating from the epigastrium to the back and chest. She is nauseated and says that her abdomen feels bloated as well as painful, and the pain is worse lying down. During the physical examination, the physician notes tachycardia, a low-grade fever, absence of bowel sounds, guarding, and an exquisitely tender abdomen. The remainder of the physical examination is noncontributory. Further questioning reveals that the patient drank excessive amounts of alcohol last night; she has no prior medical or family history of cardiac disease. A plain radiograph of the abdomen shows no air under the diaphragm. Which of the following processes is most likely in this patient?

(A) Perforated duodenal ulcer
(B) Myocardial infarction
(C) Abdominal aortic aneurysm
(D) Acute pancreatitis
(E) Renal colic

31 Which of the following is one of the criteria for diagnosing alcoholism?

(A) Aggressive behavior while under the influence of alcohol
(B) Loss of memory while using alcohol (blackouts)
(C) Quantity of alcohol consumption
(D) Frequency of alcohol consumption
(E) Two or more arrests related to alcohol

32 Which one of the following is a form of parenteral drug administration?

(A) Sublingual
(B) Intramuscular
(C) Oral
(D) Rectal

33 Which one of the following is a general anesthetic given intravenously?

(A) Halothane
(B) Ketamine
(C) Ether
(D) Procaine
(E) Nitrous oxide
(F) Lidocaine

34 The reactivation of acetylcholinesterase is caused by which one of the following cholinergic agonists?

(A) Isoflurophate
(B) Edrophonium
(C) Neostigmine
(D) Acetylcholine
(E) Pilocarpine
(F) Pralidoxime

35 Which of the following statements concerning α_1-antitrypsin deficiency is correct?

(A) Liver disease is always preceded by lung disease
(B) It may be a common but unrecognized cause of many cases of neonatal hepatitis
(C) Direct restriction fragment length polymorphism (RFLP) analysis of the gene is the only means of definitive diagnosis
(D) Of those who are homozygous for the deficiency and who survive into adulthood, about 33% develop panacinar emphysema
(E) There is no interaction between smoking and the protein deficiency

36 Which of the following symptoms is most consistent with chronic renal failure?

(A) Elevated triglycerides, uremic fetor, and normochromic, normocytic anemia
(B) Elevated triglycerides, uremic fetor, and hypokalemia
(C) Elevated triglycerides and macrocytic anemia
(D) Decreased triglycerides, uremic fetor, and hyperkalemia
(E) Decreased triglycerides, uremic fetor, and macrocytic anemia

37 Which of the following statements correctly characterizes the role of the kidneys in acid–base homeostasis?

(A) Cells of the proximal tubule are the only cells in the body with the complete enzymatic machinery for urea biosynthesis, an important route for excreting acid
(B) Carbonic anhydrase, located on the brush border of tubule cells, splits carbonic acid into a bicarbonate anion and a hydrogen ion; the hydrogen ion is pumped into the cell
(C) Bicarbonate is actively synthesized from pyruvate in the distal tubule cells
(D) Tubule cells actively secrete bicarbonate anion as a potassium salt
(E) The tubule cells secrete ammonia as one of the mechanisms to excrete excess acid

38 A 75-year-old woman with a 35-year history of non-insulin-dependent (type II) diabetes mellitus is admitted to the hospital for mental status changes. The physician considers a diagnosis of chronic renal failure and investigates the possibility of dialysis. Arterial blood gas analysis reveals a pH of 7.26, and the patient's anion gap is 12. Which of the following statements correctly describes this metabolic acidosis due to renal failure?

(A) A large anion gap indicates good compensation
(B) The metabolic acidosis is caused by excessive production of ammonia in the tubule cells
(C) The large anion gap indicates that the plasma bicarbonate is elevated
(D) This patient has probably already passed the hyperchloremic phase of acidosis
(E) Longstanding metabolic acidosis is not related to renal osteodystrophy

39 Which of the following statements regarding definitions of biostatistics terms is true?

(A) Mean is the sum of values divided by the square root of the number of values
(B) Median is the point where the number of observations above equals the number below
(C) Mode is always greater than 1
(D) Standard error is numerically greater than the standard deviation
(E) Range is the lowest-to-highest value of the average difference of individual values from the mode

40 An 11-year-old boy with a history of episodic dyspnea associated with wheezing has the following spirometric tracings in the pulmonary function laboratory. Which of the following is the most likely description of curves *(1)* and *(2)* in the figure below?

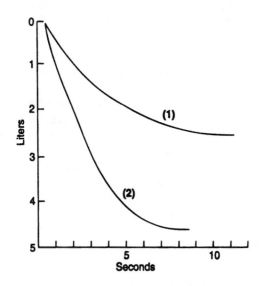

(A) Before *(1)* and after *(2)* inhalation of methacholine

(B) Before *(1)* and after *(2)* inhalation of metaproterenol

(C) Before *(1)* and after *(2)* inhalation of cromolyn sodium

(D) Before *(1)* and after *(2)* inhalation of beclomethasone

(E) Curves *(1)* and *(2)* arise from normal variation of forced expiratory maneuvers within a subject

41 Which of the cranial nerves that emanate from the pons contains only motor components?

(A) Trigeminal nerve

(B) Abducens nerve

(C) Facial nerve

(D) Vestibulocochlear

(E) Glossopharyngeal

42 Inhalation of an irritant that stimulates nonmyelinated C fibers near epithelial cells lining the airway lumen produces reflex bronchoconstriction via the

(A) sympathetic nerve endings

(B) hypoglossal nerve

(C) phrenic nerve

(D) vagus nerve

(E) intercostal nerve

43 A previously healthy 60-year-old man collapsed while playing with his grandchildren. Although he quickly regained consciousness and became fully alert, his family called an ambulance. The emergency medical team found no abnormalities on the electrocardiogram or on physical examination. However, the patient was admitted to the coronary care unit of the local hospital. During the evening, the patient was noted to have a fast rhythm with a wide complex on his monitor, followed by hypotension and loss of consciousness. After electrical cardioversion with 200 watt-seconds of direct current, possible therapy may include

(A) intravenous propranolol

(B) digitalis

(C) intravenous lidocaine

(D) intravenous diltiazem

(E) epinephrine

44 Blood is drawn serially over 8 to 48 hours from a patient in the coronary care unit, and serum enzyme studies are consistent with a diagnosis of myocardial infarction. The most likely change noted was

(A) a decrease in aspartate aminotransferase

(B) an elevation in creatine kinase muscle brain isoenzyme (CK-MB)

(C) an increase in lactate dehydrogenase

(D) a decrease in pseudocholinesterase

(E) a decrease in alkaline phosphatase

45 A possible pharmacotherapeutic approach to controlling asthma may include which one of the following?

(A) Antihistamine

(B) Propranolol

(C) Ibuprofen

(D) Theophylline

(E) Bethanechol

46 Having been discharged from the hospital after successful coronary artery bypass surgery, a patient is prescribed low-dose aspirin therapy. The rationale for selecting this therapy includes

(A) lowering the patient's body metabolism

(B) decreasing anxiety

(C) inhibiting endothelial cell prostacyclin metabolism

(D) inhibiting platelet thromboxane A_2 synthesis

(E) decreasing circulating leukotriene D_4

47 Which one of the following adrenergic agonists is both a direct-acting agent and an indirect-acting agent?

(A) Clonidine
(B) Dopamine
(C) Ephedrine
(D) Ritodrine
(E) Amphetamine
(F) Tyramine

48 Which one of the following adrenergic agonists is a catecholamine?

(A) Clonidine
(B) Dopamine
(C) Ephedrine
(D) Albuterol
(E) Amphetamine
(F) Metaproterenol

49 A 28-year-old woman with a family history of skin cancer presented with a rapidly growing (3 to 6 months) asymptomatic lesion on her right scapular area. The lesion was brown with a bluish-red (violaceous) color, and its border was palpably elevated. The lesion described is likely to be

(A) hemangioma
(B) pigmented basal cell carcinoma
(C) pigmented dermatofibroma
(D) melanoma
(E) subungual hematoma

50 Which of the following is most appropriate for the treatment of delirium tremens?

(A) Monitor vital signs for autonomic depression
(B) Treat with disulfiram
(C) Limit administration of intravenous fluids
(D) Administer vitamin B_{12} injection
(E) Treatment with benzodiazepines

Answer Key

1-B	11-A	21-C	31-E	41-B
2-C	12-A	22-D	32-B	42-D
3-E	13-D	23-C	33-B	43-C
4-E	14-C	24-D	34-F	44-B
5-A	15-D	25-E	35-B	45-D
6-B	16-C	26-D	36-A	46-D
7-C	17-B	27-B	37-E	47-C
8-D	18-D	28-E	38-D	48-B
9-B	19-A	29-C	39-B	49-D
10-D	20-B	30-D	40-B	50-E

Answers and Explanations

1 **The answer is B** *Skin and related connective tissue / Microbiology / Sepsis following severe burn*

P. aeruginosa is a major cause of sepsis in burn patients. It is ubiquitous in the environment and is a member of the indigenous flora of some people. Once it gains entry through the physical barrier of the skin, *P. aeruginosa* causes significant tissue damage. It is capable of invading the epithelium of blood vessels, leading to repeated seeding of the bloodstream.

Patients with burns over more than 20% of their body lack chemotactic activity of mononuclear leukocytes 15 to 45 days after thermal injury. Inhibition of activity corresponds to the appearance of a chemotactic inhibitor in the serum. An inability to produce opsonins antibodies and a decrease in the production of IgM are associated with splenectomy. A decrease in the number of circulating segmented neutrophils occurs during bone marrow failure. Bruton's agammaglobulinemia is a sex-linked genetic dysfunction.

2 **The answer is C** *Skin and related connective tissue / Microbiology / Sepsis following severe burn*

P. aeruginosa and other pseudomonads frequently display multiple drug resistance. The mortality rate in pseudomonas septicemia approaches 80%. A new group of antibiotics, the quinolones, have shown good in vitro activity against *P. aeruginosa*; the number of cases of disease successfully treated with the quinolones is increasing. Imidazole antibiotics and amphotericin B are antifungal agents; the imidazoles are now considered alternatives to amphotericin B therapy in some mycoses. Immune modulators, such as thymosin and interferon, have shown potential in treating infections controlled by the cell-mediated immune system.

3 **The answer is E** *Hematopoietic and lymphoreticular system / Pathology / Carcinoembryonic antigen analysis*

Carcinoembryonic antigen (CEA) is associated with carcinoma of the colon and pancreas; however, because CEA also occurs in nonmalignant conditions (e.g., as a result of cigarette smoking), it is not considered to be diagnostic but merely suggestive of a cancerous condition. Assays for CEA show their greatest promise in monitoring for the recurrence of certain malignancies after surgery or chemotherapy.

4 **The answer is E** *Endocrine system / Anatomy / Lymph node drainage*

At the time of tumor resection it is very important for the surgeon to excise the lymph nodes that would be expected to drain the tumor bed to help properly stage the cancer. The most common site of breast cancer metastasis to lymph nodes is the axillary nodes, with the pectoral group being most often involved. It is not, however, a guarantee giving the medial location of this tumor. Medial tumors most often drain to the ipsilateral parasternal lymph nodes whereas some more inferior tumors may metastasize to abdominal lymph nodes.

5 **The answer is A** *General principles / Immunology / HIV, AIDS*

ELISA for anti-HIV antibody is the mainstay in screening for HIV. ELISA is relatively sensitive (as any screening should be), but its low specificity requires confirmation with a Western blot for the anti-HIV antibody. A Western blot for viral proteins is not effective. Although viral proteins do circulate in the serum of infected individuals, the concentration of antigen is not detectable. The absolute number of CD4+ lymphocytes is used to monitor the progress of HIV-infected patients but is not particularly useful as a screening tool. In most cases, any substantial loss of T4 cells occurs many years after infection. Polymerase chain reaction (PCR) techniques, which allow extremely sensitive detection of a small fragment of viral (or any) DNA sequence, are being investigated as a possible tool for screening for HIV infection. A complete blood count with standard differential is not useful in the diagnosis of HIV infection because decreases in the number of white blood cells differentiated by routine light microscopy occur only late in the disease. Furthermore, elevations in the white cell count can indicate any of a host of inflammatory processes that may or may not be related to HIV.

6 **The answer is B** *Central and peripheral nervous system / Pathology; neurobiology / Generalized seizures*

Status epilepticus is prolonged or repetitive seizures without a period of recovery between attacks. When tonic–clonic seizures are involved (e.g., in tonic–clonic status), this state can be life-threatening. Myoclonic seizures are primary, generalized seizures that are sudden, brief, single, or repetitive muscle contractions involving one body part or the entire body. Infantile spasms are primary, generalized seizures that occur in infants between birth and 12 months of age. These seizures consist of several types of brief, synchronous contractions of the neck, torso, and both arms (usually in flexion). They can occur in an otherwise normal infant, but they often occur in infants with underlying neurologic disease. Absence (petit mal) seizures are primary, generalized seizures that consist of a sudden cessation of ongoing conscious activity or loss of postural control. Partial seizures, on the other hand, involve discrete regions of the brain. Simple-partial seizures involve motor, sensory, autonomic, or psychic symptoms in the absence of a change of consciousness. Complex-partial seizures involve focal seizure activity accompanied by an impairment of consciousness.

7 **The answer is C** *Central and peripheral nervous system / Pathology / Neuromuscular disease*

Myasthenia gravis, which is rare, has a bimodal age distribution; it occurs in women in their teens and 20s and in men aged 60 years or older. It presents with proximal weakness, especially ptosis and diplopia that fatigues with use and recovers with rest. Myasthenia gravis is an autoimmune disease. Patients with myasthenia gravis produce antibodies that destroy the ACh receptor of the muscles. Although myasthenia gravis and Lambert–Eaton myasthenic syndrome strongly resemble each other clinically, Lambert–Eaton myasthenic syndrome does not involve extraocular muscles. Therefore, patients with Lambert–Eaton syndrome do not have ptosis and diplopia.

8 **The answer is D** *General principles / Immunology / HIV, AIDS*

The HIV-1 virus is a cytopathic member of the lentiviruses; it lyses T lymphocytes in culture, whereas its sister virus human T cell lymphotrophic virus (HTLV) transforms them into an immortal cell line. The two viruses are related by the enzyme reverse transcriptase, which uses the viral RNA genome to synthesize linear DNA. The DNA is incorporated into the cellular genome via recombination and forms a template for normal mammalian replication processes. Once incorporated, the viral DNA is replicated and given to all of the cell's progeny. New strategies for intervention are focused on more effective chronic therapy for infected people and vaccination for uninfected people. Lysis of an infected cell results in a prolific release of viral progeny that are capable of infecting a large number of uninfected T4 helper cells. Direct contact is not required, and research efforts toward binding these free particles with soluble CD4 antigen may prove fruitful. The envelope proteins, including gp 120, are important in the binding, entry, and uncoating of the virus. The gp 120 envelope protein is involved in the recognition of the CD4 antigen. Efforts to develop an effective vaccine have been elusive because the envelope antigens are subject to frequent mutation. This high rate of mutation is probably the result of selection pressure, which favors a viral transcriptase prone to frequent error. Most other DNA-synthesizing enzymes, including all of the DNA synthases in healthy mammalian cells, have extensive proofreading mechanisms, which HIV reverse transcriptase lacks.

9 **The answer is B** *General principles / Immunology / HTLV*

HTLV-1 is a retrovirus related to HIV whose transmission usually requires cell-to-cell contact. Patients infected with HTLV-1 are at risk for developing adult T cell leukemia or lymphomas later in life. HIV infection is associated with the development of Burkitt's lymphoma (small, noncleaved cell lymphoma), immunoblastic lymphoma, primary central nervous system lymphoma, and Kaposi's sarcoma.

10 **The answer is D** *Hematopoietic and lymphoreticular system / Hematology / Glucose 6-phosphate dehydrogenase deficiency hemolytic anemia*

Pallor under the tongue, delayed capillary refill in the nailbeds, and, in white people, general lack of color indicate anemia. The acute onset, obvious signs of jaundice, the patient's race, and the recent prescription of primaquine indicate acute hemolytic anemia resulting from glucose 6-phosphate dehydrogenase deficiency. The patient's tachycardia and tachypnea are a reflection of the sympathetic activation produced by inadequate tissue oxygenation. Such sympathetic activation is fairly common, and some patients with chronic hemolytic anemia develop prominent, high-output S_3 flow murmurs as a result of chronic hypoxia. Wilson's disease is a complex of symptoms, primarily liver and pancreatic failure, related to the inappropriate storage of copper; jaundice (but not hemolysis) develops over time in a patient with Wilson's disease. Polycythemia vera is the neoplastic growth of hematopoietic stem cells, which gives rise to an unregulated excess of the cellular components of blood; platelets, erythrocytes, and lymphocytes can be elevated individually or in combination. Disseminated intravascular coagulation occurs when the clotting cascade is inappropriately activated and platelets (not erythrocytes) are depleted to a dangerous low. Hereditary spherocytosis does cause hemolytic anemia, but the disease is not generally triggered but, rather, is present early in adulthood. The anemia is lifelong and secondary to a defect in the plasma membrane of the erythrocytes. The name spherocytosis reflects the odd appearance of the erythrocytes in the peripheral smears from these patients.

11 **The answer is A** *Hematopoietic and lymphoreticular system / Genetics / β-Thalassemia*

Hb A is the normal hemoglobin tetramer with a subunit stoichiometry of $\alpha_2\beta_2$, and most individuals' Hb composition has 97% Hb A. Hb A_2 has a subunit stoichiometry of $\alpha_2\delta_2$ and normally accounts for less than 3% of total hemoglobin. Normal adults usually have less than 1% of their total hemoglobin composed of Hb F, which has the subtypes $\alpha_2\gamma_2$. Infants with β-thalassemia major usually present after the sixth month, when the hemoglobin promoters gradually switch from γ-subunit production for Hb F to β-subunit production for Hb A. White people of Mediterranean descent have the highest carrier frequency, and the heterozygous state is relatively common in people from central Africa, Asia, and parts of India. Jaundiced skin, icterus, elevated unconjugated bilirubin, and pallor under the tongue are a relatively specific indication of hemolytic anemia. The infant's failure to thrive indicates a chronic course that is now emerging. The peripheral smear indicates hypochromic anemia but specifically lacks evidence of spherocytosis or sickle cell anemia. Spherocytosis has a much more chronic course that often emerges in the second or third decade of life. Iron deficiency is a possibility, but ineffective erythropoiesis is not the only problem; iron deficiency does not cause hemolysis. The unconjugated bilirubin and teardrop cells indicate active destruction as well as ineffective erythropoiesis; therefore, iron deficiency is not a sufficient explanation. The inherited form of methemoglobinemia causes anemia that is much less severe than the one described and would probably not be noted except as an incidental finding on routine evaluation.

12 **The answer is A** *General principles / Cell biology / Cell cycle*

Rb is a tumor suppressor gene that binds to several important gene regulatory proteins, but its binding capacity depends on its state of phosphorylation. When Rb is dephosphorylated, it binds a set of gene regulatory proteins (e.g., the transcription factor E2F), which causes a G_1 arrest. Phosphorylated Rb releases the E2F and other proteins, allowing them to act. Rb does not bind to the cyclin-dependent kinase (cdk) inhibitor p21, nor does it arrest cells in the G_2 of the cell cycle. Rb can be phosphorylated in vivo by several kinases, such as the cdk complexes (e.g., cyclin-cdk2, cyclin D/cdk4), but not by the cyclin B/cdc2 kinase complex.

13 The answer is D *Cardiovascular system / Pathology / Tetralogy of Fallot*

Congenital heart disease occurs in 1% of births and falls into two categories: cyanotic and noncyanotic. An infant with cyanotic heart disease generally begins to show signs of oxygen desaturation within hours to days after birth, depending on the severity of the lesion. The cyanosis results from poor oxygenation in the blood and peripheral tissues. Generally speaking, cyanosis indicates a lesion that causes a substantial right-to-left shunt or a lesion in which the lungs are left out of the circulation. Patent ductus arteriosus and coarctation of the aorta are typically noncyanotic lesions at birth, although a patent ductus can lead to cyanosis later. Truncus arteriosus is a cyanotic lesion in which the aorta and pulmonary artery have fused into one large vessel that overrides both chambers; typically, there is also a ventricular septal defect to accommodate the combined outflow. The diagram clearly shows two outflow vessels. Transposition of the great arteries is a cyanotic lesion in which the right ventricle sends its output to the system and the left ventricle sends its output to the lungs. Because the return flows are not switched in the common variety of transposition, the result of transposition is two entirely separate circulations unless the ductus arteriosus remains patent. The systemic circulation is never oxygenated, and the pulmonary circulation is never deoxygenated.

14 The answer is C *Cardiovascular system / Pathology / Congenital heart defects*

The abnormal flow patterns associated with most congenital heart defects cause local jet streams, that is, local regions of fluid with rapid, turbulent flow. Unlike laminar flow that normally predominates, jet streams can be directed at tissue, especially the valves, resulting in tiny lesions to the delicate endocardium. The intact endocardium is resistant to most organisms, but the damaged endocardium provides a rough surface that is ideal for bacterial or viral attachment. Infectious endocarditis is an important source of morbidity and mortality in infants with congenital heart disease. Because it involves coronary artery disease in more than 90% of cases, myocardial infarction is highly unusual in men younger than 20 and women younger than 30 years of age, even when the patients have a family history of cardiac disease. Mitral valve prolapse is a common finding, occurring in about 7% of adults aged 20 to 40 years. Mitral valve prolapse is unusual in children, and its incidence is not increased in infants with congenital heart defects unless they also have coincidence of valvular endocarditis. By definition, rheumatic heart disease always follows a streptococcal infection, usually of the pharynx, and the pathophysiology is thought to be related to immune dysregulation, not structural abnormalities of the heart. Valvular calcification is generally related to endocardial damage, but calcification is a process of long-term inflammation and calcium deposit.

15 The answer is D *General principles / Biochemistry / Fatty acid metabolism*

Carnitine is important for transporting long-chain fatty acids into the mitochondria where β-oxidation occurs. Flavin adenine dinucleotide (FAD) is the coenzyme that is required for the formation of carbon–carbon double bonds in virtually all metabolic pathways. Free fatty acids are acetylated with acetyl CoA on the outer surface of the mitochondria; then carnitine is exchanged for acetyl CoA, and the carnitine-complexed fatty acid is moved into the mitochondria. A different enzyme catalyzes the second exchange, this time freeing the carnitine by replacing it with acetyl CoA. Acyl carrier protein is the pantothenate derivative that holds the growing fatty acid during synthesis. Very-low-density lipoprotein is the carrier for fatty acids being exported by the liver to adipose tissue.

16 The answer is C *General principles / Biochemistry / Fatty acid oxidation*

The discovery that oxidation occurs in cycles that release two carbon units in the form of acetyl CoA was a major advance in understanding fatty acid metabolism. The hydrolysis of pyrophosphate following formation of acyl CoA commits a fatty acid to degradation in the oxidative pathway. Adenosine triphosphate (ATP) molecules are not directly synthesized in the oxidative sequence; rather, energy is stored in reduced equivalents of both NADH and $FADH_2$. Because malonyl CoA is a substrate for fatty acid synthesis, high levels of malonyl CoA inhibit the fatty acid oxidation pathway to prevent a futile cycle of synthesis and oxidation. Understanding that fatty acid degradation cannot result in glucose is absolutely fundamental in understanding how various metabolic pathways are integrated by the body. Because the body cannot make pyruvate, the building bock for glucose, from any of the products of fatty acid or ketone breakdown, the β-oxidative pathway can produce only reducing equivalents and acetyl CoA units.

17 **The answer is B** *Musculoskeletal system / Biochemistry / Carnitine deficiency*

Carnitine deficiency is a relatively rare hereditary disorder with two forms. The form illustrated in this question is systemic, whereas the other variant is confined only to muscle and tends to manifest itself in older people after they exercise strenuously. Carnitine is important for transporting long-chain fatty acids into the mitochondria where β-oxidation occurs.

Oral carnitine replacement therapy should always be tried, but patients are not uniformly responsive. Because short- and medium-chain fatty acids do not require carnitine for their transport into mitochondria, a diet that excludes long-chain fatty acids may provide a great deal of relief. However, designing such a diet is far from easy, and most patients find it difficult to comply. In the nonsystemic form, muscle biopsies are often taken to determine the cause of muscular weakness. The reasons for the lipid accumulation remain obscure. Because carnitine is a carrier that is attached and then immediately cleaved following fatty acid transfer, a deficiency in the enzymes for attachment or for cleavage mimics a substrate carnitine deficiency almost identically. There are two separate enzymes, one for attachment and one for cleavage, named carnitine palmitoyltransferase I and II, respectively.

18 **The answer is D** *General principles / Biochemistry / Compartmentalization of metabolism*

To allow for integration of different metabolic pathways, some key substrates are found in several pathways. For some reactions, the energy state of the cell regulates the direction that a substrate like acetyl CoA follows. In other pathways, the entrance of a substrate is mainly regulated by substrate availability; in these cases, if a substrate is available to the enzymatic machinery, it is used. Thus, pathway compartmentalization within the cells keeps substrates from being available to the wrong pathway and helps prevent futile cycles of synthesis and degradation. Oxidative phosphorylation and fatty acid oxidation occur in the mitochondria; glycolysis and fatty acid synthesis occur in the cytosol. The pathways for gluconeogenesis and urea synthesis have enzymes in both the cytosol and mitochondria. Gangliosides and other complex lipid–carbohydrate molecules are degraded in the acidic lysosome. In several lysosomal storage disorders, particular lysosomal enzyme activities are deficient, which results in a buildup of substrate.

19 **The answer is A** *Hematopoietic and lymphoreticular system / Hematology / Differential diagnosis of acquired anemia*

Nutritional deficiencies, drugs, and several gastrointestinal disorders can give rise to acquired anemia. The principal classification of anemias is based on the size and color of the circulating red blood cells. Megaloblastic anemias are generally hyperchromic and macrocytic. In the bone marrow, the maturation of the cytoplasm proceeds at a normal rate, whereas cell division is slow, and thus the cells are especially large. The slow cell division is a result of inefficient DNA synthesis. Deficiencies in either folate or cobalamin are a common cause of megaloblastic anemia; both of these nutrients serve essential roles in nucleotide biosynthesis. However, this woman's anemia is not megaloblastic. Schilling's test reveals the exact cause of cobalamin deficiency in a patient with low levels of serum cobalamin by determining the body's secretion of intrinsic factor and measuring the ileum's ability to absorb the intrinsic factor–cobalamin complex. Iron deficiency is a common cause of new onset hypochromic, microcytic anemias, and TIBC and serum ferritin provide confirmation. TIBC is a measure of transferrin (the serum's iron transfer protein), which is increased in patients who are iron-deficient because the body attempts to trap all available iron for hematopoiesis. Ferritin, the body's storage form of iron, is usually low in patients who are iron-deficient and high in patients who are iron overloaded. Glucose 6-phosphate dehydrogenase deficiency is generally restricted to people of Asian, African, or Mediterranean descent, and the acute anemia is almost always traceable to a new prescription or infection. In addition, the anemia is hemolytic and is thus accompanied by signs of acute hemolysis (e.g., jaundice, icterus, elevated unconjugated bilirubin). Hemoglobinopathy becoming clinically significant this late in life is unusual; in addition, hemoglobinopathies are not common in white people.

20 **The answer is B** *General principles / Cell biology / Cell cycle*

The cdk family consists of at least seven members, many of which are involved with the cell cycle. The cyclin B/cdc2 complex, also called the mitosis-promoting factor, functions at the G_2/M checkpoint. The cyclin D/cdk4 complex regulates the G_1/S checkpoint called the restriction point, at which the cell commits to replicating its DNA. Mutations in cyclin D can lead to parathyroid adenomas and breast, esophageal, and hepatocellular carcinomas. Mutations in cdk4 can cause glioblastoma, sarcoma, and melanoma. p53 is a tumor suppressor gene that can bind DNA, act as a transcription factor, and induce the production of proteins (e.g., p21 cdk inhibitor), which is induced by DNA damage. However, p53 is not a cdk inhibitor itself. The cyclin levels do not remain constant throughout the cell cycle. The retinoblastoma gene product Rb plays a major role in cell cycle regulation and is under exquisite control by several cdks.

21 **The answer is C** *Hematopoietic and lymphoreticular system / Biochemistry / Regulation of trans-ferrin and ferritin synthesis*

The iron-binding protein of liver illustrates a classic case of coordinated protein synthesis; levels of transferrin and ferritin are regulated in opposite fashions by a single mechanism that is posttranscriptional, that is, following synthesis of mRNA. Transferrin mRNA is normally degraded rapidly, but in the presence of the activated (i.e., iron-free) iron-binding protein, a 3′ stem–loop structure is stabilized and the mRNA is no longer susceptible to degradation. Ferritin, the storage form of iron, has a 5′ stem–loop structure that is recognized by the activated iron-binding protein. Binding of the activated protein to the stem–loop prevents initiation of ferritin translation. Therefore, when there is no iron to inactivate the iron-binding protein, the transferrin message is stabilized, transferrin synthesis increases, and ferritin translation is blocked. When iron binds to the protein and inactivates it, ferritin translation begins proportional to the amount of message, and the transferrin message rapidly degrades prior to translation.

22 **The answer is D** *Gastrointestinal system / Pharmacology / Peptic ulcer disease*

The H_2-histamine receptor blockers (e.g., ranitidine and cimetidine) are the mainstay of peptic ulcer disease treatment. They competitively block the receptors and powerfully downregulate parietal cell acid production, providing adequate therapy for most patients with peptic ulcer disease. Sucralfate and omeprazole are relatively new drugs whose efficacy is being demonstrated as their use continues to grow. Sucralfate specifically targets the ulcer bed and coats it for up to 12 hours; it shows very little affinity for normal mucosa, and it is not absorbed systemically. Omeprazole is absorbed systemically, although it is not associated with any substantial systemic toxicities. The irreversible mechanism of action of omeprazole makes it especially useful in the treatment of refractory cases due to Zollinger–Ellison syndrome. Colloidal bismuth is another coating agent whose mechanism of action may also involve antibiotic effects against the organism *Helicobacter pylori*, which can be identified in a substantial majority of patients with chronic peptic ulcer disease. There is evidence to indicate that *H. pylori* may destroy the mucosal lining and therefore make patients susceptible to gastritis as well as to peptic ulcer disease. Atropine blocks the muscarinic receptors on the parietal cells, but it is not as efficacious as the histamine receptor blockers. Furthermore, oral or intravenous atropine is associated with a myriad of systemic side effects and is therefore not commonly used for chronic medical conditions. There are no clinically useful gastrin receptor blockers available for prescription in the United States.

23 **The answer is C** *Central and peripheral nervous system / Biostatistics / Cross-sectional study of severity of disability in cerebrovascular accident and personality type*

The patients participating in this study were simultaneously classified according to the severity of their disability and their personality type. Therefore, this is an example of a cross-sectional study. A stochastic process pertains to a series of random events.

24 **The answer is D** *Respiratory system / Anatomy / Intercostal neurovascular bundles*

In order to avoid damage to the intercostal neurovascular bundles, the surgeon must avoid the lower edge of each rib. The neurovascular bundles are located inferior to each rib and are oriented vein, artery, then nerve (VAN) from superior to inferior.

25 The answer is E *Hematopoietic and lymphoreticular system / Hematology / Differential diagnosis of acquired anemia*

Cobalamin deficiency is probably the most serious cause of anemia, because cobalamin deficiency can also result in irreversible damage to the nervous system. The neurologic complications begin with demyelination and can eventually include damage to the cerebral cortex. Cobalamin deficiency also has a more insidious onset due to the low daily requirement and the relatively large stores of cobalamin in the liver. Thus, patients can cease to absorb new cobalamin and not show symptoms for years. In some cases, the anemia is not noticeable until after the neurologic complications because the anemia emerged too slowly to become symptomatic. Pernicious anemia is the most common cause of cobalamin deficiency. In pernicious anemia, atrophy of the gastric mucosa leads to decreased secretion of intrinsic factor (IF). Because IF is required for ileal absorption of cobalamin, the cobalamin deficiency that results from gastric atrophy can be quite severe. Both ileal resection and Crohn's disease can interfere with sufficient absorption of the cobalamin-IF complex and cause a similar deficiency. Although neither cobalamin nor folate deficiency is directly associated with chronic liver damage, folate deficiency is relatively common in alcoholics, who may have associated cirrhosis. The liver's store of folate is relatively small in relation to the daily requirement of folate. Since most alcoholics are malnourished, the stores can be depleted rather quickly (i.e., in months), resulting in a relatively sudden onset of symptomatic folate deficiency. In contrast, cobalamin stores are relatively large in relation to the daily requirement, and a malnourished person is able to use the stored reserve of cobalamin for 1 to 2 years. Women are more susceptible to iron deficiency because they menstruate, which drains their iron stores each month. Even a short period of poor nutrition can result in relatively quick depletion of iron stores, especially in a woman with insufficient starting reserves.

26 The answer is D *Cardiovascular system / Pharmacology / Management of shock*

Dobutamine is the agent of choice for a hypovolemic crisis. Other adrenergic-activating agents have two drawbacks. Many (e.g., epinephrine) are not β-receptor specific, and therefore they cause vasoconstriction, which is undesired because in these patients vasoconstriction is already severe and may be causing intestinal or renal damage. Other β-specific agents (e.g., isoproterenol) are chronotropic as well as inotropic. Because increased chronotropism carries a greater risk of ischemia and because increased inotropism is a more efficient way to increase cardiac output, the selectively inotropic agent dobutamine is best suited. As an added benefit, dobutamine also activates an unusual class of dopaminergic receptors in the kidneys, causing vasodilation at a time when the kidneys may be suffering clinically significant ischemia. Albuterol is a relatively selective agonist of the β_2-class of adrenergic receptors and is commonly prescribed to relieve the acute bronchoconstrictive symptoms during episodes of asthma and chronic obstructive pulmonary disease. Because the cardiac receptors are principally representatives of the β_1-subtype, albuterol would not offer any substantial cardiac effects. Propranolol is a nonselective β-adrenergic receptor antagonist used as a class II antiarrhythmic as well as an antianginal agent. It decreases cardiac output and is not indicated for the management of shock. Furosemide is a loop diuretic that can induce rapid and large increases in urine output and is strictly contraindicated in this patient. Tubocurarine blocks neurotransmission at nicotinic cholinergic synapses and is used to provide muscular paralysis prior to intubation. It may be necessary to intubate patients during hypovolemic crisis, but tubocurarine does not support the man's cardiovascular system.

27 The answer is B *Renal/urinary system / Pathology / Management of shock*

The kidneys are especially sensitive to hypovolemic shock that lasts 30 minutes to 1 hour. Acute tubular necrosis is the most common kidney lesion seen in patients recovering from hypovolemic shock, and hyperalkemia quickly ensues, primarily as a result of oliguria. In the absence of a substantial external potassium load, most patients have only modest potassium accumulation, with rises in serum potassium of about 0.4 mM in a 24-hour period. As with all causes of kidney failure, serum BUN and creatinine are markedly elevated (creatinine as high as 8 to 12; normal = 0.8 to 1.5). An antinuclear antibody screen is useful in diagnosing systemic lupus erythematosus. A positive ASO titer is generally adequate evidence to demonstrate a recent streptococcal infection and is especially useful in diagnosing acute rheumatic fever as well as poststreptococcal glomerulonephritis. A complete blood count provides information that may be important in diagnosing infection, anemia, or neoplasia. A digoxin level is important if digoxin toxicity is suspected. However, digoxin is most commonly prescribed to support patients with congestive heart failure, which is unlikely in this 29-year-old man. Furthermore, digoxin toxicity is usually manifested in cardiac conduction disturbances and arrhythmias, not in renal failure.

28 **The answer is E** *General principles / Biostatistics / Bias*

Bias is a process at any stage of inference tending to produce results that systematically, not randomly, depart from the true values. It is not the result of random variation. Measurement bias occurs when the methods of measurement are consistently dissimilar among groups of patients. Confounding bias occurs when two factors or processes are associated or travel together, and the effect of one is confused or distorted by the effect of the other. Selection bias occurs when comparisons are made between groups of subjects that differ with respect to determinants of the outcome other than those under study.

29 **The answer is C** *Renal/urinary system / Pathology / Poststreptococcal glomerulonephritis*

Poststreptococcal glomerulonephritis is a relatively common complication of pharyngitis in children 6 to 10 years of age. Most cases are caused by group A β-hemolytic streptococci with specific types of M antigen. The child's puffiness is due to dramatically decreased glomerular filtration and the resultant oliguria with salt and water retention. As with all cases of nephritis, there is significant hematuria and proteinuria. The loss of protein combined with the salt and water retention produces the characteristic edema, and the increased blood volume is sufficient to explain her modest hypertension. Although systemic lupus erythematosus can be associated with glomerulonephritis, renal symptoms characteristic of the nephrotic syndrome are more common in the early stages, and it would be unusual for an 8-year-old to have lupus. Acute tubular necrosis can be associated with water retention, edema, and high blood pressure, but hematuria is not common in these patients. Furthermore, most cases of acute tubular necrosis are preceded by an identifiable ingestion of some acutely nephrotoxic agent or ischemic damage secondary to shock. Juvenile-onset diabetes frequently causes renal symptoms, but these changes are usually nephrotic rather than nephritic in nature (i.e., lack of hematuria and more substantial proteinuria). The onset of diabetes is generally more gradual, and significant edema would probably evolve over a longer period. Finally, all cases of diabetes manifest with polyuria, and salt and fluid retention are rarely seen prior to the onset of chronic renal failure late in the disease. Isolated hyperaldosteronism is rare and not associated with hematuria.

30 **The answer is D** *Endocrine system / Pathology / Pancreatitis*

The description of abdominal pain with guarding and hypoactive bowel sounds is classic for pancreatitis. Other causes of an acutely painful abdomen must be considered, however. The absence of free air under the diaphragm eliminates visceral perforation from the differential diagnosis in this patient with an acutely painful abdomen. Myocardial infarction is very unlikely in a 35-year-old woman with no family history of cardiac disease; furthermore, most patients describe the pain on infarction not as stabbing but rather as crushing. Similarly, aortic aneurysm generally occurs in older adults and is the result of chronic hypertension and atherosclerosis, which are unlikely in a 35-year-old woman. The pain of renal colic differs greatly from the pain this patient described. Located primarily in the flank, it radiates to the groin in classic cases and is almost always described as coming severely in 10- to 20-minute waves. Renal colic is not usually worsened by lying supine.

31 **The answer is E** *Gastrointestinal system / Behavioral science / Alcoholism*

Making a diagnosis of alcoholism is the responsibility of all physicians, because alcohol is one of the most important causes of morbidity and mortality in the United States. Clinical diagnosis of alcohol abuse relies on documenting the pattern of difficulties associated with alcohol use and does not depend on the quantity or frequency of alcohol consumption. Blackouts are often described by individuals who have drunk alcohol excessively on one or two occasions but in themselves are not sufficient for a diagnosis of alcohol dependence. According to *Diagnostic and Statistical Manual IV (DSM-IV)*, alcohol abuse is diagnosed when an individual demonstrates repetitive problems with alcohol in any one of the following four life areas: (1) inability to fulfill major obligations, (2) use in hazardous situations, (3) legal problems, and (4) social or interpersonal difficulties. The key unifying factor in all four of these problems is that socially significant, undesirable repercussions of drinking have no effect on subsequent drinking.

32 **The answer is B** *General principles / Pharmacology / Drug administration*

There are two main routes of drug administration: enteral and parenteral. Parenteral administration is used for drugs that are poorly absorbed from the gastrointestinal tract and for agents that are unstable in the gastrointestinal tract. Intramuscular drug delivery is an example of parenteral drug administration. The intramuscular route is used for depot preparations and when rapid onset of action is required (e.g., epinephrine in anaphylaxis). Sublingual administration is enteral; the drug is placed under the tongue, allowing the drug to diffuse into the capillary network and enter the systemic circulation directly. The oral route (enteral) is when the drug is given by mouth. It is the most common route of administration, but it is the most complicated pathway to the tissues. Rectal administration (enteral) is when the drug is placed in the rectum for absorption. Half of the drainage of the rectal region bypasses the hepatic portal circulation; thus, the biotransformation of drugs that are metabolized by the liver is minimized.

33 **The answer is B** *Central and peripheral nervous system / Pharmacology / Anesthetics*

Ketamine is an intravenous general anesthetic. It is also a dissociative anesthetic in that patients appear awake but are unconscious and do not feel pain. Ketamine is not widely used because it increases cerebral blood flow and induces postoperative hallucinations. Halothane, ether, and nitrous oxide are inhaled general anesthetics. Inhaled general anesthetics are used primarily for the maintenance of anesthesia after administration of an intravenous agent. Procaine and lidocaine are local anesthetics. Local anesthetics are applied locally and block nerve conduction of sensory impulses from the periphery to the central nervous system. These drugs inhibit sodium channels of the nerve membrane.

34 **The answer is F** *General principles / Pharmacology / Cholinergic agonists*

Pralidoxime is a synthetic compound that can reactivate inhibited acetylcholinesterase. It binds to the inhibitor of acetylcholinesterase and pulls it off the inhibited enzyme. Isoflurophate covalently binds to acetylcholinesterase and irreversibly inhibits this enzyme. Edrophonium and neostigmine reversibly inhibit acetylcholinesterase. Acetylcholine is the neurotransmitter of parasympathetic and cholinergic nerves and is a cholinergic agonist. Pilocarpine is also a cholinergic agonist and is unaffected by acetylcholinesterase.

35 **The answer is B** *Gastrointestinal system / Pathology / α_1-Antitrypsin deficiency*

α_1-Antitrypsin deficiency may first appear as acute hepatitis with impressive jaundice, elevated serum transaminases, and compromised blood clotting, especially in children. However, the phenotypic expression of this genotype is variable, even in persons who are homozygous for the deficiency. Some patients with heterozygous genotypes and even individuals with homozygous mutations may have emphysema and symptoms of chronic obstructive pulmonary disease before liver disease, especially if they smoked. All homozygous individuals who live into adulthood have panacinar emphysema by their early 40s. Although RFLPs are useful in providing information for genetic counseling of the patient, the definitive diagnosis can be made by directly assaying the serum for protein activity. The pathophysiology seems to involve a deficiency of the protein's normal inhibitory effect on the serine proteases released by the neutrophils residing in the lung and liver. Because both tissues have antigen-presenting cells that are regularly active, there is a small population of neutrophils normally releasing proteases, nucleases, and elastases. In unaffected individuals, the antitrypsin protein irreversibly inhibits the destructive effects of elastases and proteases, thus checking the level of local tissue inflammation. In affected individuals, this small amount of inflammation grows unchecked, causing significant tissue destruction and the recruitment of more inflammatory effector cells. Since it is known that individuals who smoke have an increased number of neutrophils and macrophages in their lung tissue, smoking results in a significantly greater amount of damage than it would in an unaffected individual.

36 **The answer is A** *Renal/urinary system / Pathology / Chronic renal failure*

Chronic renal failure is characterized by increased glomerular filtration rate, proteinuria, and the systemic symptoms of urinary protein loss. Because the kidneys have a tremendous reserve for maintaining potassium balance, neither hypokalemia nor hyperkalemia is common in patients with renal failure. However, when potassium balance is lost, hyperkalemia, generally resulting from acidosis, oliguria, or excess potassium ingestion, is more common. Proteinuria is one of the earliest findings in many types of kidney disease; the compromised glomeruli have leaky basement membranes, and albumin and other small proteins are lost from the serum. The liver increases production of all serum proteins in response to the loss. The mechanism that causes triglyceride elevation is complex and poorly understood, but it is thought that the liver's production of lipoproteins is inappropriately increased in addition to the necessary increase in albumin production. Red blood cell production depends on the kidneys' synthesis of the growth factor erythropoietin. Although the reserve production of erythropoietin is substantial, most patients with end-stage disease have clinically significant anemia. Normochromic, normocytic anemia used to be a much more serious problem in patients with renal failure. With the development of recombinant erythropoietin, this problem can be treated easily. Patients with renal failure have uremic fetor, a pungent odor in their sweat and on their breath, as a result of their elevated serum urea and creatinine.

37 **The answer is E** *Renal/urinary system / Physiology / Acid–base homeostasis*

Ammonia is one of the nontitratable acids in the urine and is a major route of acid excretion. Ammonia is synthesized in the cells of the kidney tubules and diffuses freely into the tubule fluid. Any free hydrogen ions are bound by the ammonia, making the charged ammonium ion, which does not diffuse back into the cells. Amniogenesis is tightly regulated by the kidney and is the major factor in the kidney's ability to handle large acid loads. The complete enzymatic pathway for urea synthesis is found only in hepatocytes. Urea synthesis plays no significant role in acid–base homeostasis; excretion of urea is the major route for disposal of nitrogenous wastes. Bicarbonate recycling by the tubule cells synthesizes carbon dioxide and water from bicarbonate and hydrogen ions in the tubule fluid. The carbon dioxide diffuses into the cell, where another carbonic anhydrase synthesizes the bicarbonate anion from the incoming molecule and hydroxyl anion. The bicarbonate is transported with sodium into the bloodstream, whereas the hydrogen ion is secreted into the tubule fluid, resulting in a net reabsorption of bicarbonate. Pyruvate is a substrate for gluconeogenesis in the liver, and potassium is secreted in exchange for sodium reabsorption in the distal tubules.

38 **The answer is D** *Renal/urinary system / Pathology / Metabolic acidosis and chronic renal failure*

In the initial phases of metabolic acidosis, the anion gap is small because the deficiency in serum bicarbonate is replaced by chloride anion. This phase is called hyperchloremic acidosis and reflects the initial stage in which some level of compensation is maintained. As the active transport of bicarbonate by the kidneys continues to drop, unmeasured anions, such as phosphate and sulfate, begin to fill the gap. Because they are unmeasured, the apparent gap between the measured cations (sodium and potassium) and the measured anions (bicarbonate and chloride) starts to increase. The source of phosphate that fills the anion gap is most likely the bone. Thus, hydrolysis of calcium salts in the bone provides the anions to compensate for the failure of the kidneys to synthesize ammonia and reabsorb bicarbonate. It is thought that metabolic acidosis plays a significant role in the pathophysiology, which leads to renal osteodystrophy. The synthesis of ammonia in the kidney tubules is important in acid secretion and, as discussed earlier, it is seriously compromised in patients with renal failure.

39 **The answer is B** *General principles / Biostatistics / Definitions of terms*

Standard deviation is the absolute value of the average difference of individual values from the mean. It is always more than the standard error of the mean, which is equal to the standard deviation divided by the square root of the population number. The mean is the sum of values divided by the number of values. Mode is the most frequently occurring value. However, it is not greater than 1 if each value in a set of measurements occurs only once or if the most frequent value is less than 1. The median is the point where the number of observations above equals the number below. Range is difference between the lowest and highest value in a distribution.

40 **The answer is B** *Respiratory system / Pharmacology; physiology / Asthma diagnosis*

Asthma is a possible underlying cause of episodic dyspnea associated with wheezing in an 11-year-old boy. Although it is often difficult to establish a diagnosis of asthma in the laboratory, a reduction in forced expiratory volumes *(curve 1)* that is reversible after the inhalation of a bronchodilator, such as metaproterenol *(curve 2)*, is consistent with a diagnosis of hyperreactive airway disease. Although variability in spirometric testing is common, a forced expiratory volume in 1 second (FEV_1) of less than 1 L/minute is a concern, even in a patient of this age. Methacholine is a useful provocative agent that will reduce FEV_1 at a lower dose in an asthmatic patient than in normal subjects. Although cromolyn sodium and beclomethasone are useful in the therapy of asthma, neither is likely to produce acute reversal of airway obstruction.

41 **The answer is B** *Central and peripheral nervous system / Anatomy / Cranial nerves*

The nuclei of the trigeminal (CN V), abducens (CN VI), facial (CN VII), and vestibulocochlear (CN VIII) nerves are located in the pons, with an exception being that the sensory nuclei of the trigeminal nerve extend from the midbrain to the spinal cord. The nuclei of the glossopharyngeal (CN IX) nerve is located in the medulla. The trigeminal, facial, and glossopharyngeal nerves contain both motor and sensory components. The vestibulocochlear nerve is purely sensory. The abducens nerve is the only purely motor nerve that originates in the pons.

42 **The answer is D** *Respiratory system / Physiology / Hyperreactive airway disease*

Stimulation of irritant receptors leads to reflex bronchoconstriction via a vagal reflex. Indeed, normal resting tone is set by the parasympathetic nervous system, and some aspects of hyperreactive airway disease are thought to involve a relatively high influence of vagal tone at the expense of sympathetic efferent bronchodilator activity. The intercostal and phrenic nerves are important nerves to the accessory respiratory muscle and diaphragm, respectively.

43 **The answer is C** *Cardiovascular system / Physiology / Myocardial infarction*

A fast rhythm with a wide complex is usually consistent with a ventricular tachycardia. It is highly likely that the 60-year-old man described in the question had a myocardial infarction associated with ventricular tachycardia. The treatment of choice for ventricular tachycardia associated with myocardial ischemia is lidocaine. Lidocaine is typical of a group of antiarrhythmic agents that block sodium ion channels, the current-carrying processes responsible for depolarization in fast fibers of the heart (ventricular and atrial). It suppresses these channels in the infarct area in cells with abnormal resting membrane potential. Although the mechanism underlying this selectivity is poorly understood, it is thought that abnormal tissue ion channels tend to be in inactivated states, which would increase the binding and efficacy of use-dependent agents, or that damaged myocardial tissue tends to accumulate agents such as lidocaine to a greater extent. Agents such as diltiazem, propranolol, and digitalis affect electrical propagation and conduction in sinoatrial and atrioventricular nodal tissue, where parasympathetic input predominates, and calcium is the current-carrying ion. Although propranolol has been shown to have some utility in reducing damage after myocardial infarction, it is contraindicated in patients with hypotension and potential poor left ventricular function. Epinephrine increases oxygen demands on the heart by directly stimulating β-receptors as well as increasing afterload, and in this case, it appears to be contraindicated.

44 **The answer is B** *Cardiovascular system / Physiology / Myocardial infarction*

Creatine kinase (CK) is an enzyme that catalyzes the transfer of high-energy phosphates and is found largely in tissues that use large amounts of energy. The two most common isoforms are CK-MM (muscle) and CK-BB (brain). An isoform that contains both M and B subunits (CK-MB) is found only in the myocardium. In the heart, CK is approximately 85% CK-MB. An increase in both total CK and CK-MB secondary to myocardial injury has proved to be highly sensitive and specific for the diagnosis of myocardial infarction. Lactate dehydrogenase (LDH) is often elevated 48 to 72 hours after injury.

45 **The answer is D** *Respiratory system / Pharmacology / Asthma treatment*

Theophylline is one of a number of methylxanthines useful for chronic therapy of asthma. Although it can increase intracellular levels of cyclic adenosine monophosphate (cAMP) via phosphodiesterase inhibition and can relax bronchial smooth muscle, theophylline appears to affect symptoms of asthma via other mechanisms, including affecting adenosine receptors or intracellular calcium homeostasis. Propranolol is a β-adrenergic receptor antagonist that is contraindicated in patients with asthma because it may exacerbate their symptoms. Although local concentrations of histamine contribute to the pathogenesis of asthma, antihistamines do not have an accepted role in the therapy of asthma except to manage associated rhinitis. Bethanechol is a moderately long-acting parasympathomimetic and as such is contraindicated in asthmatics. Ibuprofen and other NSAIDs (which inhibit cyclo-oxygenase) may also narrow the airway, perhaps by shuttling arachidonic acid via the bronchoconstricting lipoxygenase pathway, and are often contraindicated in a subset (e.g., aspirin hypersensitive) of asthmatics.

46 **The answer is D** *Cardiovascular system / Pharmacology / Myocardial infarction*

Low-dose aspirin has become an important component of pharmacotherapeutic approaches to reducing the risk of recurrent myocardial infarction. The desired effect is irreversible inhibition of platelet cyclo-oxygenase that reduces platelet-derived thromboxane A_2 while allowing for resynthesis of endothelial cell cyclooxygenase and maintaining useful production of prostacyclin. Aspirin does not affect lipoxygenase activity, and therefore it does not decrease circulating levels of any of the leukotrienes. Aspirin does not reduce normal body temperature.

47 **The answer is C** *Central and peripheral nervous system / Pharmacology / Adrenergic agonist*

Ephedrine is a mixed-action adrenergic agent. It releases stored norepinephrine from nerve endings, and it directly stimulates both α- and β-adrenergic receptors. Clonidine, dopamine, and ritodrine are direct-acting adrenergic agents that directly bind α- or β-adrenergic receptors, producing effects similar to those that follow stimulation of sympathetic nerves or release of the hormone epinephrine from the adrenal medulla. Amphetamine and tyramine are indirect-acting agonists that cause the release of norepinephrine from the cytoplasm or vesicles of adrenergic neurons. The norepinephrine release traverses the synapse and stimulates the α- and β-adrenergic receptors.

48 **The answer is B** *Central and peripheral nervous system / Pharmacology / Adrenergic agonist*

Dopamine is a catecholamine. Sympathomimetic amines that contain the 3,4-dihydroxybenezene group are catecholamines because 3,4-dihydroxybenezene is known as catechol. Catecholamines share the following properties: (1) they have a rapid onset of action, (2) they have a brief duration of action, (3) they are not administered orally, and (4) they do not penetrate the blood–brain barrier. Noncatecholamines (e.g., clonidine, ephedrine, albuterol, amphetamine, and metaproterenol) have a longer duration of action than catecholamines and can be administered orally.

49 **The answer is D** *Skin and related connective tissue / Pathology / Melanoma*

The lesion is a superficial, spreading melanoma. This form of melanoma often involves a rapidly expanding, superficial lesion that contains shades of brown mixed with bluish-red or black. The border of the lesion is visible or palpably elevated. It is grossly distinguishable from other common pigmented lesions based on color, shape, and rate of growth. Although the back and extremities are common sites for detection of such a lesion, melanomas can arise in other areas of the body.

50 **The answer is E** *Central and peripheral nervous system / Pathology / Acute neurologic management; alcohol withdrawal*

Benzodiazepines are cross-tolerant with barbiturates and ethanol and permit controlled withdrawal from ethanol. Disulfiram (Antabuse) has been used as a deterrent to further drinking; it is not a treatment for alcohol withdrawal. Hydration is important to prevent cardiovascular collapse. Changes in vital signs, including increased blood pressure, heart rate, and temperature, accompany ethanol withdrawal and should be monitored. Vitamin B_{12} is a treatment for pernicious anemia, which is characterized by ataxia, megaloblastic anemia, and neurologic disturbances.

test **9**

Questions

Directions: Single best answer questions consist of numbered items or incomplete statements followed by answers or by completions of the statement. Select the ONE lettered answer or completion that is BEST in each case.

1 Which of the following statements about multiple endocrine neoplasia (MEN) type IIb is correct?

(A) Pheochromocytomas associated with MEN type IIb are never malignant

(B) MEN is hereditary, and the gene has been mapped to chromosome 10

(C) The pancreas, the pituitary gland, and the parathyroid gland are most commonly affected

(D) Neuromas of the conjunctival, labial, and buccal mucosa are unusual

(E) Zollinger–Ellison syndrome is present in about 20% of cases

2 Which of the following statements concerning hemoglobin genes and thalassemia is correct?

(A) Normal individuals inherit two copies of the α-chain, one from each parent

(B) α-Thalassemias are sex-linked because the α-chain genes are on the X chromosome

(C) α-Thalassemias vary in severity with the location of the mutation within the α-chain genes

(D) Most α-thalassemias involve deletions of α-chain genes owing to a nonhomologous crossover

(E) The unique structure of the α-chain gene precludes confirmation of structural abnormalities by restriction endonucleases

3 Which of the following is most characteristic of nephrotic syndrome?

(A) Hypocoagulability
(B) Hyperlipidemia
(C) Hyperalbuminemia
(D) Hematuria
(E) Dehydration

4 Which of the following may result from chronic alcohol abuse?

(A) Wilms' tumor
(B) Esophagitis and Mallory–Weiss tears
(C) Menorrhagia
(D) Mild to moderate hypotension and decreased serum triglycerides
(E) Bronchogenic carcinoma

5 Which of the following is most closely associated with acute pancreatitis?

(A) Chest pain
(B) Lowered serum triglycerides
(C) α_1-Antitrypsin deficiency
(D) Biliary tract disease
(E) Lowered serum lipase

6 Which of the following statements most closely describes the biologic properties of immunoglobulin (Ig) E?

(A) It can cause agglutination of particulate antigens

(B) Low levels of circulating IgE are due in part to the high-affinity binding of the Fc portion to T cells

(C) It has the shortest half-life of all classes of immunoglobulins

(D) It efficiently fixes complement

7 A patient hospitalized for multiple fractures was prescribed a prophylactic antibiotic. Two days prior to discharge, the patient developed diarrhea requiring intravenous rehydration. The antibiotic was changed to a broad-spectrum cephalosporin, but diarrhea continued and the patient's condition deteriorated. Which of the following actions is most appropriate?

(A) Halting all antibiotic treatments and maintaining intravenous fluids

(B) Changing the antibiotic to clindamycin

(C) Testing for toxin in the urine

(D) Sigmoidoscopic examination

8 Which of the following sets of complications are common in patients with chronic hemolytic anemia?

(A) Emphysema and clubbing

(B) Pulmonary embolism, deep vein thromboses, and edema

(C) Congestive heart failure, severe infection by encapsulated organisms, chronic liver failure, and cardiac arrhythmias

(D) Problems digesting fats, thick sputum, difficulty breathing, and frequent pulmonary infections

(E) Progressive muscle wasting and loss of voluntary movement of muscles

9 Which one of the following cholinergic antagonists is an antimuscarinic agent?

(A) Nicotine

(B) Tubocurarine

(C) Succinylcholine

(D) Scopolamine

(E) Gallamine

(F) Pancuronium

10 Figure 46 in the color plate section is a renal biopsy from a patient with lower extremity edema proteinuria. Which of the following clinical presentations is most likely?

(A) Acute renal failure

(B) Nephritic syndrome

(C) Nephrotic syndrome

(D) Chronic renal failure

11 The irreversible inactivation of acetylcholinesterase is caused by which one of the following cholinergic agonists?

(A) Neostigmine

(B) Edrophonium

(C) Isoflurophate

(D) Carbachol

(E) Pilocarpine

(F) Bethanechol

12 A 68-year-old woman suddenly develops a fever of 38.2°C and a severe headache one evening. The following morning she also has a stiff neck and uncharacteristic drowsiness. At the emergency department, her temperature is 38.8°C, and there is pain and resistance on flexion of her neck. The patient is noted to be mentally competent although lethargic. A cerebrospinal fluid sample is obtained by lumbar puncture. On the basis of the history and physical examination of this patient, what is the most probable diagnosis?

(A) Viral meningitis

(B) Fungal meningitis

(C) Bacterial meningitis

(D) Viral encephalitis

(E) Brain abscess

13 A 22-year-old man sustains a head injury in an automobile accident. Upon secondary review in the emergency department he is found to have the following papillary irregularities. When light is shown into the left eye the pupil does not constrict. When light is shown into the right eye both pupils constrict. Where is the defect?

(A) Left CN II (optic)

(B) Right CN II (optic)

(C) Left CN III (oculomotor)

(D) Right CN III (oculomotor)

(E) Left CN II and CN III

14 A 48-year-old homeless man appears ataxic and confused in the emergency department. He is unshaven and mildly jaundiced, and he has a bleeding scalp wound over the right frontotemporal area. The physical should first

(A) ask the nurse to shower him, using antilice treatment

(B) suture his head wound

(C) order skull films

(D) obtain a serum ethanol level

(E) perform a neurologic examination

Color Plates

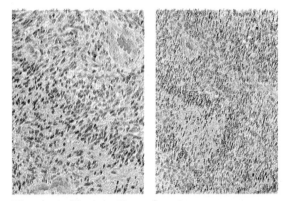

Figure 1: Test 1, Question 2

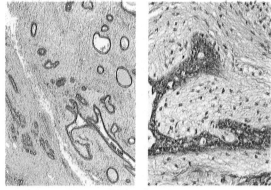

Figure 5: Test 1, Question 31

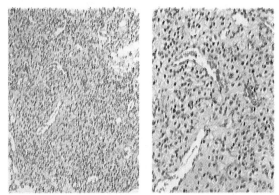

Figure 2: Test 1, Question 10

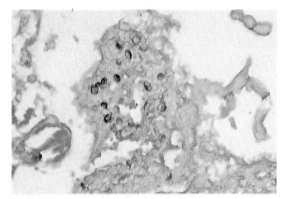

Figure 6: Test 1, Question 42

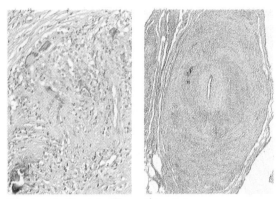

Figure 3: Test 1, Question 14

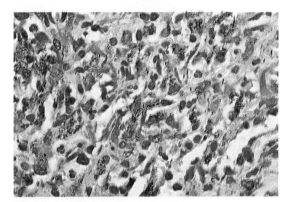

Figure 7: Test 2, Question 7

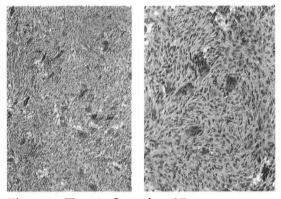

Figure 4: Test 1, Question 27

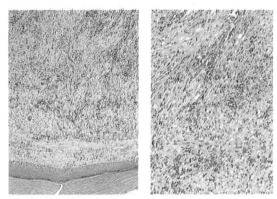

Figure 8: Test 2, Question 17

Color Plates

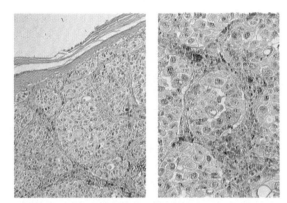

Figure 9: Test 2, Question 26

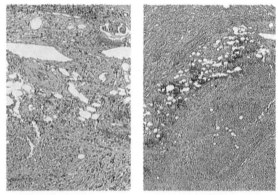

Figure 13: Test 2, Question 47

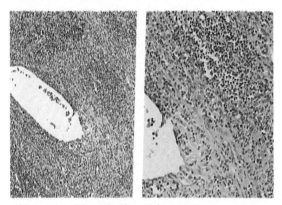

Figure 10: Test 2, Question 32

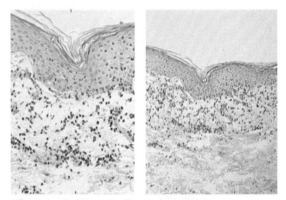

Figure 14: Test 3, Question 11

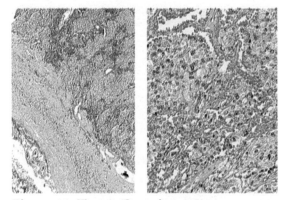

Figure 11: Test 2, Question 41

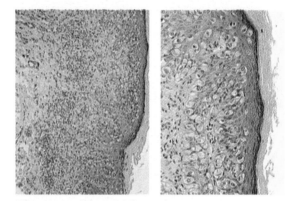

Figure 15: Test 3, Question 26

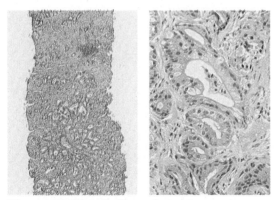

Figure 12: Test 2, Question 44

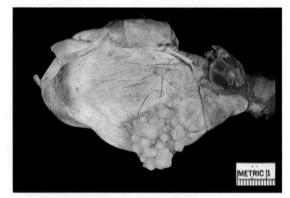

Figure 16: Test 3, Question 27

Color Plates

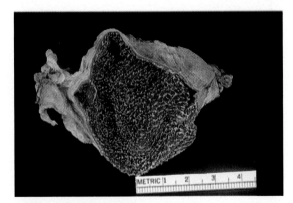

Figure 17: Test 3, Question 37

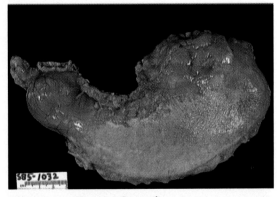

Figure 21: Test 4, Question 11

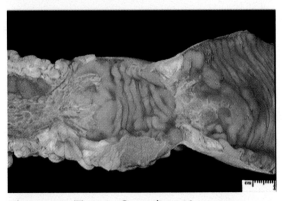

Figure 18: Test 3, Question 40

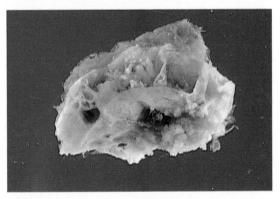

Figure 22: Test 4, Question 23

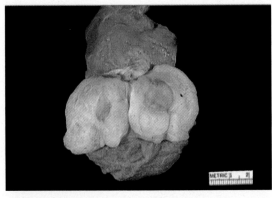

Figure 19: Test 3, Question 43

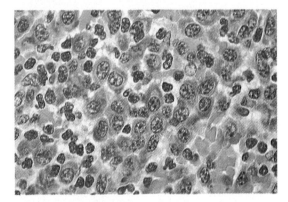

Figure 23: Test 4, Question 35

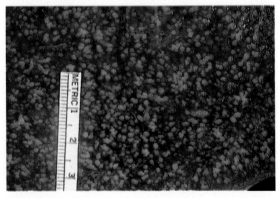

Figure 20: Test 3, Question 46

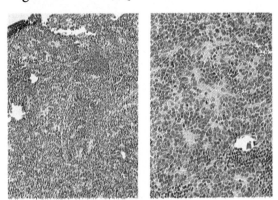

Figure 24: Test 4, Question 44

Color Plates

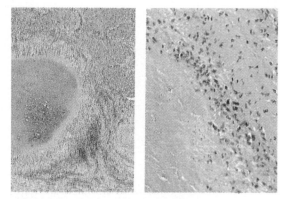

Figure 25: Test 4, Question 46

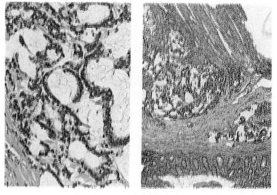

Figure 28: Test 5, Question 23

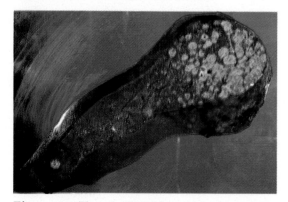

Figure 26: Test 4, Question 49

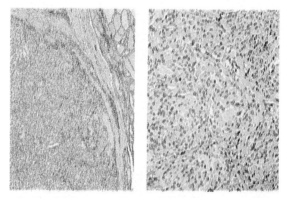

Figure 29: Test 5, Question 29

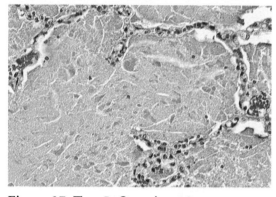

Figure 27: Test 5, Question 10

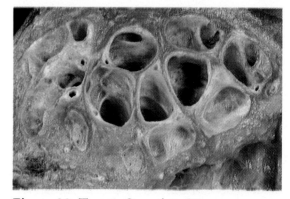

Figure 30: Test 5, Question 39

Color Plates

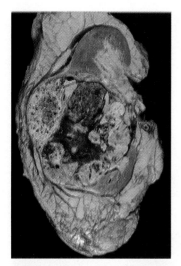

Figure 31: Test 5, Question 41

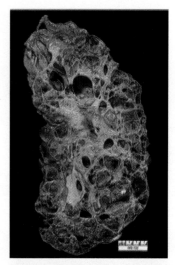

Figure 32: Test 5, Question 47

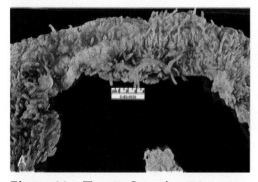

Figure 33a: Test 5, Question 50

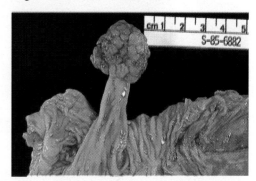

Figure 35: Test 6, Question 28

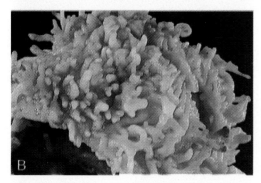

Figure 33b: Test 5, Question 50

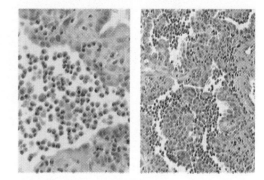

Figure 36: Test 6, Question 32

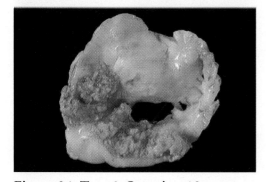

Figure 34: Test 6, Question 19

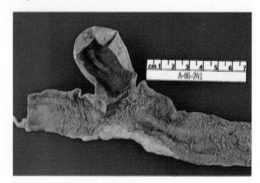

Figure 37: Test 6, Question 38

Color Plates

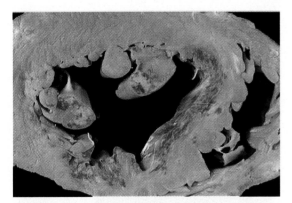

Figure 38: Test 6, Question 41

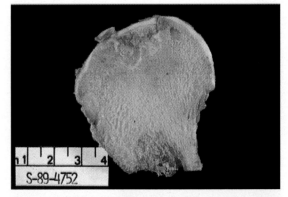

Figure 42: Test 7, Question 12

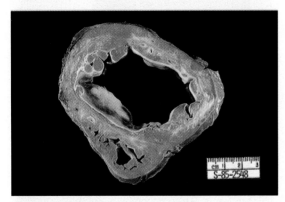

Figure 39: Test 6, Question 45

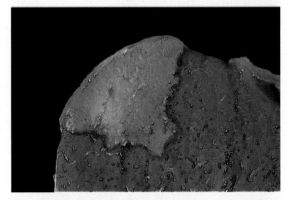

Figure 43: Test 7, Question 22

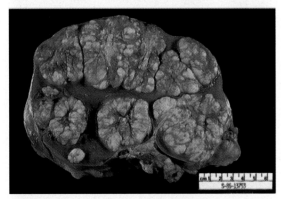

Figure 40: Test 6, Question 46

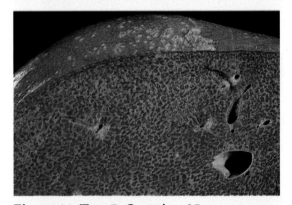

Figure 44: Test 7, Question 25

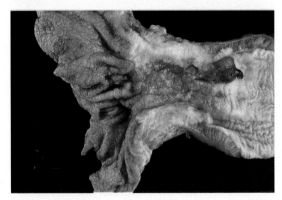

Figure 41: Test 7, Question 8

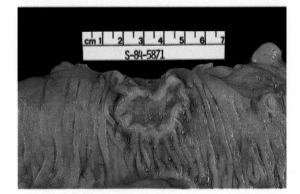

Figure 45: Test 7, Question 31

Color Plates

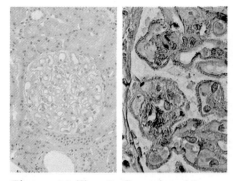

Figure 46: Test 9, Question 10

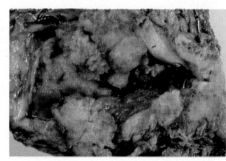

Figure 50: Test 10, Question 31

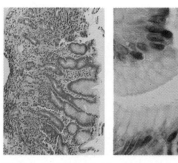

Figure 54: Test 12, Question 26

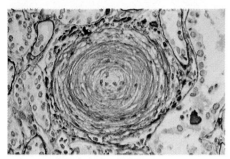

Figure 47: Test 9, Question 41

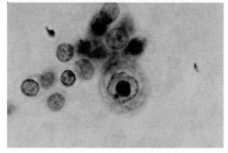

Figure 51: Test 11, Question 16

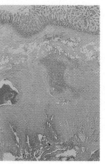

Figure 55: Test 12, Question 45

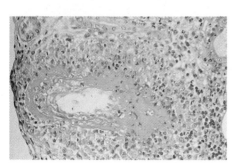

Figure 48: Test 10, Question 5

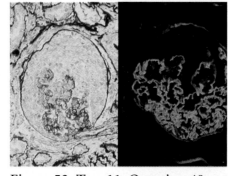

Figure 52: Test 11, Question 40

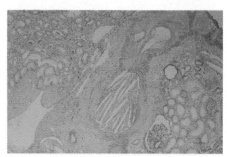

Figure 56: Test 12, Question 46

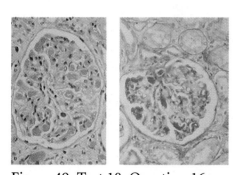

Figure 49: Test 10, Question 16

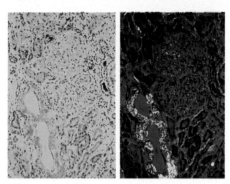

Figure 53: Test 12, Question 12

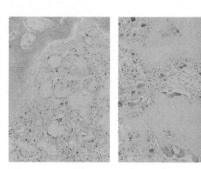

Figure 57: Test 13, Question 19

Color Plates

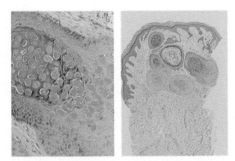
Figure 58: Test 13, Question 47

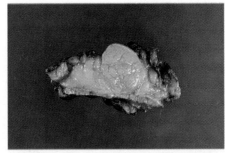
Figure 62: Test 15, Question 33

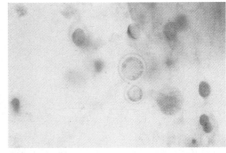
Figure 66: Test 17, Question 4

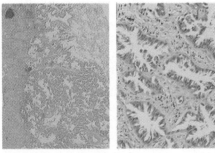
Figure 59: Test 14, Question 14

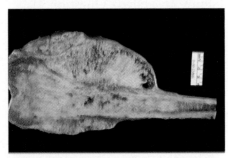
Figure 63: Test 16, Question 16

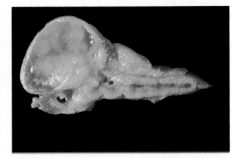
Figure 67: Test 17, Question 23

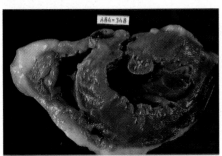
Figure 60: Test 15, Question 7

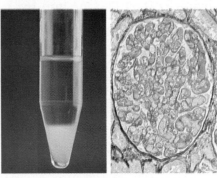
Figure 64: Test 16, Question 27

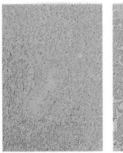
Figure 68: Test 17, Question 34

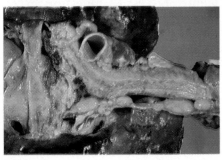
Figure 61: Test 15, Question 18

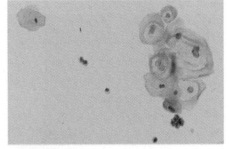
Figure 65: Test 16, Question 41

15 Which of the following concerning nucleotide repeat expansion disorders is true?

(A) All nucleotide repeat disorders are based on increased numbers of trinucleotide repeats

(B) Nucleotide repeat expansions have been described in promoter, exon, intron, 5′ untranslated, and 3′ untranslated sequences

(C) Nucleotide repeat disorders only manifest in patients when the repeat expansions are contained within coding sequences

(D) Nucleotide repeat expansion disorders are autosomal recessive genetic mutations

(E) All nucleotide repeat expansions are transmitted in an x-linked dominant or autosomal dominant manner

16 Which of the following characteristics of warfarin is correct?

(A) It is useful in pregnant women because it does not cross the placenta

(B) It affects hepatic synthesis of clotting factors present in blood

(C) It must be given parenterally

(D) It is used primarily in acute therapy

(E) Therapy cannot be reversed by the administration of vitamin K

17 Which of the following enzymes is most important in protecting red blood cells from the hydrogen peroxide generated in vivo?

(A) Pyruvate dehydrogenase

(B) Transketolase

(C) Nitric oxide synthase

(D) Glutathione peroxidase

(E) Cyclooxygenase

18 Zidovudine (ZDV), formerly known as azidothymidine (AZT), has which of the following properties?

(A) ZDV reduces the chance of progression to AIDS in asymptomatic HIV-infected subjects

(B) ZDV does little to improve the clinical symptoms of immunologic function, survival period, and quality of life of patients with advanced cases of AIDS

(C) ZDV is not toxic to the bone marrow

(D) ZDV is a protease inhibitor

(E) One of the benefits of ZDV is that prolonged treatment (1 to 3 years) with it does not result in resistance to this drug

19 Which of the following mediators released during mast cell activation causes a direct increase in vascular permeability?

(A) Eosinophil chemotactic factor (ECF)

(B) Serotonin

(C) Interleukin (IL) 1

(D) Prostaglandin E_2

(E) Tumor necrosis factor-α

20 Which of the following is a major risk factor for the development of chronic obstructive pulmonary disease (COPD)?

(A) Living at a high altitude

(B) History of pneumonia

(C) Occupational exposure to irritant gases and particles

(D) Intravenous drug abuse

(E) Pre-existing heart disease

21 Which of the following findings is most characteristic of Duchenne's muscular dystrophy?

(A) Accumulation of a dominant negative form of dystrophin

(B) Atrophy of affected muscle groups

(C) Sarcomere hypercontraction and contraction band formation

(D) Most of the cases resulting from spontaneous mutation

(E) Autosomal dominant inheritance via mutated chromosome 20

22 Agnogenic myeloid metaplasia with myelofibrosis is characterized by which of the following features?

(A) Hypercellular bone marrow

(B) Decreased levels of leukocyte alkaline phosphatase

(C) Teardrop-shaped erythrocytes

(D) Hepatomegaly without splenomegaly

(E) Erythrocytosis

23 A young child develops pharyngitis, a fever, and a rash. β-Hemolytic gram-positive cocci in chains are isolated from the throat and are found to be catalase-negative. Which of the following statements about the virulence factors of this pathogen is correct?

(A) Hemolysis results from autoimmune destruction of red blood cells

(B) The organism is not encapsulated

(C) The organism produces hyaluronic acid, which is necessary for attachment to mucosa

(D) The organism produces membrane-bound protein (M protein), which has antiphagocytic properties

(E) The rash is produced by the streptolysins

24 Which one of the following equations best describes the odds ratio?

	Cases	Non cases	
Exposed	A	B	A+B
Not exposed	C	D	C+D
	A+C	B+D	

(A) [A/(A + B)]/[C/(C + D)]
(B) (A/D)/(B/C)
(C) (A + B)/(C + D)
(D) AD/BC

25 Which one of the following statements best describes a cohort study?

(A) It is a prevalence survey of a group of individuals with a particular disease performed at a single point in time
(B) It compares the frequency of a purported risk factor in a group of cases and a group of controls
(C) Subjects are free of disease at the beginning of the observation but are exposed or not exposed to risk factors
(D) It presents in detail a single case or handful of cases

26 Which of the following is appropriate pharmacologic management of routine delirium tremens (i.e., alcohol withdrawal)?

(A) Haloperidol therapy for up to 3 weeks
(B) Phenytoin (Dilantin) tapered over 10 days
(C) Chlordiazepoxide (Librium) tapered over 5 days
(D) Morphine for up to 1 month
(E) Nortriptyline for up to 6 months

27 Which of the following is an example of confounding bias?

(A) Assessment of general health in the United States was made by distributing personal health questionnaires at an American Medical Association meeting
(B) Serum triglycerides are a risk factor for coronary heart disease but not independently of serum cholesterol
(C) The control and experimental groups of animals in a study are being taken care of by two different persons
(D) An observed association between oral contraceptives and thrombophlebitis is caused by the way in which the history of exposure was reported

28 Which of the following statements about the G_0 phase of the cell cycle is true?

(A) G_0 is a specialized, growing state of the cell cycle
(B) The rate of protein synthesis is drastically increased in G_0
(C) The cells can remain in G_0 for weeks or even years
(D) Cells can enter G_0 only directly after mitosis
(E) The cells in G_0 have more cyclin-dependent kinases and G_1 cyclins than do cells in G_1

29 Which of the following statements concerning fatty acid synthesis is correct?

(A) Palmitoyl CoA helps regulate the committed step in fatty acid synthesis through feedback inhibition of acetyl CoA carboxylase
(B) Hormone-dependent enzyme phosphorylation, which is important in gluconeogenesis, is not important in fatty acid synthesis
(C) Low levels of citrate increase the synthesis of malonyl CoA by reducing substrate inhibition of acetyl CoA carboxylase
(D) The growing fatty acid chain is elongated by a series of enzymes that exist as separate polypeptides in the mitochondrial matrix
(E) Niacin is the precursor for a coenzyme that is important in the addition of carboxyl groups to the growing fatty acid chain

30 A 40-year-old woman with refractory peptic ulcer disease consults a gastroenterologist for a complete evaluation. She is a nonsmoker and drinks only infrequently. Endoscopy reveals ectopic ulcers in the esophagus and numerous ulcers in the stomach and duodenum. The physician considers a diagnosis of Zollinger–Ellison syndrome. Which of the following problems characterizes the cause of peptic ulcer disease in most patients with Zollinger–Ellison syndrome?

(A) Increased vagal tone in the gastric branch
(B) Increased release of histamine
(C) Increased secretion of gastrin
(D) Increased secretion of pepsin
(E) Decreased mucous production

31 A 20-year-old man originally presented to his PCP with complaints of vision problems. Over the next 10 years he completely lost his vision. His only sister has not developed similar symptoms. The PCP suspected a rare genetic disease, Leber hereditary optic neuropathy. Which of the following statements concerning his disease is correct?

(A) The disease is x-linked dominant
(B) The disease is autosomal recessive and therefore the patient's father should also undergo genetic testing
(C) The disease is autosomal dominant and caused by a dominant negative mutant gene product
(D) The mutation is carried by mitochondrial DNA
(E) This disease displays incomplete penetrance

32 Which of the following statements about generalized absence seizures is correct?

(A) They may consist of staring and altered mental state
(B) They are also called grand mal seizures
(C) They are almost exclusively seen in adults
(D) There is a significant postictal state

33 Which of the following criteria would most likely establish a diagnosis of multiple sclerosis?

(A) Ages 10 to 50, more than one attack, more than one white matter lesion
(B) Ages 10 to 50, one or more attacks, one or more white matter lesions
(C) Any age, more than one attack, more than one white matter lesion
(D) Any age, one or more attacks, one or more white matter lesions

34 The accompanying figure shows flow–volume curves after inhalation to total lung capacity (TLC) and a forced expiratory maneuver to residual volume (RV) from a normal person and a patient. Absolution volume of gas within the thorax was determined independently in a body plethysmograph. The patient was a middle-aged man with a history of chronic cough with expectoration and complaints of shortness of breath, and an increasing inability to exercise. In addition, a chest radiograph revealed an enlarged heart and congested lung fields with increased markings attributable to old infections. From the following flow–volume curve, which of the following statements is correct regarding the patient?

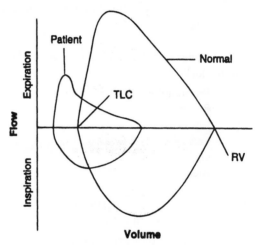

(A) TLC is greatly reduced
(B) RV is reduced
(C) Vital capacity is greatly increased
(D) Flow rate over most of expiration is less than predicted
(E) Elastic recoil of lung is likely to be greater than predicted

35 Which of the following statements correctly characterizes the secretion of acid by parietal cells?

(A) Carbonic anhydrase in the parietal cell splits carbonic acid into a bicarbonate ion, which is secreted into the blood, and a hydrogen ion
(B) Hydrogen ions are secreted passively down their gradient into the gut
(C) cAMP levels are elevated in response to either gastrin or muscarinic receptor stimulation
(D) H_2-histamine receptor activation causes elevation of intracellular calcium levels
(E) Gastrin and acetylcholine stimulate parietal cell acid production but histamine inhibits it

36 A preterm female infant is delivered at a residential hospital with a birth weight of 1,400 grams. Which of the following statements concerning this patient is true?

(A) Her risk of neonatal sepsis is 1,000 times that of a full-term infant

(B) Most cases of neonatal sepsis at this birth weight develop in the first 3 days after birth

(C) Most cases of neonatal sepsis at this birth weight will include both gram-positive and gram-negative organisms

(D) Gram-negative bacteria are implicated in more than 50% of cases

(E) Fungal infections are more common than bacterial infections due to intrapartum antibiotic treatment

37 Which one of the following adrenergic blockers is an α-blocker?

(A) Propranolol

(B) Reserpine

(C) Cocaine

(D) Prazosin

(E) Guanethidine

(F) Atenolol

38 Which of the following statements concerning the Arthus reaction is most correct?

(A) It requires only small amounts of antibody and antigen

(B) It results in systemic and widespread rupture of vessel walls followed by tissue necrosis

(C) It is the most common type III reaction seen in humans

(D) Neutrophils and platelets are present at the site of the reaction

39 Cushing's syndrome is a complex array of symptoms that are due to excess glucocorticoid levels. Which of the following statements about Cushing's syndrome is correct?

(A) It may be associated with hyperactive secretion of posterior pituitary hormones

(B) It may be secondary to abnormal hypothalamic function with excessive release of corticotropin-releasing factor (CRF)

(C) It may be due to ectopic GnRH synthesis

(D) Some aspects of it are secondary to long-term insulin therapy

(E) Increased long bone length prior to puberty is common in these patients

40 Which of the following statements about protein synthesis is true?

(A) One transfer RNA (tRNA) can bind many different amino acids

(B) The addition of aminoacyl tRNA to the growing peptide chain and subsequent translocation constitute an energy-independent process

(C) The formation of the peptide bond is catalyzed by serine kinase

(D) Synthesis occurs in the mitochondria as well as in the cytoplasm of cells

(E) Synthesis can occur in the absence of RNA

41 The lesion depicted in Figure 47 in the color plate section is most frequently associated with

(A) microangiopathic hemolytic anemia with renal involvement

(B) hypotension

(C) low fibrinogen levels early in the course

(D) antineutrophil cytoplasmic antibodies

42 Asymptomatic bacteriuria is noted in a 35-year-old pregnant woman in her second trimester. Five years ago, during her first pregnancy, she developed acute pyelonephritis that required hospitalization and parenteral antibacterial therapy. Since then, recurrent sexual intercourse-related urinary tract infections have been prevented by a single dose of nitrofurantoin after coitus. Which of the following agents would you recommend for this patient during the remainder of her pregnancy for prevention of acute pyelonephritis?

(A) Trimethoprim–sulfamethoxazole

(B) Minocycline

(C) Amoxicillin

(D) Gentamicin

43 Thymomas are associated most closely with which of the following diseases?

(A) Graves' disease

(B) Rheumatoid arthritis

(C) Addison's disease

(D) Myasthenia gravis

(E) Osteoarthritis

44 Which of the following statements concerning HIV is correct?

(A) It infects lymphocytes though the T cell receptor

(B) The infective process entails endocytosis of the HIV particle into the cell

(C) Viral infection can spread between cells without the involvement of free virus

(D) Mature viral particles are released in small bursts during lysis of the infected cells

45 Assuming that a patient's language function is normal, which of the following is the most appropriate test for functional evaluation of the visual association areas of the parietal lobe?

(A) Ability to match an item in one hand with the same item in the opposite hand while wearing a blindfold

(B) Repetition of digits, forward and reversed

(C) Interpretation of proverbs

(D) Serial 7s subtraction

(E) Copying simple shapes and objects

46 For antibiotic therapy, it is useful to understand both the action of the prescribed antibiotic and the pathogenesis of the bacteria responsible for a patient's infection. For example, the aminoglycoside antibiotic gentamicin does not enter mammalian cells and therefore is ineffective against intracellular pathogens. Considering only this information, gentamicin is effective against which of the following infectious organisms?

(A) *Brucella*

(B) *Chlamydia*

(C) *Legionella*

(D) *Rickettsia*

(E) *Pseudomonas aeruginosa*

47 Which of the following concerning the characteristics of a typical virus is correct?

(A) It can reproduce itself under harsh conditions

(B) It contains either RNA or DNA as its genetic material

(C) Viruses possess their own replicative machinery

(D) It contains a protein coat called the tegument

48 Which one of the following statements is true for both prokaryotic and eukaryotic cells?

(A) They both contain extensive internal membranes unconnected to the plasma membrane

(B) They both contain organelles

(C) They both contain a membrane-bound nucleus

(D) They both use membrane transporters to allow passage of macromolecules

(E) Most of the cellular DNA is in the form of a single circular molecule

49 Which of the following statements about β_1-adrenergic receptors is true?

(A) They decrease heart rate upon binding agonists

(B) They bind catecholamines

(C) They induce relaxation of smooth muscle in bronchial passages on binding agonists

(D) The rank order of affinities for agonists is isoproterenol > epinephrine > norepinephrine

(E) They suppress cAMP levels by activation of adenylate cyclase

50 The essential transcriptional binding factor that binds directly to the TATA box initiating RNA polymerase II transcription in mammalian cells is

(A) TFIID

(B) TFIIE

(C) TFIIB

(D) TFIIS

Answer Key

1-B	11-C	21-C	31-D	41-A
2-D	12-C	22-C	32-A	42-C
3-B	13-A	23-D	33-A	43-D
4-B	14-E	24-D	34-D	44-C
5-D	15-B	25-C	35-A	45-E
6-C	16-B	26-C	36-D	46-E
7-D	17-D	27-B	37-D	47-B
8-C	18-A	28-C	38-D	48-D
9-D	19-B	29-A	39-B	49-B
10-C	20-C	30-C	40-D	50-A

Answers and Explanations

1 The answer is B *Endocrine system / Pathology / Multiple endocrine neoplasia*

The primary components of MEN IIa are pheochromocytoma and medullary carcinoma of the thyroid, whereas MEN IIb is characterized by pheochromocytoma and medullary carcinoma as well as the unusual neural tumors of the facial mucosal surfaces. Pheochromocytomas are malignant approximately 10% of the time.

MEN I is characterized by parathyroid tumors, pituitary adenomas, and pancreatic islet cell tumors. Zollinger–Ellison syndrome is a gastrin-secreting pancreatic islet cell tumor that is often associated with MEN I. All three types of MEN are hereditary, and the genes have been tentatively assigned to chromosome 10 for type II and chromosome 11 for type I. The patterns of inheritance are variable, as is the expression of disease phenotypes. Some patients have all of the characteristic tumors, whereas others have only one or two of the classically described neoplastic growths. The medullary cells (e.g., adrenal and thyroid) and the glia involved in the neuromas arise embryologically from the neural crest. Thus, it is thought that a neoplastic clone may give rise to all three types of tumors.

2 The answer is D *Hematopoietic and lymphoreticular system / Hematology / α-Thalassemias*

None of the common hemoglobinopathies are sex-linked because none of the subunits are encoded on the X chromosome. Two copies of the α-globin subunit gene are on chromosome 16, and there are two chromosomes from each parent. On each chromosome, the proximity of the two identical α-subunit genes results in a high frequency of recombination that in turn leads to an increased frequency of nonhomologous recombination and deletion. Thus, deletions are the most common cause of α-thalassemia. Because restriction fragment length polymorphisms are very sensitive to deletions, they are useful in identifying the genotypes for genetic counseling. The α-thalassemias are most common in Asians and African Americans, with the most severe cases occurring in Asians. The severity is governed by the number of normal genes remaining; when one of the genes is missing, it is a completely silent carrier state. Deletion of two genes results in mild hypochromic anemia, clinically silent and detected only by a routine complete blood count. The more severe forms of the disease, such as hemoglobin (Hb) H disease and hydrops fetalis, result from a loss of three or four of the genes, respectively. Hb H is the abnormal hemoglobin composed of four β-subunits instead of two β-subunits and two α-subunits. Hb H disease causes hemolytic anemia that is generally well-compensated. Hydrops fetalis is incompatible with life, and these infants usually die in utero. The severe forms are most common in Asians because Asians most often carry the homozygous deletion haplotype $(\alpha\alpha/-)$; therefore, they can pass on a chromosome that has no functional α genes. African Americans with the carrier state are more frequently heterozygous in both alleles $(\alpha-/\alpha-)$.

3 The answer is B *Renal/urinary system / Pathology / Nephrotic syndrome*

Nephrotic syndrome is the name given to the set of clinical symptoms that includes proteinuria, generalized edema, hypoalbuminemia, hypercoagulability, and hyperlipidemia. The leaky glomerulus leads to massive protein loss, hence to hypoalbuminemia and hypercoagulability from the loss of anticoagulant factors and antiplasmin activity. Edema also results and is accompanied by sodium and water retention. Any of several pathologic lesions of the kidney can be seen when a renal biopsy is performed on a patient with nephrotic syndrome, but the most common is focal segmental glomerulosclerosis. People with systemic diseases (e.g., diabetes and systemic lupus erythematosus) can also have nephrotic syndrome. Nephrotic syndrome specifically excludes hematuria, microscopic or gross, which indicates a more serious lesion of the glomerular filtration apparatus and indicates nephritis, not nephrosis.

4 **The answer is B** *Gastrointestinal system / Pathology / Effects of chronic alcohol abuse*

Alcoholism is a major source of morbidity and mortality in the United States. Esophagitis associated with vomiting and chronic reflux is a common complaint of alcoholics. The more serious Mallory–Weiss tears (usually secondary to fierce retching) involve the rupture of a submucosal vein resulting in acute, voluminous blood loss. Testicular atrophy and amenorrhea are often the result of liver degeneration and the concomitant reduction in steroid metabolism. High estrogen levels result in feedback inhibition of hypothalamic gonado-tropin-releasing hormone (GnRH) secretion. Chronic alcohol abuse also results in mild hypertension for reasons that are still unclear. Protein malnutrition and the synthesis of fatty acids from ethanol combine to produce the commonly seen elevation in serum triglycerides. Wilms' tumor, a childhood renal tumor, and bronchogenic carcinoma are not associated with alcoholism.

5 **The answer is D** *Gastrointestinal system / Pathology / Acute pancreatitis*

α_1-Antitrypsin deficiency is commonly associated with damage to the liver and lungs, but not the pancreas. About 80% of pancreatitis cases are associated with biliary tract disease and alcoholism. Acute pancreatitis leads to the elevation of pancreatic enzymes, including amylase and lipase, in the blood and urine. Clearly, alcohol ingestion can cause acute pancreatitis, and several bouts of alcohol-induced subacute pancreatitis may allow chronic pancreatic failure to emerge without a clinically symptomatic episode of acute pancreatitis. Elevated serum triglycerides are found more often in people with pancreatitis than in the general population, but the reason for this phenomenon is not understood. The backup of bile into the pancreatic duct may be the reason for pancreatitis associated with biliary tract disease, but the complete sequence of events is poorly understood. Cholestasis is probably part of the reason for the increased incidence of pancreatitis following abdominal surgery, but again, the exact mechanism is not clear. Trauma or surgery leading to damaged pancreatic tissue almost invariably causes some level of pancreatitis, because the pancreas is full of digestive enzymes that are extraordinarily destructive if inappropriately released. Abdominal pain, which often radiates to the back, but not chest pain, is the primary manifestation of acute pancreatitis, with pain ranging from mild to severe.

6 **The answer is C** *General principles / Immunology / Immunoglobulins*

Immunoglobulin IgE has a serum half-life of 2 days, making it the shortest-lived immunoglobulin. The low serum levels of this class of immunoglobulin are due to both a high affinity for mast cells and basophils and a low rate of synthesis. It is elevated in certain parasitic infections, such as *Ascaris* infections, and is not an agglutinating or complement-fixing antibody.

7 **The answer is D** *Gastrointestinal system / Microbiology / Antimicrobials and pseudomembranous colitis*

The patient is likely to have antibiotic-associated pseudomembranous colitis owing to *Clostridium difficile*, which are gram-positive bacilli (note the patient's diarrhea and deterioration following antibiotic therapy). Sigmoidoscopic examination, Gram stain of feces for white blood cells, testing for *C. difficile* toxin in the stool, and isolating the patient are appropriate. However, changing the antibiotic from a cephalosporin to clindamycin is inappropriate because *C. difficile* is not sensitive to clindamycin.

8 **The answer is C** *Hematopoietic and lymphoreticular system / Hematology / Chronic hemolytic anemia and iron overload*

Patients with a long-standing history of chronic hemolytic anemia (e.g., sickle cell disease or β-thalassemia major) generally have a substantially enlarged spleen, which exacerbates their condition by destroying abnormal but functional erythrocytes. Splenectomy, however, greatly increases the patient's susceptibility to infection by encapsulated organisms because the spleen is a major site of antigen presentation. Congestive heart failure can result from many factors, including iron overload, chronic high-output demand, and mild hypoxia. The heart rate is typically fast and has an enlarged stroke volume in an effort to increase tissue oxygenation. These increased demands are made in the presence of blood, which is poor at delivering oxygen to the overworked myocardium. Increased absorption and regular transfusions combine to cause fairly severe iron overload. Cardiac myocytes, particularly in the conducting system, undergo damage principally related to iron toxicity. The liver and pancreas are also susceptible to the effects of systemic iron excess. Emphysema is not related to iron toxicity, high-output cardiac failure, or chronic hypoxia.

9 **The answer is D** *General principles / Pharmacology / Cholinergic antagonists*

Scopolamine blocks muscarinic receptors, causing inhibition of all parasympathetic functions. It also prevents motion sickness. Nicotine, a ganglionic blocker, acts at the nicotinic receptors in the autonomic ganglia to depolarize ganglia, resulting in stimulation of ganglia followed by paralysis of all ganglia. Tubocurarine, gallamine, and pancuronium are nondepolarizing (competitive) blockers of the cholinergic transmission between motor nerve endings and the nicotinic receptors on the neuromuscular end plate of the skeletal muscle. Succinylcholine is a depolarizing neuromuscular blocking drug that attaches to the nicotinic receptor and acts like acetylcholine to depolarize the junction. However, unlike acetylcholine, succinylcholine persists at high concentrations at the synaptic cleft because it is resistant to acetylcholinesterase.

10 **The answer is C** *Renal/urinary system / Pathology / Membranous glomerulonephropathy*

Membranous glomerulonephropathy (MGN) is depicted via hematoxylin, eosin, and methenamine silver stains and is characterized by the deposition of subepithelial immune complex deposits (ICDs). Subepithelial ICDs may reduce the negative charge in the glomerular basement membrane (GBM) and injure podocytes, resulting in glomerular protein loss and nephrotic syndrome (i.e., proteinuria, lipiduria, hypoalbuminemia, hyperlipidemia, and edema). In the early stage of the disease, glomeruli have a normal appearance by light microscopy; they reflect the paucity and small size of the ICDs and the absence of the GBM reaction. When the disease progresses, the ICDs become more numerous and larger, leading to diffuse thickening of the GBM. The glomerular reaction to subepithelial ICDs (i.e., by production of a new basement membrane around individual ICDs) is represented on a silver stain (which stains the basement membrane) by spikes and later by domes and "train tracks."

There are primary (80%) and secondary (20%) forms of MGN. Primary (renal-limited) MGN is caused by GBM/podocyte autoantibodies and is associated with exclusive subepithelial ICDs that contain IgG and complement system protein, C3. In secondary forms of MGN, the glomerular disorder occurs in association with an extrarenal disease (e.g., lupus, malignant neoplasm, chronic viral hepatitis B, and drug reactions). Affected glomeruli have a predominance of subepithelial ICDs but may also have smaller numbers of mesangial or subendothelial ICDs; the ICDs may contain immunoglobulin classes other than IgG as well as both early classical (C1q, C4) and alternative pathway (properdin) complement proteins ("full house" pattern by immunofluorescence microscopy).

11 **The answer is C** *General principles / Pharmacology / Cholinergic agonists*

Isoflurophate covalently binds to acetylcholinesterase and irreversibly inhibits this enzyme. Edrophonium and neostigmine reversibly inhibit acetylcholinesterase. Carbachol, bethanechol, and pilocarpine are direct-acting, cholinergic agonists that are resistant to metabolism by acetylcholinesterase.

12 **The answer is C** *Central and peripheral nervous system / Microbiology / Bacterial meningitis*

The findings of fever, headache, nuchal rigidity, and lethargy with an acute onset and the lack of dramatic neurologic manifestations suggest acute bacterial meningitis. Viral meningitis causes much the same signs and symptoms, but the onset typically is more insidious and the patient usually is less acutely ill. Patients with viral encephalitis display the same general symptoms as those with viral meningitis, but encephalitis is differentiated by dramatic neurological manifestations and a much poorer prognosis. Fungal meningitis is more chronic and frequently is seen with other systemic signs of mycotic disease. Brain abscess usually is seen with other foci of infection, and the patient typically has deficits that reflect the location of the lesion.

13 **The answer is A** *Central and peripheral nervous system / Anatomy / Cranial nerves*

The optic nerve transmits the signal that light has been shown into the eye. Therefore, the left CN II is damaged and the right CN II is intact. Since both eyes constrict following light being shown into the right eye, the right CN II is intact. The left and right CN III are both undamaged, given that they both constrict following light stimulation of the right eye.

14 **The answer is E** *Central and peripheral nervous system / Pathology / Acute neurologic management; alcohol withdrawal*

The most important action to take with the ataxic and confused homeless man is to determine what, if any, brain injuries he may have sustained. The scalp wound can be managed with a bandage before suturing. If a fracture is suspected, skull films can be obtained after an acute neurologic condition has been ruled out. A serum ethanol level is indicated, and though important, it is not a priority. Hygiene is relevant but not urgent.

15 **The answer is B** *General principles / Genetics / Nucleotide repeat mutations*

Nucleotide repeat disorders have been described in promoter (myoclonus epilepsy), 5′ untranslated sequences (fragile X syndrome), introns (Friedereich ataxia), exons (Huntington's disease), and 3′ untranslated regions (myotonic dystrophy). Myoclonus epilepsy is actually a disease caused by repeat of a 12-mer sequence. These diseases are passed on to progeny in an x-linked dominant or autosomal dominant or recessive pattern.

16 **The answer is B** *Hematopoietic and lymphoreticular system / Pharmacology / Characteristics of warfarin*

Warfarin affects normal synthesis of clotting factors in the liver, and its coagulant effects can be reversed by vitamin K. It is well absorbed orally, and it will cross the placenta and may affect the fetus. It is used on a chronic basis for deep venous thrombosis and long-term care after postmyocardial infarction because its onset of action is slow. Another useful anticoagulant is heparin, which is a large, water-soluble polymer that must be given parenterally and does not cross the placenta. Heparin is primarily used for acute anticoagulant therapy because its onset of action is rapid. The effect of heparin can be reversed by the administration of protamine. The main action of heparin is thought to involve catalyzing the activation of antithrombin III in blood, thus inhibiting thrombin and factor Xa.

17 **The answer is D** *General principles / Biochemistry / Antioxidants*

A number of enzymes participate in the protection of red blood cells from insult by hydrogen peroxide. Glutathione peroxidase catalyzes the reduction of hydrogen peroxide to water. The reduced nicotinamide-adenine dinucleotide phosphate (NADPH) used by glutathione reductase to regenerate reduced glutathione is produced in the 6-phosphogluconate dehydrogenase reaction. Catalase results in the decomposition of hydrogen peroxide to water and molecular oxygen. Transketolase is a part of the nonoxidative phase of the hexose monophosphate shunt and has no known role in protecting red blood cells from oxygen insult. Pyruvate dehydrogenase is involved in the conversion of pyruvate to acetyl CoA. Nitric oxide synthase is involved in the production of nitric oxide and citrulline from arginine. Finally, cyclooxygenase converts arachidonic acid into prostaglandin H_2, the precursor for prostacyclin, prostaglandins, and thromboxanes.

18 **The answer is A** *General principles / Pharmacology / Zidovudine and treatment of AIDS*

Zidovudine (ZDV) remains an important agent for the palliation of AIDS. ZDV is phosphorylated to a deoxynucleoside derivative, which inhibits viral RNA-dependent DNA polymerase. Its selectivity is a function of its specificity for reverse transcriptase compared with human DNA polymerase. Granulocytopenia and anemia occur in up to 45% of treated patients, and resistance to the drug does occur after prolonged therapy. ZDV delays the development of signs and symptoms of AIDS in patients who are asymptomatic and improves the clinical symptoms of patients with AIDS at most stages in their disease. Thus, the incidence of opportunistic infections decreases, and there are some improvements in neurologic deficits and AIDS-associated thrombocytopenia, psoriasis, and lymphocytic interstitial pneumonia.

19 The answer is B *General principles / Physiology / Vascular permeability; inflammation*

Mast cell-derived serotonin increases vascular permeability by causing postcapillary venular contraction. ECF is a set of tetrapeptides that produces a chemotactic gradient to attract eosinophils but has no effect on vascular permeability. Prostaglandin E_2 by itself does not affect vascular permeability. Indeed, slow-reacting substances of anaphylaxis (leukotrienes C_4 and D_4) are the only eicosanoids that directly increase vascular permeability. IL-1, a sentinel cytokine, is not known to affect vascular permeability directly.

20 The answer is C *Respiratory system / Pathology / Chronic obstructive pulmonary disease*

Risk of COPD with various degrees of emphysema or chronic bronchitis is strongly associated with cigarette smoking and exposure to irritating substances in the environment (e.g., sulfur dioxide) or workplace (e.g., silica, cotton or grain dust, toluene diisocyanate). Usually it is associated with older age groups, especially individuals with pre-existing lung disease. A genetically linked deficiency in α_1-antitrypsin is strongly linked to premature obstructive pulmonary disease. Although intravenous drug abuse is associated with pulmonary complications, including acute respiratory failure and opportunistic infections accompanying immunodeficiency-like syndromes in certain individuals, it is not usually considered a risk factor for COPD.

21 The answer is C *Musculoskeletal system / Genetics / Duchenne's muscular dystrophy*

In Duchenne's muscular dystrophy, the amount of dystrophin (a 400-kilodalton protein of unknown function but thought to be involved in Ca^{2+} regulation) is reduced from its normal 0.002% of total protein. Derangement of Ca^{2+} homeostasis is thought to be the cause of the excessive shortening of the sarcomeres. The affected muscle groups hypertrophy because of replacement of muscle mass by fibrofatty tissue. Duchenne's muscular dystrophy is most often transmitted from a female carrier to the affected male ($\sim$1 per 3,500 liveborn males) by X-linked recessive inheritance (myotonic dystrophy is associated with mutations on chromosome 19), although approximately one-third of the cases appear to be caused by mutations that arise spontaneously.

22 The answer is C *Hematopoietic and lymphoreticular system / Pathology / Agnogenic myeloid metaplasia*

Bone marrow hypocellularity and teardrop-shaped erythrocytes are pathognomonic for agnogenic myeloid metaplasia with myelofibrosis. Leukocyte alkaline phosphatase levels are normal or elevated until the final stages of the disease. The liver does not usually undergo any significant change in size, whereas the spleen is almost always greatly enlarged, as it becomes the principal site of extramedullary hematopoiesis. Patients are often anemic because of both inadequate red blood cell production and pooling of red blood cells in the spleen.

23 The answer is D *General principles / Immunology / Group A streptococci*

The symptoms and clinical microbiology results indicate that the child has scarlet fever caused by a group A streptococcus (*Streptococcus pyogenes*) infection. This organism causes hemolysis by producing extracellular hemolysins, such as streptolysin O. Other important virulence factors of this organism include M protein, which is antiphagocytic and also helps to mediate adhesion; lipoteichoic acid, which also mediates adhesion; and a hyaluronic acid capsule. The erythrogenic toxins responsible for scarlet fever rash are not hemolytic.

24 The answer is D *General principles / Biostatistics / Odds ratio*

The odds ratio is one approach to comparing the frequency of exposure among cases and controls; it provides a measure of risk that is conceptually and mathematically similar to the relative risk. It is defined as the odds that a case is exposed divided by the odds that control is exposed with certain assumptions. This can be simplified to the number of cases exposed multiplied by the number of noncases not exposed divided by the product of the number of noncases exposed multiplied by the number of cases not exposed (AD/BC). If the frequency of exposure is higher among cases, the odds ratio will exceed 1, indicating risk. Thus, the stronger the association between exposure and disease, the higher the odds ratio. Conversely, if the frequency of exposures is lower among cases, the odds ratio will be less than 1, indicating protection.

25 **The answer is C** *General principles / Biostatistics / Cohort studies*

In a cohort study, a group of people (cohort), none of whom has experienced the outcome of interest, is assembled. People in the cohort are classified according to characteristics that may be related to the outcome. These people are observed over time to see which of them experience the outcome. A case series is a prevalence survey of a group of individuals with a particular disease performed at a single point in time. Case control studies compare the frequency of a purported risk factor in a group of cases and a group of controls. The case control design has the outcome of interest at the time that information on risk factors is sought.

26 **The answer is C** *Central and peripheral nervous system / Pharmacology / Alcohol withdrawal*

Physical dependence on alcohol implies that withdrawal of the depressant results in clinically significant physical and behavioral changes. Benzodiazepines are appropriate as a substitute for the depressive effects of alcohol while the acute physical symptoms are still active (approximately 5 to 7 days). Chlordiazepoxide, a commonly prescribed benzodiazepine, is a good choice based upon its intermediate half-life and long history of use. The drug should be prescribed at a sedative dose and tapered over a 5-day period so that the physician avoids exchanging one addiction for another. Phenytoin should not be routinely prescribed because seizures are an uncommon complication and, in the few cases involving seizures, the episode passed before adequate phenytoin levels were achieved. If the alcoholism coincides with clinically significant depression, nortriptyline may be appropriate in conjunction with appropriate counseling. However, nortriptyline is an antidepressant and is not directed at the delirium tremens. Haloperidol, a commonly prescribed antipsychotic, is not appropriate therapy for delirium tremens. Since morphine, a therapeutically useful narcotic analgesic, can be just as addictive as alcohol, it is certainly contraindicated.

27 **The answer is B** *General principles / Biostatistics / Confounding bias*

Confounding bias occurs when two factors are associated and the effect of one is distorted by the effect of the other. Serum triglycerides increasing risk of coronary heart disease but not independently of serum cholesterol is an example of confounding bias. It is not an independent cause of coronary heart disease but is confounded with other factors (e.g., serum cholesterol), which is an independent cause of coronary heart disease. A study design in which one person takes care of control animals and another tends experimental ones is subject to measurement bias because there may be a systematic difference in treatment between the two groups. The association between oral contraceptives and thrombophlebitis, owing to the way the history was reported, is also an example of measurement bias. An attempt to estimate the health of the general population in the United States from the responses of members of the American Medical Association is an example of selection bias, because its members may not provide a representative sample of the population of the United States.

28 **The answer is C** *General principles / Cell biology / Cell cycle*

The G_0 resting state of the cell cycle is a specialized, nongrowing state of the cell. The rate of protein synthesis is drastically reduced, often to as little as 20% of its value in proliferating cells. Slowly dividing cells can remain in G_0 state for weeks or years. In this state, the normal cells have lower levels of G_1 cyclins and cyclin-dependent kinases than cells in the G_1 phase of the cell cycle. Cells can enter G_0 after mitosis or from G_1, depending on the type of extracellular and intracellular signals received by the cell during G_1.

29 The answer is A *General principles / Biochemistry / Fatty acid synthesis*

Feedback inhibition of pathways is common throughout cellular metabolism. The ultimate product inhibits the committed step so that when sufficient product is available, the enzymatic sequence is completely stopped. This prevents energy from being lost by moving a substrate partly through the pathway. Enzyme phosphorylation in response to elevation of cAMP is also an important part of a variety of catabolic and anabolic pathways. Elevated levels of citrate indicate a high-energy status within the cell and therefore activate acetyl CoA carboxylase to increase fatty acid production. The enzymes that catalyze fatty acid synthesis exist as independent domains on one large polypeptide. This provides for the most efficient shuttling of substrate from one reaction to the next and obviates diffusion and random collision with the next enzyme. The acyl carrier protein is a pantothenic acid derivative that is covalently bound to the growing chain. Biotin is the main carrier of carboxyl groups in nearly every reaction that requires transfer of activated bicarbonate anions. Niacin is important in the biosynthesis of nicotinamide-adenine dinucleotide (NADH), which is essential for reactions that oxidize hydroxyl groups into carbonyl groups.

30 The answer is C *Gastrointestinal system / Pathology / Peptic ulcer disease*

Zollinger–Ellison syndrome was initially described in a person with refractory erosive peptic ulcer disease. Most cases involve a pancreatic islet cell tumor that secretes gastrin, which is the most potent physiologic stimulator of parietal cell acid production. Aggressive medical treatment is sometimes not sufficient to block the copious production of acid in these patients, and usually the gastrin-secreting tumor must be extracted surgically or treated medically. Increased vagal tone results in increased acid production, but vagal hyperactivity is rarely sufficient to account for acid production of this magnitude. Increased release of histamine also leads to hyperactivity of the parietal cells. However, histamine is produced by mast cells near the parietal cells, and mast cell tumors are not a common cause of Zollinger–Ellison syndrome. Pepsin is the proteolytic enzyme whose activation is pH-dependent; hypersecretion of pepsin is uncommon and, in any case, would not lead to the refractory ulcers in this patient. Decreased mucosal production is probably involved in many cases of peptic ulcer disease, most notably those induced by stress or NSAIDs. Locally produced prostaglandins are important in regulating the production of mucus by the cells lining the stomach, and stress as well as NSAIDs can inhibit prostaglandin production. However, peptic ulcer disease of this magnitude, particularly a condition that includes esophageal ulcers, cannot be caused by insufficient mucous production.

31 The answer is D *Central and peripheral system / Genetics / Mitochondrial DNA mutation*

Leber hereditary optic neuropathy is a rare disease caused by a mutation found in mitochondrial DNA. Ova contain large amounts of mitochondria, while sperm do not; therefore, the disease can be passed only from the mother to the children. During cell division, mitochondria and their DNA are randomly divided between cells; therefore, one ovum may contain the mutated DNA while another may not. This leads to an extremely variable pattern of disease manifestation and, while patients who develop this disease are rare, the presence of mutated DNA might be much higher than the occurrence of the disease might suggest.

32 The answer is A *Central and peripheral nervous system / Pathology / Generalized seizures*

Generalized absence (petit mal) seizures are seen almost exclusively in children. The seizures usually do not have a significant aura or postictal state but may consist of a few seconds of staring and altered mental status so brief that it escapes detection by untrained observers. Often, children are thought to be daydreaming when they are actually having a seizure.

33 The answer is A *Central and peripheral nervous system / Pathology / Multiple sclerosis*

The diagnosis for multiple sclerosis is primarily clinical, despite the variability in signs and symptoms. The following are well-proven guidelines for the diagnosis: (1) two separate central nervous system lesions, (2) two separate attacks of symptoms, (3) symptoms consistent with a white matter (myelin) lesion, (4) objective deficits on examination, (5) ages 10 to 50 years of age, (6) no other disease with similar symptoms.

34 **The answer is D** *Respiratory system / Physiology / Chronic bronchitis; emphysema*

Flow–volume curves from forced expiratory maneuvers provide useful information about the dynamic function of airways in health and disease. In the patient depicted in the figure, residual volume (and functional residual capacity) are elevated because of his underlying obstructive disease (bronchitis or emphysema). Loss of elastic recoil due to underlying disease and prolongation of expiration in association with obstruction usually lead to increased functional residual capacity and total lung capacity and a decrease in vital capacity. A common pathophysiologic finding is a reduction in the flow rate at all lung volumes during expiration.

35 **The answer is A** *Gastrointestinal system / Physiology / Gastric acid secretion*

The production of acid by parietal cells is regulated by the interplay of three main substances, histamine, gastrin, and acetylcholine, all of which can stimulate acid production. Parietal cells have receptors for all three signals, and each of the three signals can regulate release of the other signals independent of the parietal cell receptors. H_2-histamine receptor activation causes an elevation of cAMP, hence activation of cAMP-dependent protein kinases. Acetylcholine from the vagus nerve mediates its actions via muscarinic-type receptors. These muscarinic receptors, as well as their gastrin receptor analogues, mediate their signals through an elevation of free intracellular calcium. Acid production is a two-step process: In the first step, carbonic anhydrase splits the carbonic acid molecule into a bicarbonate anion and a hydrogen ion. In the second step, the movement of the bicarbonate anion into the blood causes the measurable and physiologically normal alkaline tide during meals (i.e., when the arterial pH increases slightly), and the hydrogen ion is pumped against a million-fold concentration gradient into the stomach by the hydrogen–potassium ATPase.

36 **The answer is D** *General principles / Microbiology / Neonatal sepsis*

The relative risk of a preterm child to develop sepsis is associated with birth weight. Approximately 10% of infants with a birth weight of 1,000 to 1,500 grams will develop neonatal sepsis. The risk of the development of neonatal sepsis increases to 35% for infants with a birth weight of less than 1,000 grams. Approximately 0.1% of full-term infants develop neonatal sepsis. Most of the cases of neonatal sepsis develop more than 3 days after birth (70%). The most common infectious cause of these cases of neonatal sepsis are gram-negative bacteria, which comprise somewhere in the range of 50% to 60% of cases. Gram-positive bacteria have been cultured from these cases in up to 30% of cases, while fungal infections occur at a rate of 2% to 3%. Simultaneous gram-positive and gram-negative infections are not common.

37 **The answer is D** *General principles / Pharmacology / Adrenergic blockers*

Prazosin produces a competitive block of α_1-receptors without blocking α_2-receptors. It is effective in the treatment of hypertension. Propranolol and atenolol are β-blockers and competitive antagonists. Propranolol blocks both the β_1- and β_2-receptors, whereas atenolol is a cardioselective β-blocker that preferentially blocks β_1-receptors. Cocaine, guanethidine, and reserpine affect neurotransmitter uptake or release. Cocaine blocks the Na + –K + -activated adenosine triphosphatase in the cellular membrane of the adrenergic neurons, which is required for cellular uptake of norepinephrine. Guanethidine inhibits the response of the adrenergic nerve to stimulation or to indirectly acting sympathomimetic amines by blocking the release of stored norepinephrine. Reserpine blocks the ability of adrenergic neurons to transport norepinephrine from the cytoplasm into storage vesicles. This causes depletion of norepinephrine in the adrenergic neuron, because monoamine oxidase in the neuron can degrade norepinephrine.

38 **The answer is D** *General principles / Immunology / Arthus reaction*

The Arthus reaction requires relatively large amounts of antibody and antigen, which form insoluble complexes and begin to accumulate endogenously. When the aggregates are large enough, the complement cascade is activated. The formation of complement fragments C3a and C5a causes an increase in vascular permeability with resultant edema. Neutrophils and platelets accumulate at the site of the reaction. The activated neutrophils release a host of proteases and collagenases, resulting in rupture of the vessel wall, hemorrhage, and local necrosis. Serum sickness is the most common type III reaction, and the Arthus reaction is the least common.

39 **The answer is B** *Endocrine system / Pathology / Cushing's syndrome*

Cushing's syndrome may be caused by hypothalamic or pituitary pathology (or both), adrenal adenoma (or carcinoma), and exogenous glucocorticoid administration. Children may have severe growth retardation before closure of the epiphysis during puberty. Hypersecretion of adrenocorticotropic hormone (ACTH) from the pituitary gland, due to either an underlying tumor or overstimulation from CRF of hypothalamic origin, stimulates the adrenal cortex to release excessive amounts of glucocorticoids and mineralocorticoids. Other sites of excessive ACTH secretion, including tumors of nonendocrine origin, may be important. A useful initial screen to detect Cushing's syndrome is to inject dexamethasone and monitor the expected suppression of cortisol (due to pituitary inhibition) in plasma the following day. Patients with various forms of Cushing's syndrome and a responsive adrenal cortex do not undergo the predicted suppression until considerably higher amounts of dexamethasone are administered. Subsequent tests, including urinary secretion and administration of metyrapone (cortisol synthesis inhibitor), and diagnostic procedures help to identify the source of the excessive cortisol production.

40 **The answer is D** *General principles / Biochemistry / Protein synthesis*

Protein synthesis occurs in both the cytoplasm and the mitochondria of cells and requires large amounts of energy. In addition to requiring ATP for the formation of aminoacyl tRNA, guanosine triphosphate is required for initiation, formation, translocation, and termination of the peptide bond. Protein synthesis requires messenger RNA (mRNA), tRNA, and ribosomal RNA (rRNA). Peptide bond formation involves the transfer of the nascent polypeptide chain from one tRNA to the amino group of another aminoacyl tRNA. This reaction is accomplished by the enzyme complex known as peptidyltransferase, which is an integral part of the 50S ribosomal subunits. Each tRNA binds a specific amino acid. This maintains the specificity of the genetic code whereby each codon always dictates the incorporation of the same amino acid.

41 **The answer is A** *Skin and related connective tissue / Pathology / Small artery with proliferative endarteropathy associated with systemic sclerosis*

Systemic sclerosis (scleroderma) is a systemic disorder characterized by excessive collagen deposition with diffuse forms (i.e., widespread cutaneous and widespread visceral involvement) and localized forms (i.e., limited cutaneous involvement and CREST [*c*alcinosis, *R*eynaud's phenomenon, *e*sophageal motility disorders, *s*clerodactyly, and *t*elangiectasia] syndrome). The immunologic hypothesis postulates that aberrant T lymphocyte activation results through cytokine production in recruitment of mast cells and macrophages, release of fibroblast chemotactic and growth factors, fibroblast activation, and fibrosis. The vascular hypothesis asserts that repeated cycles of endothelial cell injury followed by platelet aggregation result in intimal and periadventitial fibrosis, small vessel mural thickening and luminal narrowing, tissue ischemia, and fibrosis. Patients with renal involvement (67% of patients) have variable afferent arteriolar hypoperfusion, juxtaglomerular activation of the renin–angiotensin system, malignant hypertension, and acute renal failure (scleroderma renal crisis). These patients develop characteristic vascular changes of malignant hypertension (fibrinoid necrosis and thrombosis) associated with tissue infarction and thrombotic microangiopathic hemolytic anemia (anemia with schistocytes and thrombocytopenia).

42 **The answer is C** *Reproductive system / Pharmacology / Antibacterial drug use during pregnancy*

High levels of amoxicillin in the urine can be achieved because penicillins are eliminated mainly unmetabolized via the kidney. This and other penicillins carry minimal risk for the fetus, although these agents do cross the placental barrier. Sulfonamides should be avoided because of displacement of bilirubin from serum albumin and resultant deposition of bilirubin in the central nervous system (kernicterus) of the fetus and newborn, who do not yet have an intact blood–brain barrier. Minocycline should be avoided because tetracyclines are possibly teratogenic and can cause altered bone growth owing to high calcium binding. Gentamicin can damage the eighth nerve in the fetus, leading to hearing impairment.

43 **The answer is D** *Hematopoietic and lymphoreticular system / Immunology / Immunologic disorders*

Thymomas, 90% of which are benign, are associated with myasthenia gravis, systemic lupus erythematosus, hypogammaglobulinemia, neutrophil agranulocytosis, and polymyositis. The significance of the association with these diseases, in particular myasthenia gravis, remains obscure, although removal of the thymus sometimes leads to regression of this disease. Graves' disease is a thyroid disorder, but it is not known to be associated with thymomas. Addison's disease, which results from destruction of the adrenal glands, osteoarthritis, and rheumatoid arthritis, is also not associated with the development of thymomas.

44 **The answer is C** *General principles / Immunology / HIV*

HIV has a demonstrated ability to infect any cell with a CD4 receptor, which includes T-helper cells, macrophages, and a subset of brain cells. The virus particle attaches to the cell via the CD4 receptor and gains entry through membrane fusion; it does not require endocytosis. During replication, a large amount of viral glycoprotein is produced and it is integrated into the host cell membrane. This can lead to either a budding of new virus or fusion with another uninfected CD4+ cell. One infected cell can fuse in this fashion with a large number of uninfected cells, rendering them immunologically inactive.

45 **The answer is E** *Central and peripheral nervous system / Neuroanatomy / Brain function evaluation*

The copying of a design requires many areas of the brain, namely, the visual or occipital cortex, the parietal association areas, and the prefrontal and frontal cortices. The ability to match an item in one hand with the same item in the opposite hand while blindfolded is a test for intact corpus callosum function. The repetition of digits exercise tests for attention and requires an intact reticular activating system in the pons and midbrain. Interpretation of proverbs requires intact higher cortical functions, namely the analytic and conceptual skills based in the prefrontal cortex. The serial 7s subtraction test depends on the calculating abilities in the left parietal lobe and recall of mathematical facts in memory storage areas.

46 **The answer is E** *General principles / Microbiology / Antibiotic therapy*

Gentamicin is effective against *Pseudomonas aeruginosa* infections. *Brucella* inside phagocytic cells is protected from antibodies and many antibiotics. *Legionella* is a facultative intracellular pathogen of monocytes and macrophages against which gentamicin is ineffective. *Legionella* is most commonly treated with erythromycin. *Rickettsia* is an obligate intracellular pathogen and, as such, is resistant to gentamicin treatment. It is commonly treated with vancomycin or chloramphenicol. *Chlamydia trachomatis* cannot synthesize ATP or oxidize the reduced form of NADH and is an obligate intracellular parasite. *Chlamydia* organisms are internalized by host cells but evade destruction by preventing lysosomal fusion with the phagosome. *Chlamydia* infections can be treated with tetracyclines, erythromycin, sulfonamides, sulfamethoxazole–trimethoprim, or rifampin.

47 **The answer is B** *General principles / Cell biology / Viruses*

A virus is a cellular parasite and therefore cannot reproduce itself. A virus must infect a host cell and use the host cell's transcription machinery to replicate itself. The infectious viral particle, known as a virion, consists of either RNA or DNA (not both) and is surrounded by a protein shell known as a capsid. A virus interacts with a host cell by binding to a specific cellular receptor and transferring its genetic material into the host. The virus can then manipulate the host's transcription machinery to allow synthesis and replication of its own viral proteins.

48 **The answer is D** *General principles / Cell biology / Prokaryotes and eukaryotes*

Both prokaryotic and eukaryotic cells are surrounded by a phospholipid bilayer to form a plasma membrane. The internal membranes in prokaryotic cells are all connected to the outer plasma membrane, whereas eukaryotic cells contain extensive internal membranes that are unconnected. These internal membranes of eukaryotes enclose subcellular structures known as organelles. The outer plasma membrane acts as a barrier to the cell, which allows only certain substances to enter (e.g., oxygen, carbon dioxide, water). To obtain the essential macromolecules, a cell must use membrane transporters that allow substances (e.g., inorganic ions, sugars, and amino acids) to permeate the cell. Prokaryotic cellular DNA is in the form of a single, circular molecule within a single chromosome. In contrast, eukaryotic DNA is a single, linear, double-stranded molecule divided between two or more chromosomes contained in a membrane-bound nucleus.

49 **The answer is B** *General principles / Cell biology / β-Adrenergic receptors*

β-Adrenergic receptors bind catecholamines (e.g., epinephrine and isoproterenol) to activate adenylate cyclase and elevate levels of cAMP within a cell. There are two types of β-adrenergic receptors: typically β_1- and β_2-receptors. β_1-Receptors bind catecholamines, and the order of affinities is isoproterenol > norepinephrine > epinephrine, whereas the affinities for the β_2-receptors are isoproterenol > epinephrine > norepinephrine. β_1-Receptors are located on cardiac muscle cells, whereas β_2-receptors are typically found on smooth muscle cells in bronchial airways. Upon agonist binding, β_1-receptors induce increased heart rate and contractility. This effect can be blocked by antagonists (e.g., practolol, a known β-blocker) to slow heart contractions in patients with cardiac arrhythmias and angina. β_2-Agonists (e.g., terbutaline) open air passages in patients with asthma by relaxing bronchial smooth muscle.

50 **The answer is A** *General principles / Cell biology / Transcription*

Many protein transcription factors are required to form a preinitiation complex at the TATA box to initiate RNA polymerase II transcription. However, only TFIID binds directly to the TATA box region of the DNA. This transcription factor must bind to the TATA box first, forming a stable complex between TFIID and the DNA. A second transcription factor, TFIIB, then binds to RNA polymerase II and associates with the DNA at the TFIID–TATA box site. TFIIB acts as an ATPase, which induces melting of the DNA to form an open complex. Transcription then begins in the presence of TFIIE and is assisted in elongation by the transcription factor TFIIS.

test 10

Questions

Directions: *Single best answer questions consist of numbered items or incomplete statements followed by answers or by completions of the statement. Select the ONE lettered answer or completion that is BEST in each case.*

1 Which school of family therapy is associated with the technique of clarification of transgenerational relationship patterns?

(A) Behavioral–psychoeducational approaches
(B) Structural–strategic approaches
(C) Intergenerational–experiential approaches
(D) Sociobiological approaches

2 Based on the accompanying figure, which of the following statements accurately describes events in the cell cycle?

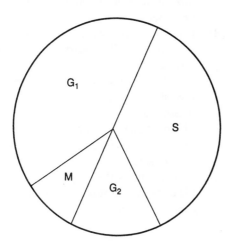

(A) Cytokinesis occurs at the end of the G_2 phase
(B) Replication of nuclear DNA occurs during the M phase
(C) G_1 phase is the interval between completion of nuclear division and the beginning of DNA synthesis
(D) Nuclear division leading to the moment of cell division occurs during G_2 phase
(E) A DNA damage checkpoint occurs at the transition between the late M and early G_1 (M/G_1) phase

3 Benzodiazepines are antianxiety medications that can be used for various purposes. Which of the following benzodiazepines is used to treat seizures?

(A) Clonazepam
(B) Amitriptyline
(C) Clomipramine
(D) Midazolam
(E) Oxazepam

4 Which of the following statements about immunoglobulin (Ig) classes is correct?

(A) IgD antibodies against IgG are present in high titers in many patients with rheumatoid arthritis
(B) IgG cannot cross the placenta
(C) IgM, frequently found as a pentamer, cannot efficiently activate the complement cascade
(D) IgA is found in mucosal secretions from the breast, gut, and respiratory tract
(E) IgE mediates type II hypersensitivity by activating mast cells and basophils

5 The biopsy depicted in Figure 48 in the color plate section is from a 60-year-old man with hemoptysis and palpable purpura on his lower extremities and trunk. Evaluation revealed new-onset hypertension, microscopic hematuria, azotemia (creatinine: 6.5 mg/dL), and normal serum complement levels. Which of the following is the most likely explanation for this patient's symptoms and laboratory values?

(A) Seropositivity for antinuclear antibodies
(B) Seropositivity of streptolysin-O antibodies
(C) Seropositivity for antineutrophil cytoplasmic antibodies
(D) Immune complex deposit-mediated disorder

6 A 22-year-old man complains of a urethral discharge and urethral itching. The patient claims to have had only one sexual partner in the past 3 years, but he has had similar symptoms on two other occasions during this period. The discharge is noted to be whitish. The result of the Gram stain is negative; however, leukocytes are present. The patient is told that he has nongonococcal urethritis and is given a prescription for penicillin. Which of the following statements is correct?

(A) The infection is always accompanied by conjunctivitis, polyarthritis, and genital infection in chronic cases

(B) The sexual partner need not be examined, because women are rarely asymptomatic carriers

(C) The selected antibiotic is appropriate for this case

(D) The organism that most likely causes this disease can produce serious complications, including death, in women

(E) The organism that is most likely causing this disease is an extracellular pathogen

7 Which of the following diseases is properly matched with its most common type of genetic mutation?

(A) Duchenne's muscular dystrophy—point mutation

(B) Cystic fibrosis—large coding sequence deletion

(C) Fragile X—mitochondrial DNA mutation

(D) Huntington's disease—unbalanced translocation

(E) Tay–Sach's—trinucleotide repeat expansion

8 During mitosis, which of the following events occurs at anaphase?

(A) The nuclear envelope begins to break down

(B) Chromosomes align halfway between the spindle poles

(C) Mitotic spindle begins to form

(D) The two sister chromatids separate into independent chromosomes

(E) The nucleolus becomes visible again

9 An air-conditioner repairman presents to his primary care physician (PCP) with complaints of shortness of breath and flu-like symptoms that have been present for more than 2 weeks. A chest x-ray is performed that shows alveolar infiltrates. Cultures of lung sputum grow microorganisms that are gram-negative, catalase-positive, and motile. Stool cultures are positive for the same microorganism. What is correct diagnosis?

(A) Klebsiella pneumonia

(B) *Escherichia coli* pneumonia

(C) Legionella pneumonia

(D) Staphylococcus pneumonia

(E) Streptococcal pneumonia

10 Bioterrorism and political unrest have brought about renewed and heightened concerns about so-called nerve gases such as sarin. Which of the following statements is correct?

(A) Prompt administration of atropine and pralidoxime are still contemporary therapeutic approaches

(B) Concerns about sarin are unfounded because it is not readily absorbed in the lungs or through the skin

(C) Anticholinergics such as atropine are useful in reversing respiratory muscle paralysis in sarin poisoning

(D) The quaternary amine, pralidoxime, is useful in counteracting the central nervous system effects of sarin

(E) Pralidoxime is the only therapy available for the delayed neurotoxicity that may accompany surviving sarin

11 A 6-year-old boy is brought to the emergency department by his mother. He has a fever and a petechial hemorrhage on his ankles and wrists. He is admitted directly to the pediatric intensive care unit. A blood culture is taken and a rapid Gram stain is performed. What would be seen on microscopic examination?

(A) Single-cell bacterium without a cell wall

(B) Gram-negative rods

(C) Gram-negative diplococci

(D) Gram-positive cocci in groups

(E) Gram-positive diplococci in strands

12 A 15-year-old boy develops insulin-dependent diabetes mellitus (IDDM). His parents want to know the risk of their other children developing diabetes. Use the accompanying pedigree.

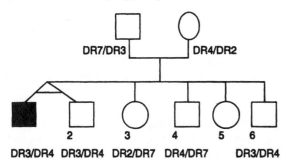

Which of the following is the risk for the proband's sister for whom no human leukocyte antigen (HLA) typing is available (II-5)?

(A) 2%
(B) 5%
(C) 20%
(D) 50%
(E) 100%

13 A 35-year-old HIV-positive man presents to his local emergency department with a stiff neck, confusion, and vomiting. A spinal tap was performed and encapsulated yeast was visualized. What is the proper treatment?

(A) Fluconazole
(B) 5-Flurocytosine
(C) Amphotericin B
(D) Amphotericin B and 5-fluorocytosine, then fluconazole
(E) Fluconazole and 5-fluorocytosine

14 A 47-year-old obese white man goes to the emergency department with a swollen and very painful right toe. He has no recollection of injuring his foot. Plasma urate levels are greatly elevated. Which of the following is the most likely diagnosis?

(A) Lyme disease
(B) Septic arthritis
(C) Rheumatoid arthritis
(D) Osteoarthritis (degenerative joint disease)
(E) Gout

15 Which of the following statements about heavy-metal toxicity is true?

(A) The inorganic form of tin is commonly used in pesticides
(B) Lead exposure has produced epidemic levels of disease in preschool children; with chronic exposure, lead causes cognitive impairment, language dysfunction and, when severe, mental retardation
(C) Tin uncouples oxidation and phosphorylation in glycolysis
(D) Chronic exposure to arsenic vapors leads to neurologic symptoms, including insomnia, excitability, memory loss, and seizures
(E) The kidney is highly resistant to cadmium toxicity

16 The patient whose renal biopsy is shown in Figure 49 from the color plate section stained by hematoxylin and eosin and Fraser–Lendrum (fibrin) stains presented with fever, headache, stiff neck, and altered sensorium. She was hypotensive and had petechial hemorrhages on physical examination. Bacteria were found within neutrophils in the peripheral blood and in the cerebrospinal fluid (CSF). The patient died within 24 hours of presentation, and an autopsy was performed. Which of the following laboratory findings is likely to be associated with this woman's clinical presentation and subsequent death?

(A) Gram-positive sepsis
(B) Fibrin split products
(C) Thrombocytosis
(D) Elevated plasma fibrinogen levels

17 The best treatment for a patient with lead poisoning is

(A) flumazenil
(B) pralidoxime
(C) deferoxamine
(D) dimercaprol
(E) naloxone

18 Which of the following statements concerning the role of luteinizing hormone (LH) in ovulation is correct?

(A) LH levels peak in luteal phase
(B) LH directly mediates endometrial vasospasm before the onset of menses
(C) LH stimulates androstenedione production in granulosa cells
(D) LH secretion is controlled by estrogen levels
(E) LH decreases progesterone production during the midcycle

19 A 27-year-old woman who is 2 months postpartum has weakness that has worsened over several weeks and progressed from the legs to the trunk and then to the arms and face. The weakness is hyporeflexive but there is no significant sensory loss. The best diagnosis is

(A) myasthenia gravis
(B) Lambert–Eaton myasthenic syndrome
(C) Guillain–Barré syndrome
(D) syphilis

20 Which of the following enzyme deficiencies in the steroid hormone synthesis pathway causes pseudo-hermaphroditism in a 46(XX) individual?

(A) 17α-Hydroxylase
(B) 21-Hydroxylase
(C) 17,20-Lyase
(D) 17β-Hydroxysteroid dehydrogenase
(E) Cholesterol side chain cleavage enzyme

21 An elderly man wakes up with severe pain from a swollen ankle. Fluid drained from the ankle is cloudy and hypercellular. Polarizing light analysis reveals numerous negatively birefringent crystals. Which of the following is the most likely diagnosis?

(A) Septic arthritis
(B) Osteoarthritis (degenerative joint disease)
(C) Lyme disease
(D) Reiter's syndrome
(E) Gout

22 Which of the following statements concerning glucose-6-phosphatase deficiency is true?

(A) It is more common in adults than in children
(B) It often causes hypoglycemia and hepatomegaly
(C) It often causes hypouricemia and splenomegaly
(D) It is a lysosomal storage disease
(E) Pathologic findings are rare in liver biopsies

23 The serum electrolytes for a patient who is being treated for lung cancer are notable for elevated calcium levels. Which of the following best supports the fact that the malignancy is causing the hypercalcemia?

(A) Increased levels of calcitriol
(B) Increased levels of parathyroid hormone (PTH)
(C) Decreased levels of PTH-related protein
(D) Increased serum phosphorus
(E) A calcium level that is even higher than that seen in primary hyperparathyroidism

24 Which one of the following statements accurately describes vitamin D?

(A) Conversion to the active form 25-hydroxyvitamin D in the liver depends on stimulation by PTH
(B) Conversion to the active form 1,25-dihydroxyvitamin D is regulated primarily by substrate availability and occurs in the distal tubules of the kidney
(C) Vitamin D is water-soluble
(D) The vitamin D receptor is located on the plasma membrane
(E) A major function of vitamin D is to increase the absorption of calcium and decrease the absorption of phosphorus in the intestine
(F) Vitamin D stimulates the secretion of PTH
(G) Although vitamin D is commonly converted to its active form in the kidney, it can also be activated in macrophages

25 A patient complains of headaches, and the physician notes that she seems nervous and is sweating profusely. On physical examination the physician initially finds that the patient has orthostatic hypotension. When the blood pressure measurement is repeated, the patient is found to be hypertensive. Her history includes medullary carcinoma of the thyroid, for which she had surgery several years ago. Which one of the following statements is correct?

(A) The patient likely has multiple endocrine neoplasia (MEN) syndrome type I

(B) The physician should check her cortisol level because she likely has a pheochromocytoma

(C) The patient should take a nonsteroidal anti-inflammatory drug, and no further evaluation is needed

(D) A 24-hour urinary excretion of epinephrine, norepinephrine, and their metabolites would be more useful in this case than the current plasma values of these substances

(E) Computed tomography (CT) with intravenous contrast material should be performed immediately

(F) No defects are seen in the adrenal glands on CT; therefore, the patient does not have a pheochromocytoma

26 Phospholipids are transported from the cytoplasmic leaflet of the endoplasmic reticulum (ER) to the exoplasmic leaflet by which one of the following processes?

(A) Spontaneous flipping from one leaflet to another

(B) Membrane budding

(C) Phospholipid exchange proteins

(D) Flippase protein

27 Which one of the following enzyme deficiencies is matched to the correct outcome?

(A) 3-β-Dehydrogenase deficiency—increased cortisol production and decreased androgen production

(B) 21-Hydroxylase deficiency decreased—cortisol production and increased aldosterone deficiency

(C) 17,20-Desmolase deficiency—normal cortisol production and decreased aldosterone production

(D) Aromatase—decreased cortisol production and increased androgen production

(E) 18-Hydroxylase deficiency—decreased cortisol production and increased aldosterone production

(F) 17-α-Hydroxylase deficiency—decreased cortisol production and increased deoxycorticosterone and corticosterone production

28 In the United States, the most common tumor in men is found in which one of the following organs?

(A) Kidney
(B) Colon
(C) Prostate gland
(D) Liver
(E) Testis

29 Correct statements concerning toxic exposure to organophosphates include which one of the following?

(A) Aminophylline is the agent of first choice in reversing the respiratory symptoms

(B) Atropine and pralidoxime are useful antidotes

(C) Exposure must be inhalational, since organophosphates are not well-absorbed through the skin

(D) Immediate injection of epinephrine is a useful antidote

30 In general, tolerance to self-antigens exists, even if the antigens are not expressed in the thymus. For example, antigens on the pancreatic islet cells produce insulin. Which of the following statements is a reasonable explanation for this?

(A) Pancreatic antigens are shed and are transported to the thymus via the circulation; at the thymus, they are associated with the major histocompatibility complex (MHC) and induce positive selection of immature T cells

(B) Immature CD4 + CD8 + thymic T cells are transported to the pancreas, where they undergo negative selection; they then return to the thymus for final maturation

(C) Mature T cells circulate to the pancreas, recognize pancreatic antigen in context of self-MHC, which stimulates them via the T cell receptor; however, no interleukin-1 is produced, so T cells are inactivated

(D) T cell progenitors in the bone marrow circulate to the pancreas before being transported to the thymus; they undergo negative selection at the pancreas and then proceed to the thymus, where T cell differentiation occurs

31 Which of the following statements about the disease represented by the cystoprostatectomy specimen in Figure 50 of the color plate section is correct?

(A) Smoking is not a risk factor

(B) Low-grade lesions are infrequently missed by urinary cytology

(C) Clinical investigation for upper tract involvement is the standard of care, particularly in patients with multiple lower tract lesions

(D) Squamous cell carcinoma is the most likely histologic subtype for this tumor

32 Which of the following statements accurately matches the developmental milestone with the appropriate age range if the child is progressing normally?

(A) Successfully reaches for objects not in the immediate range of grasp at 0 to 2 months of age

(B) Can use two- and three-word phrases at 1 to 3 years of age

(C) Can group objects on the basis of common features; understands that mass or volume is conserved despite a change in shape or form (i.e., fixed volume of water is the same regardless of whether it is in a tall glass or a short glass) at 3 years of age

(D) Begins to fear strangers at 0 to 3 months of age

33 Which of the following structural motifs is important for the transcriptional activation produced by some steroid-bound hormone receptors?

(A) Zinc fingers

(B) EF hands

(C) β-Pleated sheets

(D) Immunoglobulin folds

(E) Gly-X-Y repeats

34 Which of the following statements is correct concerning retroviruses?

(A) Each viral particle contains one copy of the retroviral genome

(B) The particles contain an RNA-dependent RNA polymerase

(C) Integration into the host genome is not essential for viral replication

(D) The retroviral group antigens are highly reactive between strains

(E) The RNA has minus polarity

35 Which one of the following drugs is a barbiturate?

(A) Diazepam

(B) Thiopental

(C) Lorazepam

(D) Ethanol

(E) Buspirone

(F) Hydroxyzine

36 Topoisomerase enzymes are important in the replication of DNA because they

(A) anneal Okazaki fragments

(B) relax supercoiled DNA

(C) degrade histone proteins

(D) "proofread" newly synthesized DNA

(E) synthesize the RNA primer fragment

37 Which of the following statements about the termination of messenger RNA (mRNA) translation is true?

(A) It is recognized by the stop signal codon AUG

(B) It requires the aid of RNA polymerase II

(C) The complete polypeptide is released

(D) It is followed by degradation of the two ribosomal subunits

(E) It does not require guanosine triphosphate (GTP) hydrolysis

38 Which of the following situations is an example of negative reinforcement?

(A) A woman buys new clothes each time she loses 10 lb of excess body weight

(B) A boy stops teasing his sister when she no longer chases him in response to the teasing

(C) A teenager washes the dishes to avoid losing her driving privileges

(D) A man obeys the speed limit while driving to work after his fifth speeding ticket

39 Which of the following defense mechanisms is correctly defined?

(A) Projection—mental processes are separated to different identities

(B) Sublimation—feelings are transferred to an unassociated object or person

(C) Dissociation—unacceptable feelings or desires are expressed in socially appropriate ways

(D) Splitting—events or people are categorized as entirely good or bad due to refusal to accept ambiguity

(E) Displacement—one's own desires are seen as being another's

40 A 10-year-old boy with type I diabetes mellitus has vomiting and abdominal pain. His glucose level was tested after a large meal, and it was elevated. He appears dehydrated and is breathing with sighing respirations. Which one of the following statements is correct?

(A) Although hypokalemia is a concern in this patient, the physician does not need to worry about diabetic ketoacidosis (DKA) because that only occurs in type II diabetes mellitus

(B) This patient took too much insulin

(C) Initial laboratory results indicate that his potassium level is within normal limits; therefore, the physician can proceed with the treatment without risk of causing hypokalemia

(D) If the patient is mildly acidotic, a single bolus of bicarbonate should be given to correct the acid–base imbalance

(E) This patient's condition could not have been prevented because it is an inevitable complication of type I diabetes mellitus

(F) Rehydration can be started before the patient is given any insulin

41 Given the following blood types of a couple planning to have children, which of the following must be an offspring of the couple?
Mother: AB, MN, Rh −
Father: O, MN, Rh −

(A) O, MN, Rh −

(B) O, M, Rh −

(C) AB, MN, Rh −

(D) B, MN, Rh −

(E) B, MN, Rh +

42 A woman at 8 weeks' gestation of her first pregnancy is in an automobile accident and requires a blood transfusion. Her blood type is determined to be A, MN, Rh −. She thinks that the fetus's father is Rh +. Which of the following blood types is best suited for transfusion into this patient?

(A) A, MN, Rh +

(B) AB, M, Rh −

(C) B, MN, Rh −

(D) O, MN, Rh −

(E) AB, MN, Rh −

43 A new patient complains of loss of balance and reports a diagnosis of pernicious anemia from his previous PCP. You confirm the diagnosis by looking at the peripheral blood smear. Which of the following do you see under the microscope?

(A) Psammoma bodies

(B) Microcytic, hypochromic red blood cells

(C) Hypersegmented granulocytes and megaloblastic red blood cells

(D) Helmet cells

44 Which of the following is a probable mechanism for the development of pernicious anemia?

(A) Folate deficiency

(B) Overabundance of intrinsic factor

(C) Iron deficiency

(D) Thyroid hormone deficiency

(E) Vitamin B_{12} deficiency caused by depleted intrinsic factor

45 Patients with hereditary retinoblastomas have several hundred-fold greater risk than the general population of developing what other type of cancer?

(A) Chrondroblastoma
(B) Fibrous histiocytoma
(C) Glioblastoma multiforme
(D) Medulloblastoma
(E) Osteosarcoma

46 Which statement places the cellular event in the correct intracellular location?

(A) O-linked glycosylation and acylation and sorting of many proteins occur in the ER
(B) Translation of hexokinase occurs in the rough ER
(C) Transcription of mRNA occurs in the nucleolus
(D) The lysosome is the ultimate destination for proteins with mannose 6-phosphate signals
(E) Translation of proteins with signal sequences occurs on cytosolic ribosomes

47 An 80-year-old man with a progressive dementia, diagnosed with Alzheimer's disease, dies in his sleep. The family requests an autopsy. Which of the following neuropathologic findings is most likely to be found in the histologic sections?

(A) Prions
(B) Hippocampal neurofibrillary tangles
(C) Multinucleated giant cells
(D) Argentophilic intraneuronal inclusions
(E) Lewy bodies

48 A 28-year-old who has been hospitalized with AIDS dies. An autopsy is performed. Which of the following findings is the most likely neuropathologic feature?

(A) Hippocampal neurofibrillary tangles
(B) Amyloid plaques
(C) Argentophilic intraneuronal inclusions
(D) Lewy bodies
(E) Multinucleated giant cells

49 A 68-year-old man with bradykinesia and tremor is diagnosed with Parkinson's disease. Which of the following neuropathologic features would be expected in a section of his hippocampus?

(A) Lewy bodies
(B) Hippocampal neurofibrillary tangles
(C) Argentophilic intraneuronal inclusions, or Pick's bodies
(D) Prions
(E) Multinucleated giant cells

50 A young woman with anorexia nervosa is determined to be in late starvation (>3 weeks). Which of the following findings would be expected?

(A) Increased protein breakdown
(B) Increased gluconeogenesis
(C) Increased cardiac output
(D) Decreased levels of follicle-stimulating hormone and LH
(E) Decreased fatty acid oxidation
(F) Increased resting energy expenditure

Answer Key

1-C	11-C	21-E	31-C	41-D
2-C	12-B	22-B	32-B	42-D
3-A	13-D	23-E	33-A	43-C
4-D	14-E	24-G	34-D	44-E
5-C	15-B	25-D	35-B	45-E
6-D	16-B	26-D	36-B	46-D
7-A	17-D	27-F	37-C	47-B
8-D	18-D	28-C	38-C	48-E
9-C	19-C	29-B	39-D	49-A
10-A	20-B	30-C	40-F	50-D

Answers and Explanations

1 **The answer is C** *General principles / Behavioral science / Family therapies*

The family therapies can be roughly divided into three schools. The behavioral–psychoeducational approaches are grounded in social learning theory and often instruct patients in the principles of this theory during treatment. The structural–strategic therapies view family problems as misguided and dysfunctional attempts to adapt to life circumstances. Clarification of relationship patterns, such as alliances and coalitions, and cognitive reframing are techniques associated with these therapies. The intergenerational–experiential therapies view family problems as rooted in the family's fixation at a particular stage of development; therapy attempts to discover the cause of this fixation by examining transgenerational patterns and elaborating the family's identity.

2 **The answer is C** *General principles / Cell biology / Cell cycle*

The cell cycle is divided into several distinct phases. Replication of the nuclear DNA usually occupies only a portion of interphase, called the S phase of the cell cycle. The interval between the end of DNA synthesis and the beginning of mitosis is the G_2 phase. The G_2 phase provides a safety gap, allowing the cell to ensure that DNA replication is complete before going into mitosis. Mitosis, or M phase, is the next phase. Nuclear division occurs during this phase, leading up to the moment of cell division. The interval between the completion of mitosis and the beginning of DNA synthesis is the G_1 phase. During the G_1 phase, the cell monitors its environment and its own size; when the time is right, the cell takes the step that commits it to DNA replication and completion of the division cycle. DNA damage checkpoints occur at the G_1/S transition, the S phase, and the G_2/M transition point. Phases S, G_2, M, and G_1 are the subdivisions of the standard cell cycle.

3 **The answer is A** *Central and peripheral nervous system / Pharmacology / Antianxiety medication*

Clonazepam has an intermediate length of action and is used to treat absence seizures and panic disorders. Midazolam is used as an anesthetic and has a short duration of action. Oxazepam also is short-acting but is used in the treatment of alcohol withdrawal. Amitriptyline and clomipramine are heterocyclic antidepressants, not benzodiazepines. Amitriptyline is used to treat depression accompanied by insomnia, whereas clomipramine is used to treat obsessive–compulsive disorder.

4 **The answer is D** *General principles / Immunology / Immunoglobulin properties*

IgA is especially important in defending against enteric pathogens, and IgE-mediated hypersensitivity results in allergic rhinitis. The biologic significance of IgD remains obscure. It has no properties that set it apart from any other Ig, and it has not yet been implicated in any specific disease states. IgM antibodies against IgG are known as rheumatoid factors and are frequently seen in various autoimmune-related diseases. IgG is the main serum antibody, and it remains elevated long after the antigen has disappeared. IgM is the first responder in the body's production of humoral immunity and is found in the highest titers during the first 10 days following antigen presentation.

5 **The answer is C** *Skin and related connective tissue / Pathology / Pauci-immune, necrotizing, leukocytoclastic small vessel vasculitis*

This small vessel has concentric fibrin deposition in the inner wall adjacent to the lumen, surrounded by a mixed inflammatory infiltrate containing histiocytes, neutrophils, and cellular debris. There are immune complex-mediated (e.g., Henoch–Schönlein purpura) and pauci-immune forms of small vessel leukocytoclastic vasculitis. The pauci-immune forms are commonly associated with circulating antineutrophil cytoplasmic autoantibodies (ANCA). Primed neutrophils exposed to ANCA undergo complement-independent degranulation with release of hydrolytic enzymes and free radical oxygen; in the microcirculation, this results in leukocytoclastic small vessel vasculitis and frequently necrotizing or crescentic glomerulonephritis. The major ANCA-mediated systemic vasculitides include microscopic polyangiitis and Wegener's granulomatosis. Microscopic polyangiitis is associated with antimyeloperoxidase antibodies [perinuclear (p)-ANCA] and typically involves small vessels of the skin, mucous membranes, lungs, brain, heart, gastrointestinal tract, kidneys, muscle, and/or nerves. Wegener's granulomatosis is associated with antiproteinase 3 antibodies [cytoplasmic (c)-ANCA] and characteristically presents with upper and/or lower respiratory tract and/or renal involvement and necrotizing granulomatous vasculitis.

6 **The answer is D** *Reproductive system / Microbiology / Chlamydia*

Chlamydia trachomatis is the most common cause of nongonococcal urethritis. This organism exists in two forms: (1) reticulate bodies, which are the metabolically active intracellular form, and (2) elementary bodies, which are the extracellular infectious form. The organism is spread by sexual contact, and it may exist in asymptomatic women. Untreated carriers may continue to reinfect their partners. In some men, the disease may cause a triad of symptoms, including conjunctivitis, polyarthritis, and genital infection, known as Reiter's syndrome. It is also capable of causing serious harm to women, including salpingitis and pelvic inflammatory disease, which can lead to infertility, ectopic pregnancy, and death. Tetracycline and other antibiotics (e.g., erythromycin, doxycycline) that can penetrate into eukaryotic cells are appropriate treatments, because this organism is metabolically active only inside cells.

7 **The answer is A** *General principles / Genetics / Genetic mutations*

The most common genetic mutation responsible for Duchenne's muscular dystrophy and cystic fibrosis are point mutations in the dystrophin gene and cystic fibrosis transmembrane conductance regulator (CFTR) gene. Fragile X is caused by a trinucleotide repeat expansion in the 5′ untranslated region of the FMR-1 gene. Huntington's disease is also a trinucleotide repeat expansion disease with the expansion found in one of the exons of the Huntington gene. Tay–Sach's disease is associated with several single mutations, polymorphism and complex mutations of the hexosaminidase A gene.

8 **The answer is D** *General principles / Cell biology / Mitosis*

Cellular genetic material is equally distributed during cell division by mitosis, which is divided into several stages: prophase, metaphase, anaphase, and telophase. During early prophase, centrioles begin moving toward opposite poles of the cell as the nuclear membrane begins to disaggregate. As the cell reaches middle and late prophase, chromosomes are condensed and can be visualized as two chromatids joined at the centromeres. Microtubular spindles also begin to form. In metaphase, the chromosomes move toward the equator of the cell. The two sister chromatids separate into independent chromosomes at anaphase (not at telophase). Each chromatid contains a centromere bound by a spindle fiber that links the chromatid to the pole of the cell to which it will migrate. As the cell elongates, cytokinesis begins and a cleavage furrow forms. At telophase, two new daughter cells are formed, each containing one copy of each chromosome, and the nucleolus becomes visible again.

9 **The answer is C** *General principles / Microbiology / Legionella pneumonia*

This patient should be diagnosed with legionella pneumonia. Legionella are commonly cultured from sites of standing water and the patient's history of work surrounding areas of standing water is a risk factor. In infected individuals, legionella can be cultured from a variety of lung cultures but may also be positive in stool cultures. Legionellae are gram-negative, catalase-positive, motile rods with polar or lateral flagella. Most species produce beta-lactamase and liquefy gelatin. The oxidase reaction is variable, and reactions for nitrate reduction, urease, and carbohydrate utilization are negative.

10 **The answer is A** *Central and peripheral nervous system / Pharmacology; toxicology / Cholinergic*

Sarin is a highly lipid-soluble organophosphate that is readily absorbed through the skin and lungs. Sarin irreversibly inhibits cholinesterase and its toxicity is secondary to buildup of acetylcholine (ACh) at cholinergic synapses. Pralidoxime can reactivate cholinesterases in the periphery as it does not penetrate the central nervous system. In addition, it is ineffective against aged phosphorylated cholinesterase and thus must be given rapidly after exposure. Atropine will block effects at muscarinic receptors (salivation, bronchoconstriction, bronchial secretions) but will not affect nicotinic receptors that account for skeletal muscle paralysis.

11 **The answer is C** *General principles / Microbiology / Neisseria species infection*

These symptoms are suggestive of *Neisseria meningitides*. The fact that the bacteria are isolated from the bloodstream is evidence of meningococcemia, which is a medical emergency. A Gram stain of *N. meningitides* will show gram-negative single cocci or diplococci with flattened adjacent sides.

12 **The answer is B** *Endocrine system / Genetics / Insulin-dependent diabetes mellitus*

Approximately 95% of patients with IDDM have HLA DR4. HLA DR3/DR4 heterozygotes are particularly susceptible to IDDM, and the DR3/DR4 antigens account for more than half of the genetic contribution underlying IDDM. However, the HLA haplotype alone does not underlie the genetics of IDDM, and other genes must also contribute to the development of the disease. If a proband with IDDM and his sibling share no haplotype, the risk that the sibling will develop IDDM is approximately 2%. The risk is 5% to a sibling who does share one HLA haplotype with a proband affected with IDDM. Approximately half of the normal population has HLA DR3 or HLA DR4; the empiric risk for developing IDDM is approximately 5% to a sibling for whom no HLA typing is available. If the proband and sibling both share DR3 and DR4, the risk that the sibling will develop IDDM is approximately 20%. The HLA haplotype alone is not the sole genetic determinant for IDDM, and other genes must also contribute to the development of the disease.

13 **The answer is D** *General principles / Microbiology / Fungal meningitis*

Encapsulated yeast in the CSF of immune-compromised patients is diagnostic of cryptoccal meningitis. Initial treatment for this stage (moderate to severe infection due to brain-related symptoms) of cryptococcal infection is amphotericin B and 5-fluorocytosine for 2 weeks. After initial treatment, another blood test and/or spinal tap is performed to check for cryptococcus. If the test is positive, combination treatment will be continued. If the tests are negative, both drugs are stopped and fluconazole is started to prevent recurrences. It is currently recommended that fluconazole be continued for the rest of a patient's life.

14 **The answer is E** *Musculoskeletal system / Pathology / Differential diagnosis of arthritis*

Gout is a poorly understood disease that results from urate crystal formation in joints (i.e., arthritis), renal tubules (i.e., gouty nephropathy, urate renal calculi), and soft tissues (i.e., tophi). Although hyperuricemia is usually necessary for the manifestations of gout, it is not sufficient; hyperuricemia can exist without the clinical findings of gout. The association pairing gout with diet and alcohol intake is well documented. Obesity and hyperlipidemia are common in patients with gout, and excess intake of ethanol during the course of a heavy meal may be adequate to incite a painful attack. Plasma urate levels are elevated in gout. Synovial fluid samples show negatively birefringent urate crystals that produce a bright yellow color under polarized light. The cellular infiltrate seems to be a response to the crystals, and leukocyte counts between 2,000 and 75,000/mm^3 are routine findings.

15 **The answer is B** *General principles / Toxicology / Heavy-metal poisoning*

The largest epidemic of lead poisoning in history followed the introduction of lead into paints as a color stabilizer. Each year in the United States more than 2 million preschool children are affected. Lead toxicity in all tissues is related to the disruption of sulfhydryl groups in proteins. In adults, chronic exposure leads to abdominal pain, anemia, renal disease, ataxia, and memory loss. Childhood poisoning often causes abdominal pain and anemia, but the central nervous system (CNS) effects are most important. Unfortunately, subclinical toxicity is most common; the lead poisoning retards CNS development without causing any symptoms that might bring an affected patient to medical attention. Mental retardation, language deficits, cognitive dysfunction, and abnormal behavior are all common manifestations of long-term exposure to lead during the critical preschool years.

Tin is not a common cause of heavy-metal toxicity, nor is it commonly used in pesticides. Chronic exposure to mercury, not arsenic, produces toxicity principally in the CNS. The neuropsychiatric signs commonly observed in workers making felt hats who were exposed to mercury vapor led to the expression "mad as a hatter."

The toxic metal arsenic is commonly encountered in various forms (i.e., inorganic, organic, vapor); it produces toxicity in almost every organ system by tightly binding to sulfhydryl groups as well as by interfering with oxidative phosphorylation. Exposure to arsenic vapor can lead to the rapid onset of severe hemolysis and hematuria. Exposure to the organic and inorganic forms (i.e., through skin or gastrointestinal absorption) can produce acute or chronic symptoms depending on the dose and duration of exposure. Gastric lavage, penicillamine, dimercaprol, and hemodialysis should all be considered for the effective management of arsenic toxicity.

16 **The answer is B** *Hematopoietic and lymphoreticular system / Pathology / Disseminated intravascular coagulation*

Disseminated intravascular coagulation (DIC) is a systemic coagulation disorder that is characterized by inappropriate diffuse activation of the intrinsic or extrinsic coagulation systems. This disorder has two phases: (1) widespread microvascular thrombosis followed by (2) widespread microvascular hemorrhage. Coagulation is initiated either by the release of tissue factor or thromboplastic substances into the circulation or by widespread endothelial cell injury. Common initiators of DIC include infection (particularly gram-negative sepsis), obstetric complications (e.g., amniotic fluid embolization, dead retained fetus, placental abruption), neoplasms (e.g., mucinous adenocarcinomas, acute promyelocytic leukemia), massive tissue injury (e.g., trauma, burns), and miscellaneous causes (e.g., acute intravascular hemolysis, snakebite, vasculitis, shock). Widespread microvascular platelet–fibrin thrombosis may lead to diffuse organ ischemia and to microangiopathic hemolytic anemia. As a consequence of consumption of platelets and coagulation factors and activation of fibrinolytic mechanisms, diffuse small vessel hemorrhage ensues; this hemorrhage is associated with thrombocytopenia, elevated prothrombin time and partial thromboplastin time, decreasing fibrinogen level, and fibrin split products/D-dimers. Therapy is individualized according to the clinical phase of the disease. The patient in this question had DIC in association with gram-negative septicemia.

17 **The answer is D** *General principles / Pharmacology / Lead poisoning*

The best treatment for lead poisoning is dimercaprol or CaEDTA. Flumazenil is used for benzodiazepine poisoning; pralidoxime is used for anticholinesterase poisoning; deferoxamine is used for iron poisoning; and naloxone is used to treat opioid poisoning.

18 The answer is D *Reproductive system / Biochemistry / Hormonal regulation of the menstrual cycle*

Luteinizing hormone is under feedback control by plasma estrogen levels. LH release is inhibited by low estrogen levels and is significantly enhanced by rising and/or high estrogen concentrations. In the proliferative (follicular) phase, estradiol levels begin to rise because granulosa cells produce it in the maturing follicle. Positive feedback causes a rise in LH levels until a peak, known as the LH surge, is reached late in the follicular phase. The LH surge is responsible for the final maturation of the follicle. The cellular action of LH is twofold. First, it stimulates androstenedione production in thecal cells. Androstenedione then diffuses across the basement membrane, and the granulosa cells convert it to estrogen. Second, LH acts on granulosa cells to increase progesterone secretion at midcycle. LH does not, however, mediate endometrial vasospasm, which leads to menses; this event is caused by locally synthesized prostaglandins in response to a decrease in estrogen and progesterone levels.

19 The answer is C *Central and peripheral nervous system / Pathology / Neuromuscular disease*

Guillain–Barré syndrome is acute inflammatory polyradiculopathy with inflammation of the nerve roots and peripheral nerves. It often follows viral infection, surgery, pregnancy, and other immune system-altering events. It runs a monophasic course with weakness progressing for several days to weeks, reaching a plateau, then waning over several weeks to months. Clinically, the diagnosis is confirmed by weakness, often but not always in an ascending pattern (from legs to trunk to the arms and face). The weakness is hyporeflexive, but there is no significant sensory loss. Rapidly progressive weakness with absent reflexes and no sensory change is almost always Guillain–Barré syndrome. Myasthenia gravis causes proximal weakness, especially ptosis and diplopia, that fatigues with use and recovers with rest. Myasthenia gravis and Lambert–Eaton myasthenic syndrome strongly resemble each other clinically, except that Lambert–Eaton myasthenic syndrome does not involve extraocular muscles. Syphilis does not present this ascending pattern of weakness.

20 The answer is B *Reproductive system / Biochemistry / Glucocorticoid and androgen synthesis*

Female pseudohermaphroditism in a genotypically normal female usually results from an excess of androgens during development. 17,20-Lyase and 17β-hydroxysteroid dehydrogenase are involved exclusively in androgen synthesis; therefore, a deficiency in either of these enzymes leads to androgen shortage and to male, not female, pseudohermaphroditism. 17α-Hydroxylase and cholesterol side chain cleavage enzyme are involved in the synthesis of both glucocorticoids and androgens. Deficiency in these enzymes leads to low cortisol and androgen levels. Lack of androgens results in male pseudohermaphroditism. 21-Hydroxylase is one of the two terminal enzymes in glucocorticoid synthesis; the other is 11β-hydroxylase. Deficiency in either one of these proteins impairs formation of hydrocortisone. A compensatory increase in adrenocorticotropic hormone (ACTH) secretion causes adrenal hyperplasia, which in turn leads to increased androgen production. High androgen levels lead to masculinization of female genitalia, resulting in female pseudohermaphroditism. 21-Hydroxylase deficiency accounts for 95% of congenital adrenal hyperplasia cases and is the most common cause of ambiguous genitalia in the newborn in the Unites States and Europe.

21 The answer is E *Musculoskeletal system / Pathology / Radiographic anatomy; differential diagnosis of arthritis*

Hyperuricemia leads to the formation and deposition of urate crystals in tissues, hence to gout. Urate crystal deposition in joints can lead to arthritis, whereas deposits in the soft tissues lead to tophi formation and deposits in the renal tubules can lead to gouty nephropathy; these deposits may be very painful and tender. Synovial fluid taken from such patients may be cloudy and hypercellular, with elevated leukocyte counts between 2,000 and 75,000/mm^3. Under polarized light, urate crystals appear negatively birefringent and bright yellow.

22 **The answer is B** *Gastrointestinal system / Pathology / Type I glycogen storage disease*

Glucose-6-phosphatase (G-6-Pase) deficiency, also known as type I glycogen storage disease or von Gierke's disease, is one of the most common glycogen storage diseases in children. G-6-Pase catalyzes conversion of G-6-Pase to glucose during glycogenolysis. Patients who are deficient in this enzyme cannot maintain normal glucose levels because they cannot break down glycogen stored in the liver. The disease may manifest itself in neonates with hypoglycemia and lactic acidosis. More commonly, however, the patients present at 3 to 4 months of age with prominent hepatomegaly and/or hypoglycemia. These children may have thin extremities, a protuberant abdomen, and doll-like faces with fat cheeks. Laboratory findings often include hyperuricemia and lactic acidosis owing to increased shunting of pyruvate to lactic acid. Accumulation of excess glycogen in the liver leads to characteristic pathologic findings of hepatocytes distended with glycogen and fat with prominent lipid vacuoles. von Gierke's disease is not a lysosomal storage disease, however, because (1) most hepatic glycogen is stored in the cytoplasm and (2) lysosomal glycogen is broken down by α-glucosidase.

23 **The answer is E** *Endocrine system / Pathology / Hyperglycemia of malignancy*

Certain malignancies cause hypercalcemia. Frequently, hypercalcemia is induced by elevated levels of PTH-related protein that is produced by the tumor. This protein has an amino-terminal end with many of the same actions as PTH. Thus, its effects, particularly on the bone and kidneys, cause an increase in serum calcium. PTH is rarely produced by tumors outside the parathyroid glands. In fact, PTH levels are reduced in hypercalcemia of malignancy as a result of the inhibition of the parathyroid glands by the high concentration of calcium. Calcitriol is often reduced because PTH is a major stimulus in the formation of calcitriol. However, in some lymphomas, the production of excess calcitriol causes hypercalcemia. Serum phosphorus concentrations may be low in hypercalcemia of malignancy because of increased renal excretion. The level of hypercalcemia, when caused by malignancy, may be higher than that normally caused by primary hyperparathyroidism, because the tumor often produces multiple factors that act synergistically to cause greater increases (e.g., interleukin-1, interleukin-6, and tumor necrosis factor-α).

24 **The answer is G** *Endocrine system / Biochemistry / Vitamin D metabolism*

Vitamin D is a fat-soluble vitamin that comes from diet. It is made from cholesterol with the help of sunlight. It is converted to the 25-hydroxyvitamin D form in the liver, a process that is regulated by substrate availability. Then it is converted to its most active form, 1,25-dihydroxyvitamin D (calcitriol), in the proximal tubules of the kidneys and, to a lesser extent, in macrophages and mononuclear cells. This step is stimulated by PTH and phosphate depletion. Feedback inhibition also occurs, with 1,25-dihydroxyvitamin D inhibiting both its own production and the synthesis of PTH. The actions of vitamin D are mediated by a cytosolic receptor that translocates to the nucleus on binding with vitamin D. Its functions are to increase calcium and phosphorus absorption in the intestine, to act synergistically with PTH in the bone to increase calcium and phosphate release, and to suppress helper T cells when produced locally by activated macrophages and mononuclear cells.

25 **The answer is D** *Endocrine system / Pathology / Pheochromocytoma*

The patient has a pheochromocytoma. Heart palpitations, abdominal pain, and weight loss are other symptoms associated with these tumors. Although about 10% of pheochromocytomas are associated with a familial syndrome, they are not seen in MEN syndrome type I. They may be seen in MEN type II A or B, as is medullary carcinoma of the thyroid. Pheochromocytomas are usually in the adrenal medulla but may be found elsewhere in the body. They excrete epinephrine and norepinephrine, not cortisol. The 24-hour urinary excretion is a better measure of catecholamine production than are the plasma levels because the latter is more easily affected by the emotional status of the patient and the venipuncture. Although CT is often helpful in forming the diagnosis and treatment plan for a patient with pheochromocytoma, intravenous contrast material may precipitate a hypertensive crisis; therefore, the contrast material should be avoided if possible. Because pheochromocytoma is a life-threatening disease for which there is a treatment, patients showing several of the signs and symptoms should be evaluated promptly.

26 **The answer is D** *General principles / Cell biology / Cell membranes*

The inner and outer leaflets of biologic membranes have different lipid compositions, inducing lipid asymmetry. A phospholipid cannot move spontaneously from the cytoplasmic leaflet to the exoplasmic leaflet in the ER because the hydrophilic head group cannot pass through the hydrophobic bilayer. This does not occur through membrane budding because in this process vesicles transfer phospholipids from one organelle to another. It also does not occur through phospholipid exchange proteins because these proteins also remove phospholipids from one membrane and release them to another membrane or organelle. The movement of a phospholipid in the ER into the exoplasmic leaflet is catalyzed by the flippase protein so that movement occurs within a few minutes.

27 **The answer is F** *Endocrine system / Pathology; endocrinology / Adrenal steroid hormone production*

A 17-α-hydroxylase deficiency causes decreased cortisol production and increased deoxycorticosterone and corticosterone production. The excess of the latter two hormones is due to the lack of feedback inhibition of cortisol on the pituitary and hypothalamus. A 3-β-dehydrogenase deficiency does not allow the production of either cortisol or aldosterone; only androgens are produced. A 21-hydroxylase deficiency does not allow cortisol or aldosterone production, whereas dehydroepiandrosterone (DHEA) and androstenedione are produced in excess. A 17,20-desmolase deficiency blocks androgen synthesis, not that of aldosterone or cortisol. Aromatase deficiency does not block cortisol production or lead to an increase in androgen production. An 18-hydroxylase deficiency blocks the synthesis of aldosterone, not cortisol.

28 **The answer is C** *Reproductive system / Pathology / Neoplasia of the reproductive tract*

In the United States, 25% of men have a tumor in the prostate gland. A prostatic tumor rarely occurs before age 40, but the incidence rises rapidly with advancing age. Of prostatic tumors, 75% arise in the posterior lobe, are easily palpable, and therefore are detectable.

29 **The answer is B** *General principles / Pharmacology / Organophosphate exposure*

Organophosphates are highly toxic insecticides that occasionally affect agricultural workers. They are also frequently the primary agent in chemical weapons. They are highly lipid-soluble and are absorbed through virtually all body parts, including the skin. They produce a cholinergic crisis secondary to inhibition of acetylcholinesterase, which involves nicotinic and muscarinic receptors, both centrally and systemically. Atropine decreases some of the muscarine effects, including the bronchospasm and increased secretions of the airways. Mechanical ventilation may still be required if respiratory muscles are paralyzed. Pralidoxime, if given early enough, will help regenerate new cholinesterase and ultimately hasten reversal of the overdose.

30 **The answer is C** *General principles / Immunology / Self-tolerance*

The thymus is an antigenically privileged site, and thymocytes pass through only once; therefore, peripheral tolerance may be a necessary mechanism. There is no evidence that T cells leave and then come back to the thymus. Tolerance seems to be a negative selection phenomenon, and it is believed that all selection initially takes place in the thymus.

31 **The answer is C** *Renal/urinary system / Pathology / Cystoprostatectomy specimen containing multiple papillary urothelial neoplasms within the bladder*

Urothelial neoplasia are thought to be initiated by carcinogens concentrated in the urine and promoted by chronic irritation related to recurrent infections, indwelling catheters, and so forth. The most common histologic subtype of urothelial neoplasms shows transitional cell differentiation. Early (in situ) lesions are either flat or papillary; they may be solitary or multifocal; and they may be confined to the bladder or involve the extravesical urothelium. Invasive carcinomas may arise from flat or papillary in situ carcinomas, which occur most frequently in patients with high-grade cytology. Hematuria and irritative urinary symptoms are common but nonspecific presentations. Screening includes urinary cytology, with cytoscopy and/or biopsy and upper tract studies performed in patients who have abnormal screening cytology or who are at high risk. Because exfoliated cells from low-grade urothelial neoplasms are difficult to distinguish from reactive urothelial cells, low-grade lesions are often missed by cytology but on biopsy are recognized cytoscopically as papillary lesions. The sensitivity of urinary cytology for high-grade urothelial neoplasms is much better; furthermore, because many of these lesions are flat, they are difficult to recognize cystoscopically. Random cystoscopic histology biopsies confirm flat in situ urothelial carcinoma in patients with abnormal cytology. Invasive carcinomas are usually recognizable cystoscopically, and biopsy studies are used to assess the depth of invasion. Therapy is based on the clinical stage of the disease.

32 **The answer is B** *General principles / Behavioral science / Childhood development*

Effective monitoring of childhood developmental milestones is critical for the early detection and management of developmental delay. Several helpful charts allow the PCP to make an assessment of normal cognitive development. Infants reach for objects outside of their immediate grasp as early as 3 months of age but should have achieved this task by 8 months of age. Similarly, some precocious toddlers use intelligible phrases by 2 years of age, but the sole use of single words in a child of 3 years is clearly abnormal. Anxiety with strangers usually begins between 5 and 8 months of age. Piaget described the concrete operations phase (generally from 7 to 11 years), during which children learn to categorize and mentally manipulate tangible objects. Before this stage, children are easily fooled by the short glass or tall glass trick. For some children, achievement of this milestone marks their final cognitive development, because some adults never become proficient at abstract thinking.

33 **The answer is A** *General principles / Biochemistry / Protein structure*

Many polypeptides have a distinctive tertiary structure that provides insight into their function. Zinc fingers and leucine zippers are structural motifs that seem to be crucial in most proteins with DNA-binding functions. Current research indicates that the zinc fingers insert into the major groove of DNA between the bases. EF hands are structural motifs that are important in the calcium-binding properties of molecules like calmodulin, troponin C, and the ryanodine receptor. β-Pleated sheets are frequently involved in the transport of hydrophobic molecules: a_1-microglobulin carries porphyrin rings, and apolipoproteins transfer cholesterol esters via β-pleated sheets. Gly-X-Y repeats are important in producing the tight triple-helix of collagen. Glycine has only a hydrogen as its side chain and therefore allows the individual helices to be wound tightly without a bulky structure in the center. Immunoglobulin folds are important in the superfamily, which includes immunoglobulins, epidermal and nerve growth factors, and other proteins with diverse functions.

34 **The answer is D** *General principles / Biochemistry / Retroviruses*

The retroviruses are unique in their diploid genetic structure, with two identical RNA molecules per virion. To initiate an effective infection, the virion-associated reverse transcriptase must produce a double-stranded DNA copy of the viral RNA, and that copy must be integrated into the host genome. Infectious virus is produced from the integrated copy. The various viral antigens are made from mRNA produced from the DNA copy, and these antigens include both group-specific and host-specific reactive antigens. The viral RNA has plus polarity.

35 **The answer is B** *General principles / Pharmacology / Barbiturates*

Thiopental is a barbiturate with a rapid onset of action. Barbiturates are thought to interfere with sodium and potassium transport across cell membranes, leading to inhibition of the mesencephalic reticular activating system. Polysynaptic transmission is inhibited in all areas of the CNS. Barbiturates also potentiate γ-aminobutyric acid (GABA) action on chloride entry into the neuron. Diazepam and lorazepam are benzodiazepines, anxiolytic drugs that inhibit the action of GABA (A) neurotransmitter. Ethanol is a CNS depressant, producing sedation and ultimately hypnosis with increasing dosage. Buspirone actions are mediated by serotonin receptors, although it has some affinity for dopamine receptors. Hydroxyzine is an antihistamine with antiemetic activity.

36 **The answer is B** *General principles / Biochemistry / DNA replication*

Topoisomerase enzymes are important for regulating the equilibrium between supercoiled and relaxed DNA. Okazaki fragments are annealed by the actions of a ligase, and the newly synthesized DNA is "proofread" by a subunit of DNA polymerase III. The RNA primer is required to initiate DNA synthesis and is thought to be synthesized by RNA polymerase.

37 **The answer is C** *General principles / Cell biology / Protein synthesis*

Protein synthesis in eukaryotic cells occurs by translation of mRNA in three stages: initiation, elongation, and termination. In the termination stage, a single transcription factor recognizes the stop codon UAG in the mRNA sequence and signals the release of the peptidyl transfer RNA used to add each additional amino acid. This subsequently releases the newly synthesized polypeptide chain. Once the ribosome detaches from the mRNA, GTP is hydrolyzed, which provides enough energy to divide the ribosome into two subunits. The two ribosomal subunits are not degraded after translation of the mRNA is complete. AUG, which codes for methionine, is a start codon. RNA polymerase II is important in transcription; it is not important in translation.

38 **The answer is C** *General principles / Behavioral science / Operant conditioning*

Negative reinforcement is used to increase a desired behavior by encouraging avoidance of a negative consequence. The negative consequence is losing driving privileges; the desired behavior is washing the dishes. Rewarding a behavior (e.g., losing weight) is an example of positive reinforcement. Ignoring a behavior to cause the cessation of the behavior is extinction. The issuing of speeding tickets to bring about the desired behavior is an example of punishment.

39 **The answer is D** *General principles / Behavioral science / Defense mechanisms*

Splitting is a result of someone being unable to cope adequately with ambiguous, confusing situations. Rather than accept that a good person can make mistakes, he or she will reclassify the person as bad. Projection is transferring one's own desires or impulses to another; that is, believing your neighbor is spying on you when really you want to spy on her. Sublimation is the successful channeling of negative feelings or desires in a positive, socially acceptable way. Dissociation is associated with multiple personality disorder and involves developing different identities with separate mental processes. Displacement involves venting feelings at an object or person who is not associated with the source of the feelings.

40 **The answer is F** *Endocrine system / Pathology; endocrinology / Diabetic ketoacidosis*

Diabetic ketoacidosis is a complication of type I diabetes mellitus that is preventable in a patient who is following the proper therapeutic regimen. DKA may also be a part of the initial presentation of diabetes mellitus. It is usually brought on by a precipitating event (e.g., infection, failure to take enough insulin, and possibly emotional stress). Hypokalemia is a concern in patients with DKA. The potassium level should be monitored closely, even if initially normal, because the serum concentration may drop with rehydration. The administration of bicarbonate to a patient with DKA is controversial except in severe acidosis. However, it should not be given as a bolus, as that would shift the Bohr curve strongly to the left in this setting of low bisphosphoglycerate and decrease oxygen delivery to the brain. Instead, it should be given slowly and the increase should be monitored closely. Rehydration therapy may be started before insulin is given, as this allows assessment of the effects of rehydration on glucose levels.

41 **The answer is D** *General principles / Hematology; genetics / Blood typing*

Because the father has no blood type antigen, the offspring will inherit either an A or B antigen from the mother and can never be an O blood type. Similarly, because both parents have the M and N antigen, the offspring can inherit either antigen from either parent. Both parents are Rh −, so the offspring must inherit the Rh −. As a consequence, options A, B, C, and E are all genetically impossible outcomes from the given parental genotype.

42 **The answer is D** *Hematopoietic and lymphoreticular system / Hematology / Blood transfusions; Rh factor incompatibility*

This patient has a chance of carrying an Rh + fetus. To minimize the possibility of inducing antibody formation against the Rh factor, she should be transfused with Rh − blood. Because the patient's blood type is A, MN, Rh −, the ideal match is blood of the same type. Given the answer choices, however, the preferred blood for transfusion is the universal donor type O blood with MN antigens and no Rh factor. Transfusing this patient with either type B or type AB blood would cause hemolytic anemia by destroying transfused red blood cells carrying the B antigen.

43 **The answer is C** *Cardiovascular system / Pathology / Pernicious anemia*

Hypersegmented granulocytes and megaloblastic red blood cells are characteristic of pernicious anemia. Iron deficiency anemia is characterized by microcytic, hypochromic red blood cells. Helmet cells are a result of hemolysis. Psammoma bodies are concentric spherules seen most often in papillary adenocarcinoma.

44 **The answer is E** *Hematopoietic and lymphoreticular system / Pathology / Pernicious anemia*

Pernicious anemia is a result of vitamin B_{12} deficiency caused by autoimmune destruction of intrinsic factor, which is needed to absorb vitamin B_{12} in the terminal ileum. Vitamin B_{12} deficiency causes megaloblastic anemia with hypersegmented granulocytes. Folate deficiency also causes megaloblastic anemia. Folate deficiency, however, is not the underlying pathology of pernicious anemia.

45 **The answer is E** *General principles / Pathology / Retinoblastomas*

Individuals who inherit a mutant retinoblastoma gene have a vastly increased chance of developing retinoblastoma. This mutation is also involved in the development of osteosarcomas, and thus the two diseases often affect the same individual.

46 **The answer is D** *General principles / Biochemistry / Protein synthesis, posttranslational modification, and targeting*

Proteins destined for the cytoplasm, such as hexokinase, are translated on free ribosomes. Proteins with signal sequences are targeted to the rough ER for translation. *N*-linked glycosylation occurs in the lumen of the rough ER; then the protein is sent to the Golgi complex. Although its function is still being studied, it is clear that the Golgi complex is the key site for sorting proteins that are emerging from the rough ER. The *N*-linked sugars are modified, and additional sugars are frequently added to the oxygen-based side chains of serine or threonine (O-linked glycosylation). Fatty acids and other lipid moieties are also often added in the lumen of the Golgi complex (e.g., acylation). These various modifications may contribute to the protein's function or structural stability. Sometimes they serve as signals for targeting mechanisms. Mannose 6-phosphate was the first targeting signal to be well established. Mannose 6-phosphate moieties are essential for an enzyme to be transferred into the lysosomal lumen. Patients with lysosomal storage disease often have a defect in this targeting mechanism. Usually the enzyme has a defective signal, so that it is synthesized but not concentrated in the site where it serves its degradative function. The nucleolus is where ribosomal RNA (rRNA) is synthesized and ribosomal units are assembled.

47 **The answer is B** *Central and peripheral nervous system / Pathology / Alzheimer's disease*

Hippocampal neurofibrillary tangles are not unique to Alzheimer's disease because they are also seen in Down's syndrome, normal aging, and pugilistic dementia; however, they uniquely occur in high concentrations in the hippocampus of patients with Alzheimer's disease. The presence of prions is associated with the development of Creutzfeldt–Jacob dementia, whereas multinucleated giant cells are found in cases of patients with AIDS and encephalitis. Argentophilic (silver-staining) intraneuronal inclusions are associated with Pick's disease. Lewy bodies are characteristic for Parkinson's disease.

48 **The answer is E** *General principles / Pathology / AIDS*

Multinucleated giant cells are a common pathologic feature in patients with AIDS who have encephalitis. Amyloid plaques and hippocampal neurofibrillary tangles are commonly found in patients with Alzheimer's syndrome, whereas Lewy bodies and eosinophilic cytoplasmic inclusions in the substantia nigra are characteristic of Parkinson's disease. Pick's bodies stain silver and are inclusions within neurons.

49 **The answer is A** *Central and peripheral nervous system / Pathology / Parkinson's disease*

Lewy bodies and eosinophilic cytoplasmic inclusions in the substantia nigra are characteristic of Parkinson's disease. Neurofibrillary tangles are not unique to Alzheimer's disease because they are also seen in Down's syndrome, normal aging, and pugilistic dementia; however, they uniquely occur in high concentrations in the hippocampus of patients with Alzheimer's disease. Pick's bodies stain silver and are inclusions within neurons. Prions, proteins devoid of nucleic acid that are infectious, are associated with Creutzfeldt–Jakob dementia. Multinucleated giant cells occur in patients with AIDS who have encephalitis.

50 **The answer is D** *General principles / Biochemistry / Starvation*

In late starvation, ketone bodies are produced from lipids, so there is less need for gluconeogenesis. Thus, protein breakdown decreases. Other metabolic adaptations are decreased levels of insulin, follicle-stimulating hormone, LH, decreased cardiac output, decreased ventilation, and increased risk of developing respiratory infections. Malnutrition due to starvation causes the body to decrease its resting energy expenditure; however, it may be increased in the setting of malnutrition due to metabolic stress (e.g., severe burns).

test **11**

Questions

Directions: Single best answer questions consist of numbered items or incomplete statements followed by answers or by completions of the statement. Select the ONE lettered answer or completion that is BEST in each case.

1 A child is taken to the pediatrician for evaluation of difficulty walking. Examination reveals a waddling gait, proximal muscle weakness, pseudohypertrophy of the calf muscles, and a Gower maneuver upon standing from a sitting position. A tentative diagnosis of Duchenne's muscular dystrophy (DMD) is made pending the results of serum enzyme studies, electromyography, and muscle biopsy. According to this family pedigree, the mode of inheritance of DMD is

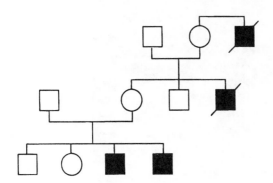

(A)   autosomal recessive
(B)   autosomal dominant
(C)   X-linked
(D)   nonpenetrant

2 A 58-year-old man is brought to the emergency department by his daughter. He appears inebriated and complains of severe pain localized over his left lower chest wall. A chest x-ray shows a bulging left lower lobe. A bloody sputum sample is obtained, which shows gram-negative rods. What is the most appropriate treatment?

(A)   Penicillin G
(B)   Penicillin G and streptomycin
(C)   Ampicillin
(D)   Amoxicillin
(E)   Cefotaxime

3 Angiotensin converting enzyme (ACE) inhibitors such as captropril or enalapril are useful in the therapy of myocardial insufficiency and congestive heart failure because they

(A)   enhance the degradation of the edematogenic substance, bradykinin
(B)   prolong the half-life of angiotensin II
(C)   indirectly decrease the release of aldosterone and arginine vasopressin
(D)   inhibit sodium- and potassium-activated adenosine triphosphate (NaK-ATPase)
(E)   elevate cyclic andenosine monophosphate (cAMP) in the myocardium

4 Which of the following statements about the cyclin B/cdc2 kinase complex is true?

(A)   Destruction of the cyclin B activates the cyclin B/cdc2 kinase activity
(B)   Freshly synthesized cyclin B blocks the reactivation of the cyclin B/cdc2 kinase complex
(C)   The cyclin B/cdc2 kinase complex is important in the cell entering mitosis
(D)   Activated cyclin B/cdc2 kinase complex causes a G_1 arrest in the cell cycle
(E)   Cyclin B/cdc2 kinase phosphorylates cell cycle proteins but is rarely phosphorylated itself

5 A 53-year-old man complains of shortness of breath when climbing stairs and a productive cough. He has had respiratory infections each of the past 2 years, has smoked two packs of cigarettes per day for the past 35 years, is obese, and looks somewhat cyanotic. Which one of the following statements is most likely correct?

(A) The patient has a low forced expiratory volume in 1 second (FEV_1) but a normal FEV_1/forced vital capacity (FVC) ratio

(B) The patient has restrictive rather than obstructive pulmonary disease

(C) The patient is likely to have emphysematous disease rather than bronchitic disease

(D) The patient has elevated hemoglobin and hematocrit levels

(E) The patient has α_1-antitrypsin deficiency

(F) The patient's history of smoking has no relation to this disease

6 The violaceous skin nodule apparent in the photomicrograph, which was taken from a young individual, is most likely

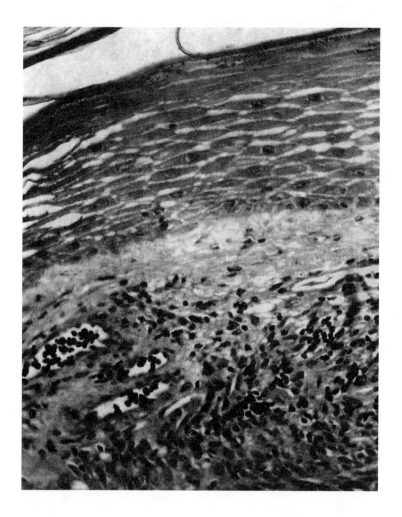

(A) seen on the back of infants' necks

(B) a highly malignant pigmented melanoma

(C) seen in men infected with HIV

(D) due to radiation therapy that was administered over 10 years ago

7 Which one of the following statements concerning referred pain is true?

(A) Pain from the transverse colon is usually referred to a midline area below the umbilicus

(B) Somatic pain is usually referred in a diffuse, poorly localized pattern

(C) Diaphragmatic pain is usually referred to the inguinal area

(D) The mechanism of referred pain is well-understood

8 An 18-year-old college freshman has been acting strangely for several months, according to his roommates. His grades are deteriorating and he avoids social interactions. He talks about being the devil's accomplice. He is unshaven, and his clothes are messy. The first diagnosis to consider with this patient is

(A) schizophrenia

(B) mania

(C) schizoaffective disorder

(D) major depression

(E) phencyclidine psychosis

9 The high metabolic needs of the heart and its relative exclusive reliance on aerobic metabolism require a high degree of regulation of coronary blood flow to maintain myocardial oxygen demands. As such, coronary perfusion

(A) is greatest during systole

(B) increases directly over a broad range of arterial pressures

(C) is controlled mainly by local metabolic factors

(D) is greatly decreased by direct sympathetic stimulation of resistance vessels

(E) is achieved primarily via collateral vessels in healthy subjects

10 A reasonable medication trial for complex partial seizures is

(A) haloperidol

(B) carbamazepine

(C) imipramine

(D) alprazolam

(E) clonidine

11 The term that describes the adherence of neutrophils and monocytes to the vascular endothelium before movement into the extravascular space is

(A) margination

(B) diapedesis

(C) pavementing

(D) migration

(E) clotting

12 A fluorescent probe that binds to glucocorticoid receptors is applied to cells. The probe is freely diffusible throughout the cell and has no effect on the glucocorticoid receptor. If the cell has not been stimulated by glucocorticoids, where is the most intense fluorescence?

(A) Cell membrane

(B) Cytosol

(C) Nuclear membrane

(D) Nucleus

(E) Nucleus and cytosol

13 A middle-aged woman has a throbbing headache and bilateral tenderness over her forehead. Knobby cords are palpated at the sides and sampled for biopsy. The tissue is pictured in the micrograph. The correct diagnosis is

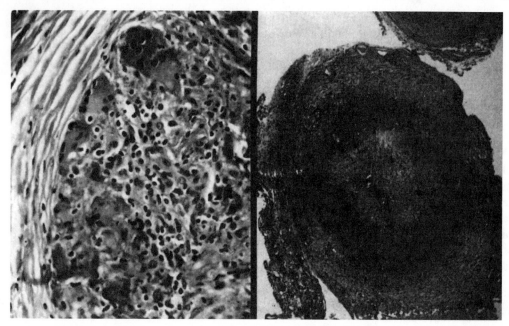

(A) temporal arteritis
(B) foreign body giant cell reaction to an injected substance
(C) Mönckeberg's arteriosclerosis
(D) Takayasu's arteritis

14 Cromolyn sodium is the first-line agent for the treatment of mild to moderate asthma, especially asthma in children associated with allergenic causes. Although its mechanism of action is unclear, cromolyn sodium's widespread use is due to its

(A) bioavailability after oral administration
(B) direct bronchodilating effect, making it useful in acute emergencies
(C) prophylactic potential due to inhibition of the release of inflammatory mediators
(D) immediate effect to reduce bronchospasm
(E) antimuscarinic effects

15 A patient presents with pleuritic chest pain, nonproductive cough, diminished breath sounds at the base bilaterally, and dullness to percussion. A chest radiograph is consistent with pleural effusion. Thoracentesis is performed. Which of the following results is interpreted correctly?

(A) The pleural fluid has high levels of protein and lactate dehydrogenase (LDH); therefore, it is a transudate
(B) The pleural fluid has a high level of LDH, but the protein level is within the normal range; therefore, the fluid is a transudate
(C) The pleural fluid has a low level of glucose (30 mg/dL) and a low pH (6.5); therefore, a chest tube should be inserted because of the likelihood of empyema
(D) The pleural fluid has an amylase level that is lower than serum levels; therefore, pancreatic disease and esophageal varices are at the top of the differential diagnoses
(E) The pleural fluid has LDH and protein levels within the normal range; therefore, the fluid is an exudate

16 A bone marrow transplant patient has dyspnea, hypoxemia, and bilateral pulmonary infiltrates on a chest radiograph. Which of the following infections is most likely, based on the bronchoalveolar lavage preparation shown in Figure 51 of the color plate section?

(A) Herpes simplex virus (HSV)
(B) Cytomegalovirus (CMV)
(C) Polyomavirus
(D) Adenovirus

17 A patient has epigastric and right upper quadrant pain. The pain is most intense 2 to 4 hours after eating and is reduced by the ingestion of antacids. The patient states that he has passed black tarry stools (melena) within the past week. Fiberoptic endoscopy reveals a yellowish crater surrounded by a rim of erythema that is 3 cm distal to the pylorus. Accordingly, an ulcer has been identified in the patient's

(A) fundus
(B) antrum
(C) duodenum
(D) jejunum
(E) ileum

18 Glyeryl trinitrate (GTN or nitroglycerin) remains a mainstay in the therapy of ischemic heart disease because it

(A) is conveniently administered orally
(B) has a long half-life
(C) is a potent coronary artery vasodilator
(D) relaxes venous capacitance vessels at therapeutic doses
(E) reverses the course of atherosclerosis

19 A patient is given 100% oxygen to breathe and his arterial oxygen tension (P_{O2}) is considerably less than that of a normal subject. The patient's hypoxemia is likely to be secondary to

(A) a shunt
(B) hypoventilation
(C) diffusion impairment
(D) ventilation perfusion abnormality
(E) retention of carbon dioxide

20 The most important prognostic factor for human cancer is

(A) the patient's age
(B) tumor stage
(C) lymphocytic infiltration
(D) vascular invasion
(E) the mitotic index

21 Growth hormone (GH; somatotropic hormone; somatotropin) is synthesized and stored in large amounts in the anterior pituitary gland (adenohypophysis). Which of the following statements accurately describes GH?

(A) It is secreted continuously
(B) Synthesis is stimulated by the action of somatostatin
(C) Receptors have a limited distribution outside the central nervous system (CNS)
(D) It stimulates cartilage and bone growth via somatomedin
(E) It has a proinsulin-like effect in addition to its other actions

22 A 29-year-old intravenous drug abuser has bilateral fluffy lung infiltrates. A transbronchial biopsy is performed. A Grocott–Gomori methenamine-silver nitrate stain of the lung tissue is pictured below. The diagnosis is

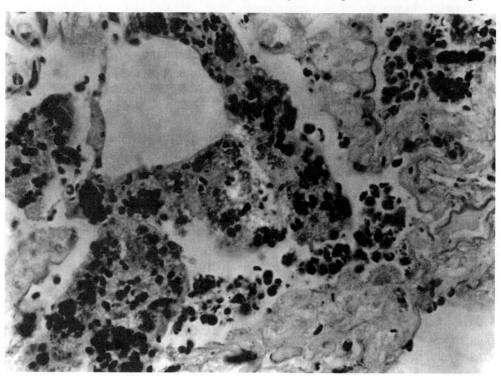

(A) atypical mycobacterial infection
(B) CMV pneumonitis
(C) nocardial abscess
(D) pneumocystis pneumonia
(E) Legionnaire's disease

23 A 24-year-old African American woman has chest pain; her chest radiograph reveals mediastinal lymphadenopathy. A lymph node biopsy from the anterior mediastinum is obtained by mediastinoscopy, and the tissue sample is portrayed in the photomicrograph. The correct diagnosis is

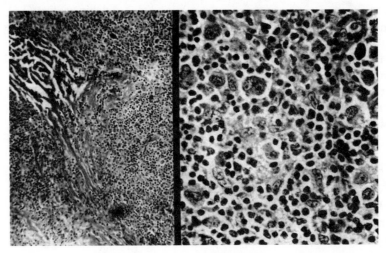

(A) sarcoidosis
(B) thymoma
(C) sclerosing mediastinitis
(D) Hodgkin's disease

24 Which of the following statements regarding the proximal tubular epithelium illustrated below is most likely to be correct?

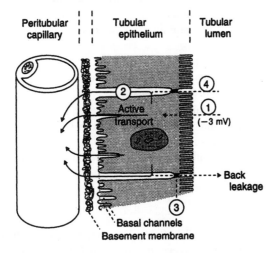

(A) The ion whose movement is depicted in (*1*) is Na+
(B) The process depicted at site (*2*) is aldosterone sensitive
(C) The cell is impermeable to water because of the tight junctions shown in (*3*)
(D) The process depicted at site (*4*) is affected by antidiuretic hormone (ADH)
(E) The intracellular potential is similar to the tubular lumen potential (− 3 mV)

25 Of the following statements regarding thoracic outlet syndrome, which one is true?

(A) It results from an irregularly shaped first thoracic rib
(B) Compression of the left phrenic nerve may occur
(C) Numbness and tingling occur along a median nerve distribution
(D) Compression of the subclavian artery may occur

26 Glucose stimulation of β cells in the endocrine pancreas subsequently causes

(A) enhancement of gluconeogenesis in the liver
(B) increased glycogenolysis by the liver
(C) stimulation of the release of glucagon
(D) decreased oxidation of amino acids in the liver

27 Which of the following statements about meiosis is true?

(A) Chiasma is the point on a chromosome that separates the long arm of the chromosome from the short arm
(B) Meiosis II is the reduction division in which the number of chromosomes is halved
(C) Homologous recombination occurs during prophase I
(D) In primary oocytes, meiosis is initiated by fertilization

28 Which of the following stages of mitosis is accurately defined?

(A) Dissolution of the nuclear envelope occurs in telophase

(B) Separation of the centromeres occurs in early prophase

(C) The first appearance of chromosomes occurs in late prophase

(D) Alignment of chromosomes in the equatorial plane occurs during metaphase

(E) Cytokinesis occurs during anaphase

29 Many antimicrobials inhibit protein translation. Which of the following antimicrobials is correctly paired with its mechanism of action?

(A) Tetracyclines inhibit peptidyltransferase

(B) Diphtheria toxin binds to the 30s ribosomal subunit

(C) Puromycin inactivates eEF-2

(D) Clindamycin binds to the 30s ribosomal subunit

(E) Erythromycin binds to the 50s ribosomal subunit

30 Which of the following statements about RNA processing is true?

(A) Capping on the 3′ end of the RNA is important for RNA stability

(B) A poly-A tail is added to the 3′ end of RNA by a special polymerase called poly-A polymerase

(C) RNA splicing removes exons from the RNA transcript

(D) RNA splicing occurs in the cytoplasm once the transcript is bound to a ribosome

31 Psychoanalysis as a form of psychotherapy relies on which form of communication between the patient and therapist?

(A) Interpretation

(B) Resistance

(C) Countertransference

(D) Free association

(E) Meditation

32 Which of the following is true about carbon monoxide (CO) poisoning?

(A) CO has 200 times as much affinity for hemoglobin as does O_2

(B) CO poisoning causes headache, confusion, and coma but rarely convulsions

(C) The best treatment for CO poisoning is penicillamine

(D) CO is a yellowish, odorless gas

33 In approximately 55% of patients with multiple myeloma, the predominant immunoglobulin (Ig) in the serum is

(A) IgM

(B) IgD

(C) IgE

(D) IgA

(E) IgG

34 Monitoring aminoglycoside serum levels is requisite for the systemic use of the drugs because

(A) they are extensively metabolized by hepatic enzymes

(B) they are rapidly eliminated

(C) they can cause severe hypersensitivity reactions

(D) their therapeutic index is low, and toxicity manifests easily

(E) they rapidly cross the blood–brain barrier

35 Tamoxifen can control the growth of some forms of female breast cancer by

(A) inhibiting estrogen synthesis

(B) inhibiting androgen-induced DNA transcription

(C) competing for estrogen receptors

(D) inhibiting the secretion of luteinizing hormone (LH)

(E) stimulating nuclear transcription

36 Propranolol, a β-blocker, may be used with nitroglycerin (glyceryl trinitrate, or GTN) in concurrent therapy for typical (exertional) angina because propranolol

(A) is a potent vasodilator of coronary arteries

(B) increases conduction in the atria and atrioventricular node

(C) blocks the reflex tachycardia that occurs with the use of GTN

(D) dilates constricted airways

(E) is positively inotropic

37 Phenytoin (Dilantin) is effective in most forms of epilepsy (with the exception of absence seizures) because it

(A) directly binds to chloride channels in the CNS
(B) enhances the inhibitory actions of γ-aminobutyric acid (GABA) at its receptor in the CNS
(C) affects Na + conductance in neurons via voltage-sensitive Na + channel inhibition
(D) is usually started concurrently with phenobarbital therapy

38 Which one of the following statements concerning the synthesis of different types of RNA molecules in eukaryotic cells is true?

(A) RNA polymerase I produces mainly transfer RNA (tRNA)
(B) RNA polymerase III produces ribosomal RNA (rRNA)
(C) RNA polymerase II produces mainly messenger RNA (mRNA)
(D) RNA polymerase IV produces mainly small RNA

39 Which one of the following drugs or chemicals has been associated with the induction of aplastic anemia?

(A) Acetaminophen
(B) Methyldopa
(C) Benzene
(D) Penicillin
(E) Thiouracil

40 A 20-year-old man has hemoptysis, acute renal failure, and hematuria; he has bilateral pulmonary infiltrates on a chest radiograph. The renal biopsy (methenamine silver and IgG immunofluorescence stains) is depicted in Figure 52 of the color plate section. Which of the following circulating antibodies is the patient likely to have?

(A) Antiglomerular basement membrane antibody
(B) Anti–double-stranded DNA antibody
(C) Antineutrophil cytoplasmic antibody
(D) Hepatitis C antibody

41 A monoclonal antibody, IgG, that neutralizes endotoxin has been produced. This antibody has tremendous therapeutic potential for patients suffering septic shock from endotoxemia, and it may be useful in treating patients who have which one of the following diseases?

(A) Pulmonary anthrax
(B) Whooping cough
(C) Cholera
(D) Leprosy
(E) Bubonic plague

42 Which of the following proteins bind to penicillin?

(A) Alanine racemase
(B) 30s Ribosomes
(C) Peptidoglycan
(D) Porin
(E) Transpeptidase

43 A medical student receives a deep laceration in an altercation at a party. He reports having had a DTP (diphtheria–tetanus–pertussis) series in childhood. The most appropriate treatment would be

(A) injection of human tetanus IgG
(B) injection of equine tetanus IgG
(C) intravenous administration of an aminoglycoside
(D) injection of tetanus toxoid

44 Which of the following statements concerning acetylsalicylic acid (aspirin), the prototype of a group of nonsteroidal anti-inflammatory agents that are also analgesic and antipyretic, is correct?

(A) Aspirin is a potent lipoxygenase inhibitor
(B) The major adverse effect of aspirin is gastrointestinal bleeding
(C) Aspirin can reduce normal body temperature
(D) Aspirin is a competitive inhibitor of platelet cyclo-oxygenase

45 Which one of the following statements concerning mRNA splicing is true?

(A) Alternate splicing, producing two different mRNA molecules from the same gene, is a common occurrence in most mammalian genes

(B) Spliceosomes are collections of small nuclear ribonucleoproteins (snRNPs) near ribosomes on the rough endoplasmic reticulum

(C) U1 snRNP binds to a nucleotide segment on the 5′ end of the intron to be spliced

(D) Spliceosomes recognize splicing sites by the large, 50 to 80 base pair sequences on the 5′ and 3′ regions of introns

46 The most common tumor of the appendix, pictured below, is

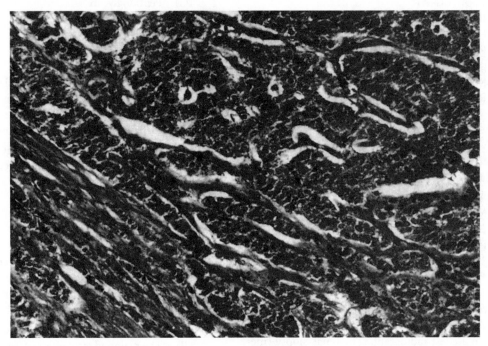

(A) a carcinoid tumor
(B) an adenocarcinoma
(C) a mucocele
(D) an inflammatory pseudotumor

47 Which one of the following conditions results in a negative nitrogen balance?

(A) Consumption of dietary proteins that are deficient in glycine

(B) Normal intake of dietary protein accompanied by defective cholecystokinin–pancreozymin (CCK–PZ) production

(C) Nitrogen consumption that exceeds nitrogen excretion

(D) A tyrosine supplement in the diet of a child with phenylketonuria (PKU)

(E) A 50% reduction in the hydrochloric acid (HCl) content of gastric juice

48 Translation of a synthetic polyribonucleotide containing the repeating sequence CAA in a cell-free protein synthesizing system produces three homopolypeptides: polyglutamine, polyasparagine, and polythreonine. If the codons for glutamine and asparagine are CAA and AAC, respectively, which of the following triplets is a codon for threonine?

(A) AAC
(B) CAA
(C) CAC
(D) CCA
(E) ACA

49 It is hypothesized that nocturnal body temperatures are linearly related to body weight in 60- to 70-year-old women. Nursing records are reviewed for weights in kilograms and 4:00 A.M. temperatures in degrees Celsius. These variables are considered to be

(A) continuous
(B) nonparametric
(C) constants
(D) reciprocal
(E) outliers

50 The most common finding associated with a myelomeningocele is

(A) Arnold Chiari type I
(B) Arnold Chiari type II
(C) rachischisis
(D) Dandy Walker malformation
(E) anencephaly

Answer Key

1-C	11-C	21-D	31-D	41-E
2-E	12-B	22-D	32-A	42-E
3-C	13-A	23-D	33-E	43-D
4-C	14-C	24-A	34-D	44-B
5-D	15-C	25-D	35-C	45-C
6-C	16-B	26-D	36-C	46-A
7-A	17-C	27-C	37-C	47-B
8-D	18-D	28-D	38-C	48-E
9-C	19-A	29-E	39-C	49-A
10-B	20-B	30-B	40-A	50-B

Answers and Explanations

1 The answer is C *General principles / Genetics / DMD*

Duchenne's muscular dystrophy, or childhood muscular dystrophy, having a pattern of X-linked inheritance, classically occurs only in boys. This pattern can be deduced from the pedigree that accompanies the question because all of the affected individuals are males, the mothers and fathers are not affected, and the affected males are on the maternal side of the family.

2 The answer is E *General principles / Microbiology / Klebsiella pneumonia*

Klebsiella pneumonia is a common infection found in alcoholics and physically disabled patients. Sputum cultures often are described as mucoid with blood present ("currant jelly sputum"). Klebsiella are gram-negative rods. Chest x-rays normally show considerable consolidation with a cavitation or necrosis found in more than 20% of cases. Although this patient shows disease involvement in the left lower lobe, this is relatively uncommon; the upper lobes are most commonly involved. Klebsiella are normally highly resistant organisms and antibiotic treatment should be tailored to local resistance profiles. Examples of agents that show high levels of activity against Klebsiella third-generation cephalosporins (e.g., cefotaxime, ceftriaxone), carbapenems (e.g., imipenem/cilastatin), aminoglycosides (e.g., gentamicin, amikacin), and quinolones. Therefore, answer (E) lists the only antimicrobial agent that should be considered.

3 The answer is C *Cardiovascular / Pharmacology / Congestive heart failure; ACE inhibitors*

Captopril or enalapril are ACE inhibitors that are commonly used for congestive heart failure. Unlike digitalis that is a positive inotrope via inhibition of sodium pump or β-adrenergic agents or phosphodiesterase IV inhibitors that elevate myocardial cAMP, ACE inhibitors block the synthesis of angiotensin II (and the degradation of bradykinin). Reduced cardiac output increases renin release and thereby increases circulating angiotensin II that increases aldosterone from the adrenal cortex and vasopressin from the pituitary. These latter actions increase peripheral vascular resistance and promote water retention. Thus, ACE inhibitors (by lowering circulating angiotensin II) decrease circulating aldosterone and vasopressin and reverse and/or inhibit the deleterious myocardial effects of the pathophysiology of congestive heart failure.

4 The answer is C *General principles / Cell biology / Cell cycle; mitosis*

The cyclin B/cdc2 complex (also known as cyclin B-cdel) controls entry into mitosis. During the S phase, cyclin B is synthesized, reaching its maximal levels at G_2 phase of the cell cycle, when most cyclin B binds cdc2. Destruction of cyclin B inactivates the cyclin B/cdc2 kinase activity, and newly synthesized cyclin B allows reactivation of the complex. The cyclin B/cdc2 complex is then phosphorylated and dephosphorylated in a complex series of events to reach activation and drive the cell into mitosis. The threonine-161 residue must be phosphorylated and the tyrosine-14 and threonine-15 residue must be dephosphorylated for cyclin B/cdc2 activation. The cyclin B/cdc2 complex is deactivated at the end of mitosis by the destruction of the cyclin B of the complex. The cyclin B/cdc2 complex has no role in the G_1 phase of the cell cycle.

5 The answer is D *Respiratory system / Physiology / Chronic bronchitis*

These symptoms are typical of chronic bronchitis. The age and smoking history make α_1-antitrypsin deficiency unlikely, as this person would have presented these symptoms sooner. His obesity, productive cough, and cyanosis are more typical of chronic bronchitis than emphysema. Both of these diseases are obstructive rather than restrictive; therefore, one would expect a FEV_1 and a low FEV_1:FVC ratio. In addition, the hemoglobin and hematocrit levels in patients with chronic bronchitis are often elevated to compensate for the chronic hypoxia due to hypoventilation. Smoking is by far the most important risk factor for this condition.

6 The answer is C *Skin and related connective tissue / Histology; pathology / Kaposi's sarcoma*

Kaposi's sarcoma was initially described as a cutaneous hemorrhagic nodule usually occurring on the lower extremities of elderly men. Kaposi's sarcoma is now recognized as being associated with HIV infection and afflicting primarily men with the virus. It is recognized histologically by irregular fascicles of spindle cells in the dermis accompanied by extravasated erythrocytes that impart a purple color. Kaposi's sarcoma is believed to be derived from endothelial cells, perhaps lymphatic endothelium. Unlike angiosarcomas, it does not form anastomosing vascular channels.

7 The answer is A *Central and peripheral nervous system / Physiology / Referred pain*

Referred pain is not well-understood. Somatic referred pain is very well-localized and intense. Visceral referred pain is the opposite and is thought to be conveyed by autonomic fibers. Diaphragmatic pain is usually referred to the shoulder.

8 The answer is D *Central and peripheral nervous system / Behavioral science / Depression*

Major depression is the first diagnosis to consider because of the subacute time course, self-neglect, social withdrawal, and psychotic symptoms. Major depression, even depression associated with psychotic symptoms, is treatable and has a good prognosis. There is no mention of drug abuse to suggest phencyclidine psychosis and no euphoria or increased sociability to suggest mania. The time during which symptoms have occurred has not been long enough to suggest schizophrenia or schizoaffective disorder.

9 The answer is C *Cardiovascular system / Physiology / Myocardial metabolism*

The high extraction ratio of oxygen across the heart (>50%), even at rest, suggests a limited reserve for further oxygen utilization and, thus, a close relationship between myocardial metabolism and underlying blood flow. Accordingly, it appears that local metabolic factors (such as adenosine) closely couple perfusion with myocardial demands. Compression of collapsible vessels within the myocardial wall result in perfusion being maximal during diastole. The heart exhibits extraordinary autoregulation and perfusion is thus constant over a broad range of arterial pressures. Although vessels are innervated by sympathetic fibers that can produce constriction in response to sympathetic activation, the concomitant increase in myocardial metabolism overrides this phenomenon and results in vasodilation in response to sympathetic stimulation. Healthy subjects have minimal collateral vessels and even in patients with severe myocardial disease, perfusion via collateral vessels is only sufficient to maintain basal metabolism and cannot enable large increases in blood flow in response to exercise or other stimuli.

10 The answer is B *Central and peripheral nervous system / Pharmacology / Epilepsy*

Carbamazepine is the preferred treatment for complex partial seizures. Haloperidol is an antipsychotic drug that can be used to treat psychotic symptoms associated with complex partial seizures only if the psychotic symptoms do not respond to the antiepileptic agent. Haloperidol and the antidepressant imipramine lower the seizure threshold. The antipanic drug alprazolam is not indicated, although some other types of benzodiazepines are used as antiepileptics.

11 The answer is C *General principles / Immunology / Inflammation and cellular margination*

As the vascular phase of the inflammatory response progresses, neutrophils and monocytes move toward the periphery of the microcirculatory vessels (margination) and adhere to, or pavement, the vascular endothelium in preparation for migration into the extravascular space. To migrate, leukocytes develop pseudopods and move, without accompanying loss of fluid, through gaps between the endothelial cells (diapedesis). In the latter part of the vascular phase, increased vascular permeability causes loss of plasma with resultant venous stasis and eventually clotting in the small capillaries local to the inflamed area.

[12] The answer is B *General principles / Cell biology / Hormone receptors*

The cytosol would contain the most fluorescence. Glucocorticoid receptors are soluble receptors and are not associated with the plasma membrane. Glucocorticoids diffuse into cells, bind to receptors in the cytosol, and then translocate to the nucleus. Inside the nucleus this hormone receptor complex regulates transcription via binding to specific sequences of DNA.

[13] The answer is A *Cardiovascular system / Histology; pathology / Temporal arteritis*

Temporal (giant cell) arteritis may be one component of the syndrome of polymyalgia rheumatica. Patients have headache, tenderness over the temporal artery, visual loss if retinal vessels are affected, and facial pain. Histologically, a granulomatous reaction is seen within the vessel wall associated with a mixed neutrophilic and lymphocytic infiltrate. Giant cells appear to phagocytize portions of elastica, and the vessel may be thrombosed in its late stage (*right*). Clinical response to steroids is excellent. Mönckeberg's arteriosclerosis shows medial calcification of arteries and is not arteritis, whereas Takayasu's arteritis (pulseless disease) involves the aortic arch and its major branches.

[14] The answer is C *General principles / Pharmacology / Asthma*

Cromolyn sodium inhibits degranulation of mast cells and, in other poorly understood ways, interferes with the inflammatory process assumed to be critical to moderate asthma caused by a variety of allergens and other conditions. Cromolyn is not absorbed from the gut and must be administered topically to the lung, where it acts prophylactically to inhibit bronchospasm caused by inhaled allergens, exercise, or altered environmental conditions. It does not directly relax bronchial smooth muscle in vivo or in vitro; hence, it is of little use in acute emergencies of bronchial hyperreactivity. However, it reduces the bronchial response to a number of spasmogens.

[15] The answer is C *Respiratory system / Physiology / Transudates and exudates*

When thoracentesis is performed, differentiation between transudates and exudates should always be an initial part of the analysis. To do this task, the protein and LDH levels of the pleural fluid and serum must be determined. If either the protein or LDH level of the pleural fluid is elevated, or if either protein or LDH ratio to the serum levels is elevated, the fluid should be classified as an exudate. All of these values should be normal in the setting of a transudate. Low glucose levels and low pH are typical of parapneumonic effusions and may indicate empyema or a grossly purulent effusion. This type of effusion with an infectious cause requires drainage with a chest tube because it may progress rapidly to become loculated. Elevated amylase in pleural effusion is often caused by either pancreatic disease or esophageal varices, so the patient should be evaluated for these complications. In addition, the appearance of blood in pleural fluid is an indication for checking the hematocrit of the fluid to determine whether there is a hemothorax. Elevated triglycerides suggest chylothorax if they are moderately elevated (50 to 110 mg/dL) and diagnostic if they are greater than 110 mg/dL. Lipoprotein electrophoresis is useful in the setting of a moderate elevation of triglycerides to determine the contribution of chylomicrons.

16 The answer is B *General principles / Pathology / Cytomegalovirus infection*

All of these viruses produce characteristic cellular inclusions. CMV and HSV are herpes viruses, a family of double-stranded DNA viruses that also includes varicella zoster virus (VZV). CMV causes either a subclinical or mononucleosis-like infection in immunocompetent individuals, latently infects white blood cells, and can be transmitted to uninfected persons via blood and body fluids. CMV may reactivate in patients with defective cell-mediated immunity, causing pneumonitis, renal tubulitis, hepatitis, esophagogastroenteritis, chorioretinitis, and meningoencephalitis. CMV produces a characteristic large, intranuclear, basophilic inclusion surrounded by a halo and variable, multiple basophilic cytoplasmic inclusions in mononucleate cells (epithelial and endothelial cells and leukocytes). HSV types 1 and 2 and VZV cause primary skin and mucous membrane infections, secondarily infecting dermatomal neurons, in which the virus becomes latent; reactivation results in reinfection of the skin and mucous membrane in the same distribution. Infected cells are often multinucleate, with nuclear molding, and the individual nuclei contain large, glassy, eosinophilic inclusions with peripheral margination of host chromatin (Cowdry type A inclusion). Adenovirus is a double-stranded DNA virus that infects glandular cells of the gastrointestinal and respiratory tracts, causing smudgy, basophilic intranuclear inclusions. Polyomavirus is a member of the double-stranded DNA papovavirus family (papillomavirus, polyomavirus, vacuolating viruses). Papillomaviruses cause cutaneous and mucosal warts and squamous cell neoplasms. Polyomaviruses cause urinary tract (e.g., BK virus) and CNS (e.g., JC virus) infections with reactivation in immunosuppressed patients and produce eosinophilic to basophilic gelatinous intranuclear inclusions in mononucleate cells. Vacuolating viruses are indigenous to animals and are encountered as contaminating agents in monkey kidney cell cultures.

17 The answer is C *Gastrointestinal system / Pathology; pharmacology / Peptic ulcer disease*

A number of physiologic, genetic, and other factors increase the risk of gastric and duodenal peptic ulcers. The evidence that *Helicobacter pylori* plays a principal role is compelling. Smoking and caffeine adversely affect the morbidity, mortality, and healing rates of peptic ulcers. In general, men and first-degree relatives of peptic ulcer patients have a threefold to fourfold increased risk of developing this disorder. Paradoxically, in gastric ulcer disease, acid secretion is not elevated. It is possible that excess secreted hydrogen ion is reabsorbed across the injured gastric mucosa. In general, a defect in gastric mucosal defense is the more important local physiologic factor promoting ulceration at this site.

18 The answer is D *Cardiovascular / Pharmacology / Ischemic heart disease; nitrovasodilator*

Glyeryl trinitrate (or nitroglycerin) is a palliative agent that does not affect the course of underlying ischemic heart disease. Most of its therapeutic affect is by increasing the compliance of venous capacitance vessels and thereby decreasing preload and myocardial oxygen consumption. Although it has a modest effect on collateral vessel tone in the heart, it generally is not a potent direct coronary vasodilator in human subjects. GTN is rapidly metabolized by enzymes in the liver and is usually taken sublingually to bypass first pass hepatic effects.

19 The answer is A *Respiratory system / Physiology / Hypoxemia*

In patients with hypoventilation, diffusion impairment or ventilation perfusion abnormality, arterial P_{O2} will usually eventually reach the level of a normal subject breathing 100% oxygen. In a subject with a shunt, although the end capillary P_{O2} may be as high as alveolar, it will mix with shunted blood that has oxygen tensions similar to mixed venous. Because the oxygen dissociation curve is basically flat at high oxygen tensions, the admixed blood oxygen tension will fall precipitously, thereby enabling a diagnosis. Most individuals with a shunt do not retain carbon dioxide because of ventilatory adjustments.

20 The answer is B *General principles / Pathology / Tumor*

In most human cancers, the stage of the disease, not the age of the patient, is the most important prognostic factor. Stage refers to the extent, or degree of spread, of the disease (i.e., local, regional, or distant). Tumor grade (i.e., differentiation), mitotic count, and extent of invasion correlate with the stage of the tumor in that high-grade (i.e., less differentiated) tumors and highly invasive tumors tend to be high-stage lesions.

21 **The answer is D** *Endocrine system / Physiology / Growth hormone*

Growth hormone stimulates cartilage and bone growth via somatomedin, an intermediary peptide. It is secreted periodically, like many other pituitary hormones, and is affected in a negative fashion by somatostatin, a hypothalamic peptide. Unlike other anterior pituitary hormones, cellular targets for growth hormone are relatively widespread. Somatomedin, synthesized in the liver and possibly other sites (e.g., muscle), is an important mediator of the growth effects of the hormone on cartilage and bone. Indeed, growth hormone has no direct effects on these cells by itself. Growth hormone has a large array of effects on amino acid, fat, and carbohydrate activities and in general displays anti-insulin-like actions.

22 **The answer is D** *Respiratory system / Microbiology / Pneumocystis pneumonia*

Pneumocystis pneumonia is caused by *Pneumocystis carinii,* a micro-organism of uncertain classification that belongs to either the protozoa or the fungi. It forms four to seven microcysts within a frothy, honeycomb-like alveolar exudate in the air spaces. These cysts contain numerous sporozoites that are released from the cysts at maturation. Pneumocystis pneumonia is commonly seen in individuals infected with HIV, a condition to be suspected in a person with a history of intravenous drug abuse.

23 **The answer is D** *Hematopoietic and lymphoreticular system / Histology; pathology / Hodgkin's disease*

The photomicrograph of the woman's biopsy shows classic features of nodular sclerosing Hodgkin's disease. The node is divided into irregular nodules by broad bands of dense collagen (*left*). In the panel on the *right,* the nodal infiltrate is composed of lymphocytes, plasma cells, eosinophils, and multilobated cells with prominent red nucleoli, called Reed–Sternberg cells. Although Reed–Sternberg cells are not pathognomonic of this disease, they are diagnostic when seen in this appropriate inflammatory milieu. The nodular sclerosis type of Hodgkin's disease usually includes a large mediastinal mass and involvement of adjacent lymph node groups (e.g., supraclavicular nodes).

24 **The answer is A** *Renal/urinary system / Physiology / Na+ transport and renal epithelial physiology*

Na+ is transported from the tubular lumen to the peritubular capillary by an electrochemical gradient that is largely generated by the action of the Na+/K+-ATPase activity at the basolateral surface. The cell is freely permeable to water and chloride, and hence reabsorbs a virtually isosmotic fraction of tubular luminal fluid. The attraction of Na+ creates a very large, intracellular negative potential, approximately -70 mV. There is no significant hormone dependence of ion transport in these cells on either aldosterone or ADH.

25 **The answer is D** *Musculoskeletal system / Anatomy / Thoracic outlet syndrome*

Thoracic outlet syndrome describes compression of the lower trunk of the brachial plexus and the subclavian artery by an anomalous thirteenth (cervical) rib. Sensory changes occur over the distribution of the ulnar nerve; the phrenic nerves are not involved.

26 **The answer is D** *Endocrine system / Biochemistry / Gluconeogenesis and glycolysis*

Stimulation of β cells by glucose results in the release of insulin. Insulin has numerous effects on virtually every tissue, and its overall effect is the conservation of body fuel supplies. It does this by promoting the uptake and storage of glucose, amino acids, and fats. In the liver it decreases gluconeogenesis and glycogenolysis and promotes glycolysis. In addition, it promotes lipogenesis in the liver and fat cells and is antilipolytic. It is also an important anabolic protein hormone that inhibits the breakdown of amino acids and the release of glucagon from neighboring α cells.

27 **The answer is C** *General principles / Cell biology / Cell division*

Chiasma is crossover between homologous chromosomes during prophase I of meiosis. Centromere is the location on a chromosome, which separates the long arm from the short arm of the chromosome. Meiosis I is the reduction division in which the amount of DNA per cell is halved. Meiosis in primary oocytes is arrested in prophase I until ovulation, which releases this arrest. Fertilization releases metaphase (in meiosis II) arrest. In meiosis, centromeres do not duplicate and divide. Thus, a reduction division is possible in meiosis I. This is in contrast with mitosis, in which centromeres do duplicate and divide during anaphase I.

28 **The answer is D** *General principles / Histology / Cell division*

The beginning of prophase is marked by the appearance of chromosomes within the nucleus. Throughout prophase, the chromosomes condense further; dissolution of the nuclear envelope marks the end of this phase. During metaphase, the kinetochore becomes attached to tubulin, the major component of the mitotic spindle. Metaphase is marked by the alignment of chromosomes along the equatorial (metaphase) plane. The next stage of cell division is anaphase, which is marked by separation of the centromeres. The addition of tubulin to the mitotic spindle draws the chromosomes toward opposite poles of the cell. Anaphase ends when the chromosomes are clustered at opposite poles of the cell. During the final stage, telophase, the chromosomes uncoil; the nuclear envelope reforms; and the cell divides. As the cell divides, the cytoplasm also divides by cytokinesis; these processes continue until two daughter cells are produced. Cell division during telophase is thought to occur by the constriction of a ring of actin filaments.

29 **The answer is E** *General principles / Biochemistry / Protein synthesis, posttranslational modification, and targeting*

Tetracyclines inhibit the 30s ribosomal subunit. (Chloramphenicol inhibits peptidyl transferase.) Diphtheria toxin binds eEF-2. Puromycin has a similar structure to aminoacyl tRNA, is incorporated into the growing chain, and inhibits any further elongation of the peptide chain. Clindamycin and erythromycin both bind the 50s ribosomal subunit.

30 **The answer is B** *General principles / Biochemistry / Protein synthesis, posttranslational modification, and targeting*

Protein synthesis begins in the nucleus, where the gene in question is first transcribed into mRNA. Posttranscriptional processing produces the final mRNA product. Such processing includes 5′ capping, which confers stability to the RNA and plays a role in the initiation of protein synthesis. In addition, a poly-A tail is added to the RNA by poly-A polymerase. This tail contributes to RNA stability and helps RNA to exit the nucleus. The nascent transcript generally contains introns, which are pieces of the transcript that do not code for amino acid sequences. The introns are removed in exon splicing. This occurs in the nucleus. The correctly spliced mRNA transcript leaves the nucleus and is bound to a free ribosome.

31 **The answer is D** *Central and peripheral nervous system / Behavioral science / Psychoanalysis*

Free association is the major method of communication in psychoanalysis. Interpretation is a method of intervention, and resistance and countertransference are processes that develop during the treatment. Meditation is not involved in the psychoanalytic process.

32 **The answer is A** *Respiratory system / Pathology / Carbon monoxide poisoning*

CO competes with oxygen for hemoglobin (Hb), forming carboxyhemoglobin. It has 200 times as much affinity for Hb as does oxygen. CO poisoning causes headache, confusion, visual disturbances, convulsions, coma, and death. Treatment consists of removing the CO exposure and administering 100% oxygen or hyperbaric oxygen. Penicillamine is used to treat poisoning caused by heavy metals. CO is a colorless, odorless gas.

33 **The answer is E** *Hematopoietic and lymphoreticular system / Immunology / Multiple myeloma; immunoglobulin abnormalities*

In approximately 55% of people with multiple myeloma, the membrane-bound protein (M protein) is IgG; in 25%, the M protein is IgA, and it is rarely IgM, IgD, or IgE. In the remaining 20%, Bence Jones proteinuria without the serum M protein is seen.

Well-demarcated (or "punched out") osteolytic lesions are almost pathognomonic for multiple myeloma. In 99% of patients with multiple myeloma, electrophoretic analysis of the serum proteins shows an increase in one of the Ig classes or light chains, approximately 23,000 daltons (Bence Jones protein), in the urine. The presence of 55,000-dalton monoclonal proteins indicates heavy-chain disease, a different type of monoclonal gammopathy that is not associated with osteolytic lesions. Although it is not specific for this disease, patients with multiple myeloma do have suppressed synthesis of normal antibodies and are thus susceptible to recurrent bacterial and viral infections.

34 **The answer is D** *General principles / Pharmacology / Aminoglycosides; therapeutic index*

Aminoglycosides can cause severe nephrotoxicity and ototoxicity. Their therapeutic index is low; peak and trough levels are commonly monitored to allow for dose adjustments or a change in timing of administration. Aminoglycosides are eliminated rapidly, with a serum half-life of 1 to 5 hours. However, rapid clearance is not the major determinant for therapeutic monitoring. Aminoglycosides are not extensively metabolized. Because they are polar molecules, they are lipid-insoluble and do not cross the blood–brain barrier. The incidence of hypersensitivity reactions is extremely low.

35 **The answer is C** *General principles / Pharmacology / Neoplasia and hormone action*

Tamoxifen has become the drug of choice for the initial endocrine management of breast cancer and a useful adjuvant therapy for the palliative management of advanced breast cancer. It is relatively nontoxic, and patients with breast tumors containing estrogen receptors are most likely to respond to the drug. The drug binds to the estrogen receptor in the nucleus but does not stimulate transcription. The tamoxifen–estrogen receptor complex does not readily dissociate, thereby affecting estrogen receptor recycling. In premenopausal women, competition with estrogen receptors in the anterior pituitary and hypothalamus disrupts normal feedback inhibition of gonadotropin-releasing hormone, thereby enhancing gonadotropin release.

36 **The answer is C** *General principles / Pharmacology / Angina therapy*

Glyceryl trinitrate is most effective by decreasing preload in angina. GTN at high concentrations provides some benefit in angina by reducing afterload. However, this effect is often accompanied by reflex tachycardia that may disrupt the improvement in myocardial oxygen consumption and supply achieved by GTN. Propranolol is useful in blocking this reflex effect because it is negatively inotropic and negatively chronotropic. Propranolol may be accompanied by coronary artery vasospasm after removing β-receptor-mediated dilation and leaving unopposed coronary artery α-receptor-mediated vasoconstriction.

37 **The answer is C** *General principles / Pharmacology / Antiepileptics*

Phenytoin decreases resting Na+ flux and the flow of Na+ currents during chemical depolarization or action potential. In the CNS, this results in depression of the generation and transmission of repetitive action potentials in epileptic foci. It is usually the drug of choice for seizures except absence seizures and in general is started alone to assess its efficacy. Phenytoin is associated with teratogenic effects (fetal hydantoin syndrome). Other agents, such as diazepam and phenobarbital, affect chloride channels by interacting with GABA at its receptor site.

38 **The answer is C** *General principles / Biochemistry / RNA synthesis*

RNA polymerase I produces rRNA. RNA polymerase II produces mostly mRNA. RNA polymerase III makes tRNA and other small RNAs. The reason mammalian cells use three different types of RNA polymerases is not known. There is no known eukaryotic DNA-directed RNA polymerase IV.

39 The answer is C *General principles / Pharmacology / Toxicology and aplastic anemia*

Benzene can induce aplastic anemia by damaging myeloid stem cells. Thiouracil is associated with agranulocytosis, primarily because of its ability to decrease production or increase destruction of neutrophils. Penicillin acts as a hapten, which produces erythrocyte destruction via warm antibody autoimmune hemolysis. In contrast, methyldopa stimulates the production of antibodies against intrinsic red blood cell antigens. Ingestion of an excessive quantity of acetaminophen is followed by the production of toxic metabolites, which first decrease hepatic glutathione levels and then cause centrilobular necrosis due to biomolecular adduct formation.

40 The answer is A *Renal/urinary system / Pathology / Crescentic glomerulonephritis secondary to antiglomerular basement membrane antibodies*

Rapidly progressive glomerulonephritis (RPGN) encompasses three categories of disorders, all of which are characterized by glomerular crescents and distinguished by their appearance on immunofluorescence microscopy. Type I RPGN includes disorders that have an autoantibody targeting a type IV collagen antigen within the basement membrane. The autoantibody is typically IgG, which binds to a uniformly distributed antigen in the basement membrane, thus producing a linear pattern of fluorescence and absence of immune complex deposits by electron microscopy. A subset of patients presents with renal limited disease characterized by progressive renal dysfunction and glomerular hematuria (i.e., antiglomerular basement membrane disease). Other patients have a pulmonary–renal syndrome (Goodpasture's disease) and concurrent intra-alveolar pulmonary hemorrhage secondary to necrotizing capillaritis of alveolar septal capillaries. Type II RPGN includes crescentic glomerulonephritides caused by immune complex deposits. All immune complex disorders have a type II RPGN variant, with lupus being the most common. Type III RPGN, or pauci-immune crescentic glomerulonephritis, includes disorders with absence or paucity of immune deposition and more frequent concurrent small vessel vasculitis. There are renal-limited and systemic (e.g., microscopic polyangiitis and Wegener's granulomatosis) forms of type III RPGN, many of which are associated with antineutrophil cytoplasmic antibodies. Some of the systemic forms are associated with a pulmonary–renal presentation. Patients with RPGN typically have a nephritic syndrome and without therapy progress to irreversible renal failure over time.

41 The answer is E *General principles / Immunology / Monoclonal antibodies and gram-negative bacteria*

A monoclonal antibody, such as IgG, is useful only against organisms producing lipopolysaccharide (i.e., gram-negative bacteria). The organism must produce a disease state through bacteremia, since IgG is present only in the circulatory system. Organisms such as *Bordetella pertussis,* the causative agent of whooping cough, and *Vibrio cholerae,* the agent of cholera, are gram-negative but do not invade the bloodstream. Pulmonary anthrax is caused by *Bacillus anthracis,* which is gram-positive. Leprosy is caused by *Mycobacterium leprae,* which is acid-fast, not gram-negative. Bubonic plague, however, is caused by *Yersinia pestis,* a gram-negative organism that multiplies in the bloodstream, spreading through to the lymphatics. *Y. pestis* has many virulence factors, including lipopolysaccharide.

42 The answer is E *General principles / Pharmacology / Mechanism of action of penicillin*

The principles of antibiotic action are perhaps best exemplified by penicillin. Antibiotics act by specifically binding to macromolecules found only in the parasite. Transpeptidase is the only penicillin-binding protein listed; it is inactivated when binding occurs.

43 The answer is D *General principles / Immunology / Passive immunity; vaccination*

The most appropriate treatment for the medical student described in the question is an injection of tetanus toxoid, which triggers an anamnestic response because of the DTP series received in childhood. If there is no history of DTP immunization, passive immunity can be induced by the administration of heterologous (e.g., equine) or homologous (i.e., human) antibodies. Types I and III reactions can result from heterologous administration. Aminoglycosides are given for infections caused by gram-negative bacteria. The tetanus toxoid is produced by *Clostridium tetani,* a gram-positive rod.

Test 11 • 265

44 **The answer is B** *General principles / Pharmacology / Adverse effects of aspirin*

The major adverse effect of aspirin is gastrointestinal bleeding. Inhibition of local cytoprotective arachidonic acid metabolites (prostaglandin E_2 and prostacyclin) in the gastric mucosa contributes to this adverse effect and can be offset by simultaneously using exogenous synthetic prostanoids. In addition, aspirin has a direct irritating effect on the mucosa. Nonsteroidal anti-inflammatory agents in general have little effect on lipoxygenase activity but do affect cyclo-oxygenase. In particular, aspirin irreversibly inhibits this enzyme in platelets and other cell types by acetylating the α-amino group of the terminal serine. This irreversible inhibition has significant implications in that platelet function is not restored to normal until a new enzyme has been synthesized. Aspirin has little effect on normal body temperature but reduces abnormally elevated body temperatures secondary to alterations in central thermoregulation.

45 **The answer is C** *General principles / Biochemistry / RNA splicing*

The splicing reaction takes place in the nucleus of the cell before capping and polyadenylation as part of the posttranscriptional modification of eukaryotic RNA. U1 snRNP recognizes a 9-base pair region of the introns involved and is thought to precipitate the organized formation of the large particle termed the spliceosome on the RNA. The splicing reaction then cuts the intron at the 5′ end and forms a lariat structure by covalently binding the cut 5′ end of the intron to a sequence on the 3′ end. The intron is cut again at the 3′ end and thus is cut out of the RNA.

46 **The answer is A** *Hematopoietic and lymphoreticular system / Pathology / Carcinoid of the appendix*

The most common tumor of the appendix is a carcinoid tumor. The neoplastic cells show neuroendocrine differentiation. The cells grow in nests and are associated with a delicate, branching vascular network. The nuclei of the cells have a salt-and-pepper chromatin distribution. Typically, the cytoplasm of the cells contains granules that are visible by special stains. Silver salts turn the granules black; thus, they are argyrophilic. The behavior of these tumors is related to their depth of invasion into the muscular wall and serosal adipose tissue.

47 **The answer is B** *General principles / Biochemistry / Nitrogen metabolism*

Negative nitrogen balance results from defective CCK–PZ production when the consumption of dietary protein is normal. Negative nitrogen balance occurs when the excretion of nitrogen exceeds the intake of nitrogen. A number of conditions can cause a negative nitrogen balance, including a deficiency in any one of the essential amino acids or a defect in the intestinal phase of protein digestion and absorption. CCK–PZ is essential for stimulating the secretion of inactive pancreatic zymogens, which become active proteases in the small intestine. The intestinal phase of digestion is essential to maintaining nitrogen balance; the gastric phase appears to have little or no effect. For example, gastric resection does not affect nitrogen balance. In PKU, tyrosine becomes an essential amino acid and must be supplied in the diet.

48 **The answer is E** *General principles / Biochemistry / Protein synthesis*

The synthetic polynucleotide sequence of CAACAACAACAA . . . could be read by the in vitro protein synthesizing system starting at the first C, the first A, or the second A. In the first case, the first triplet codon would be CAA, which codes for glutamine; in the second case, the first triplet codon would be AAC, which codes for asparagine; and in the last case, the first triplet codon would be ACA, which codes for threonine.

49 **The answer is A** *General principles / Biostatistics / Continuous variables*

The variables described in the question are continuous in that their values are along a continuum, as are age and IQ, as opposed to being categorical. Categorical variables such as sex, race, and marital status require the use of nonparametric statistical tests, such as the chi-square test.

50 **The answer is B** *Central and peripheral nervous system / Pathology / Arnold Chiari malformation*

Arnold Chiari type II malformation consists of a small posterior fossa, abnormal midline cerebellum, and extension of the cerebellar vermis through the foramen magnum. It is associated with myelomeningocele and hydrocephalus. Arnold Chiari type I malformation consists of a downward shift of cerebellar tonsils. Rachischisis is a more severe form of spinal column nonclosure. Dandy Walker malformation is characterized by absence of the cerebellar vermis, an enlarged posterior fossa, and dysplasias of the brain stem nuclei. Anencephaly is a malformation of the anterior end of the neural, grossly characterized by the absence of the brain and calvarium.

test **12**

Questions

Directions: Single best answer questions consist of numbered items or incomplete statements followed by answers or by completions of the statement. Select the ONE lettered answer or completion that is BEST in each case.

1 *Pseudomonas aeruginosa, Staphylococcus aureus,* and *Serratia marcescens* all produce which one of the following substances?

(A) Endotoxins
(B) Enterotoxins
(C) Lipoteichoic acids
(D) Mycolic acids
(E) Pigments

2 Resistance to phagocytosis is among the most important properties for virulence of many bacteria. *Mycobacterium tuberculosis* is very resistant to phagocytic killing and actually grows in macrophages. The successful antiphagocytic strategy employed by *M. tuberculosis* clearly involves which one of the following mechanisms?

(A) Production of protein exotoxins to kill or impair the phagocyte
(B) Prevention of phagosome–lysosome fusion
(C) Elaboration of immunoglobulin (Ig) A protease
(D) Production of the antiphagocytic polysaccharide capsule
(E) Escape from the phagolysosome into the cytoplasm

3 Injection of a pharmacologically effective amount of an antimuscarinic agent, such as atropine, may

(A) increase bronchial glandular secretions
(B) increase heart rate
(C) cause paralysis in some skeletal muscles
(D) constrict the pupil
(E) promote sweating

4 G proteins are involved with various cellular signaling pathways and are known to hydrolyze

(A) adenosine triphosphate (ATP)
(B) guanosine triphosphate (GTP)
(C) adenosine diphosphate (ADP)
(D) guanosine diphosphate (GDP)
(E) adenosine monophosphate (AMP)

5 Down's syndrome is most frequently caused by which of the following?

(A) An unbalanced translocation event
(B) Meiotic nondisjunction
(C) Trisomy 22
(D) Trisomy 21 mosaicism
(E) Trinucleotide repeat expansion in chromosome 21

6 Which of the following statements about the endoplasmic reticulum (ER) is true?

(A) Secreted proteins do not require a signal peptide to direct the protein to the ER membrane
(B) Translocation of proteins across the ER membrane usually occurs posttranslation
(C) Unlike the Golgi complex, the ER plays a minor role in lipid biosynthesis
(D) *N*-linked glycosylation occurs in the ER
(E) Sequestration of chloride ions from the cytosol is an important function of the ER

7 A peripheral lung nodule was resected from a 50-year-old man. The tumor, pictured here, is best classified as

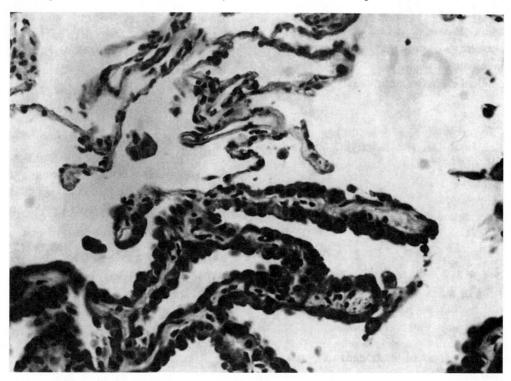

(A) small cell carcinoma
(B) undifferentiated large cell carcinoma
(C) adenoid cystic carcinoma
(D) bronchioloalveolar carcinoma
(E) diffuse large cell lymphoma

8 A lymph node removed from a 32-year-old man shows diffuse large cell lymphoma. Which of the following clinical scenarios most likely characterizes this patient?

(A) Disseminated disease at presentation; prolonged survival and eventual death owing to lymphoma or its complications
(B) Rapid development of circulating immature blasts, requiring aggressive cytotoxic therapy
(C) Greater than 90% chance of being alive 10 years after diagnosis
(D) Rapid death if therapy is unsuccessful; approximately 50% chance for long-term survival if therapy achieves complete response
(E) Spontaneous remission in 20% of patients

9 A young man visits his physician with complaints of polyuria and unexplained weight loss. Fasting plasma glucose is greater than 140 mg/dL on two occasions, and oral glucose tolerance test is consistent with a diagnosis of type I insulin-dependent diabetes mellitus (IDDM). The likely histologic site underlying this patient's disorder is

(A) pancreatic acini
(B) zymogen-containing cells of the pancreatic acinus
(C) α cells of the islets of Langerhans
(D) β cells of the islets Langerhans
(E) δ cells of the islets of Langerhans

10 Which of the following statements about the composition of amyloid is true?

(A) Is 95% composed of nonbranching fibrils of indefinite length
(B) Has a mixed α chiral/β-pleated sheet formation
(C) Ninety percent of fibrils are single fibers
(D) Is 50% composed of minor compounds, component P, proteoglycans, and sulfated glycoaminoglycans
(E) Has a variable electron microscopic structure depending on the type of amyloid deposited

11 An endogenous hormone that tends to decrease circulating blood glucose is

(A) glucagon
(B) growth hormone (GH)
(C) somatostatin
(D) epinephrine
(E) thyroid hormone

12 A 60-year-old woman with longstanding rheumatoid arthritis presents with insidious renal failure, proteinuria, hepatosplenomegaly, restrictive cardiomyopathy, and malabsorption with diarrhea. Which of the following statements about the renal biopsy shown in Figure 53 of the color plate section is correct?

(A) Deposited material consists of an α-helix protein
(B) Serum and urine immunoelectrophoresis are likely to show a monoclonal immunoglobulin, and bone marrow biopsy is likely to show a plasma cell dyscrasia
(C) Electron microscopy reveals amorphous granular electron-dense deposits
(D) Deposited material is a β-pleated sheet

13 Surfactant is a substance that is critical for normal lung function. Which of the following statements about surfactant is true?

(A) Surfactant consists mainly of proteins and a smaller percentage of lipids, the most abundant lipid being dipalmitoyl phosphatidylcholine
(B) Surfactant is synthesized by the alveolar type II epithelial cells; damage to these cells in patients with adult respiratory distress syndrome (ARDS) can lead to increased alveolar collapse
(C) Surfactant increases pulmonary compliance by increasing alveolar surface tension
(D) Surfactant forms a lipid bilayer with interspersed protein molecules that line the alveolar surface, thus preventing atelectasis and facilitating gas exchange
(E) The hydrophilic tails of the dipalmitoyl phosphatidylcholine are pointed toward the gas or air phase, whereas the hydrophobic heads are pointed toward the cell and aqueous hypophase
(F) Surfactant replacement is not yet an available therapy for neonatal respiratory distress syndrome

14 Halothane has blood:gas and oil:gas partition coefficients of 2.4 and 220, respectively. Methoxyflurane has blood:gas and oil:gas coefficients of 13 and 950, respectively. Which of the following statements regarding these volatile anesthetics is correct?

(A) Both result in faster induction than does nitrous oxide (blood:gas partition coefficient of 0.47)
(B) The minimal alveolar concentration of halothane is less than that of methoxyflurane
(C) Both agents are useful because they do not have any cardiodepressant effects
(D) Recovery from methoxyflurane is faster than that from halothane
(E) An increase in ventilatory rate makes the onset of anesthesia more rapid for either agent

15 Restriction enzymes have which one of the following characteristics? They

(A) can cleave only circular DNA
(B) generate either staggered (sticky) or blunt ends upon cleaving DNA
(C) cleave different DNAs randomly
(D) can cleave different DNAs only once
(E) can cleave both DNA and RNA

16 A chronically ill 43-year-old patient with a relapse of multiple sclerosis has been in the hospital for 4 weeks. He has angered the nurses by being very demanding, including calling them "every 5 minutes" for minor reasons and complaining that they do not respond promptly. To remedy this situation, the physician must

(A) instruct the patient to behave better
(B) order a sedating medication
(C) arrange for the nurses to visit the patient for 3 minutes every hour
(D) warn the patient that he will be transferred to another hospital if he does not straighten out

17 A 74-year-old man has hypertension, diabetes mellitus with retinopathy, and chronic obstructive pulmonary disease (COPD). He admits to drinking four bottles of beer a day. He has been living alone for the past year since his wife died. His primary care physician should be especially and immediately concerned about the risk of

(A) renal insufficiency
(B) silent myocardial infarction
(C) suicide
(D) peripheral neuropathy
(E) pneumonia

18 This graph measures the number of viable bacterial cells in a control culture and cultures of exponentially growing cells to which antibiotics were added at the point indicated by the *arrow*. The antibiotic added to the culture to produce *curve A* was which one of the following?

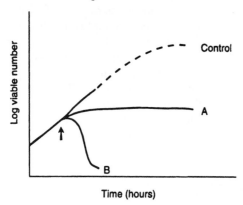

(A) Polymyxin B
(B) Cephalothin
(C) Chloramphenicol
(D) Methicillin
(E) Vancomycin

19 According to the Henderson–Hasselbalch equation:

$$pH = \frac{6.1 + \log[HCO_3]}{0.03 \times PCO_2}$$

The apparent dissociation constant, pK, in blood is 6.1, and the solubility constant for CO_2 in plasma at 38°C is 0.03 mmol/L/mm Hg. (Recall that log 10 = 1; log 20 = 1.3; log 30 = 1.5; normal values of $[HCO_3^-]$ = 25 mmol/L; PCO_2 = 40 mm Hg.) If a patient has a plasma $[HCO_3^-]$ of 37 mmol/L and arterial PCO_2 of 60 mm Hg, the patient is most likely to have

(A) respiratory alkalosis
(B) respiratory acidosis
(C) fully compensated respiratory acidosis
(D) metabolic alkalosis
(E) metabolic acidosis

20 The ability of erythrocytes to pump Na+ from the cytoplasm into the plasma compartment would be compromised most directly by a total deficiency of

(A) stearoyl coenzyme A (CoA) desaturase
(B) diphosphoglycerate kinase
(C) pyruvate carboxylase
(D) glucose 6-phosphatase
(E) malate dehydrogenase

21 A total of 25 hypertensive patients are followed for 2 weeks for the effects of a diuretic drug on K+ concentrations. The statistical test used to compare the K+ serum levels before and after medication is most likely to be

(A) discriminant analysis
(B) paired *t*-test
(C) regression analysis
(D) chi-square test
(E) Pearson correlation

22 Which of the following statements about testosterone is correct?

(A) It is synthesized from cholesterol by Sertoli cells in the testes
(B) It is sufficient for spermatogenesis and spermatid maturation
(C) It is not produced in women
(D) It is usually maintained at a constant level at all times
(E) It regulates luteinizing hormone (LH) secretion at the levels of hypothalamus and pituitary

23 A patient's symptoms lead a physician to suspect a point mutation in a portion of a gene for which the physician has polymerase chain reaction (PCR) primers. The physician amplifies this region of the patient's DNA using PCR and then performs a single-strand conformational polymorphism (SSCP) analysis on his DNA. Which one of the following statements about the interpretation of this test is correct?

(A) If the patient is heterozygous for a dominant mutation, the physician sees two bands
(B) If the physician sees four bands, the patient has multiple mutations
(C) If the physician sees two bands, the patient is either homozygous normal or homozygous for the mutation
(D) If the physician sees four bands, the patient has a point mutation that is causing his disease
(E) If the patient does not have a point mutation within the amplified region, the physician sees only one band
(F) SSCP is not useful in this situation

24 A patient has paroxysmal episodes of hypertension, tremor, weakness, and sweating. Urinary catecholamines and their metabolites are elevated, and computed tomography (CT) of the abdomen detects a mass within the adrenal gland. The tumor most likely involves which one of the following cells?

(A) Zona glomerulosa
(B) Zona fasciculata
(C) Zona reticularis
(D) Chromaffin cells of the medulla

25 If the tumor in a patient diagnosed with pheochromocytoma is deemed inoperable, pharmacotherapy of the disorder may include which one of the following drugs?

(A) Clonidine
(B) Propranolol
(C) Methyldopa
(D) Phenoxybenzamine

26 Which of the following statements applies to the organism shown in the endoscopic biopsy (hematoxylin and eosin and Giemsa stains) in Figure 54 of the color plate section?

(A) It produces bicarbonate, locally reducing gastric acidity
(B) Patients infected with it are at increased risk for developing neoplasms in the involved organ
(C) It frequently invades deep into the wall of the involved organ, resulting in perforation and peritonitis
(D) It is a gram-positive bacillus

27 Which of the following is true about insecticide poisoning?

(A) Chlorinated hydrocarbons, including dichlorodiphenyl trichloroethane, inhibit cholinesterase
(B) Treatment of cholinesterase inhibitor poisoning includes pralidoxime and atropine
(C) Symptoms associated with organophosphate poisoning include salivation, bronchoconstriction, vomiting, diarrhea, and pupil dilation
(D) Cholinesterase inhibitors have a much longer half-life than do chlorinated hydrocarbons.

28 A 22-year-old male college student visits the student health service complaining of extreme fatigue, sore throat, difficulty concentrating, and fever to 39°C over the last week. Physical examination is unremarkable except for mild lymph node enlargement in the axillary, cervical, and inguinal regions and a palpable spleen tip. A blood count shows hemoglobin of 10 g/dl, platelets of 105,000/μl, and white cell count of 22,000/μl with 60% lymphoid cells. The laboratory blood profile also shows an absolute red cell count of 2.3×10^6/μl, mean red cell volume of 125 femtoliters (fl), and mean cell hemoglobin concentration of 43 g/dl. What is the most likely diagnosis for this patient?

(A) Infectious lymphocytosis
(B) *Bordetella pertussis* infections
(C) Cytomegalovirus (CMV) mononucleosis syndrome
(D) Mononucleosis secondary to Epstein–Barr virus (EBV) infection (infectious mononucleosis)
(E) Mononucleosis secondary to *Toxoplasma golndii* infection

29 A 21-year-old female patient presents to her local emergency department complaining of "a vision problem." Upon examination she is found to have a bitemporal hemianopia. Where is the site of a potential lesion?

(A) Cranial nerve II
(B) Cranial nerve III
(C) Pituitary gland tumor
(D) Right lateral geniculate body
(E) Left occipital cortex

30 The eclipse phase of the virus replication cycle has which one of the following characteristics? It

(A) is defined as that period after which the first virus particles are assembled
(B) denotes the time between virus entry into the cell and the appearance of extracellular virus particles
(C) is the part of the replication cycle during which virus particles cannot be recovered from the infected cells
(D) is comparable to the metaphase portion of mitosis

31 Light microscopy requires the use of special techniques, such as stains, to visualize cells and cell components. Which of the following cellular components can be visualized after staining for catalase?

(A) Golgi complex
(B) Lysosomes
(C) Rough ER
(D) Smooth ER
(E) Peroxisomes

32 Dinitrochlorobenzene was applied to a patient's skin over a 1-cm² area on the right forearm. Approximately 2 weeks later, a pruritic rash occurred at the site. It can be concluded that

(A) the patient lacks all T cell–mediated immune function
(B) the patient suffers from DiGeorge's syndrome
(C) the reaction would require an additional 2 weeks to develop on subsequent exposure to dinitrochlorobenzene
(D) the reaction observed was most likely caused by CD4+ T cells

33 An ophthalmologic examination of a 60-year-old man complaining of vision problems reveals increased intraocular pressure (25 mm Hg) with optic disk changes and visual field defects. These findings strongly suggest primary open-angle glaucoma for which pharmacotherapy is considered. The underlying cause of the patient's condition is a decreased outflow facility of the aqueous humor. A primary anatomic structure involved with the histopathologic changes that account for this problem is the

(A) conjunctiva
(B) cornea
(C) canal of Schlemm
(D) ciliary process
(E) choroidal vessel

34 Pharmacotherapy for a patient with primary open-angle glaucoma is initially designed to open trabecular meshwork by contracting the ciliary muscle. A useful agent for this purpose is

(A) atropine
(B) succinylcholine
(C) pilocarpine
(D) dexamethasone
(E) tubocurarine

35 Which one of the following statements about mechanical ventilation is true?

(A) Hypoxemic respiratory failure is an indication for mechanical ventilation, but hypercarbic respiratory failure is not
(B) A backup respiratory rate is set for the assist–control but not for the synchronized intermittent mandatory ventilation mode
(C) In the assist–control mode, every breath the patient takes has a set volume
(D) Pressure support ventilation is the mode most commonly used at first for mechanical ventilation of the acutely ill
(E) A potential disadvantage of using positive end-expiratory pressure is that it may increase cardiac output but decrease oxygen delivery to the tissues
(F) With mechanical ventilation, accurate control of the oxygen concentration of the air inhaled by the patient is not possible

36 Which of the following is true about the role of cell cycle regulators in disease?

(A) Unlike the retinoblastoma gene, p53 is rarely mutated in human cancers
(B) Li-Fraumeni syndrome is caused by germline mutations in the retinoblastoma gene
(C) Neurofibromatosis II is caused by a mutation in a tumor suppressor gene, neurofibromin, on chromosome 17q
(D) Familial adenomatous polyposis coli is caused by a mutation in a mismatch repair gene
(E) Carcinoma of the uterus caused by papillomavirus is primarily caused by the E6 and E7 genes of papillomavirus, which interfere with cellular tumor suppressor proteins

37 Glucagon plays an important role in the regulation of glycogen metabolism. Which of the following statements concerning the action of glucagon is correct?

(A) It inhibits adenyl cyclase in hepatocytes
(B) It promotes branching on glycogen molecules
(C) It antagonizes the effect of epinephrine on glycogen metabolism
(D) It regulates hepatic phosphorylase
(E) It inhibits gluconeogenesis

38 A man takes his wife to the hospital because she has run through the family bank account by making lengthy long-distance telephone calls and by purchasing expensive jewelry and clothing. Which of the following most likely describes her disorder?

(A)   Histrionic personality disorder
(B)   Major depression
(C)   Obsessive-compulsive disorder
(D)   Borderline personality disorder
(E)   Bipolar I disorder

39 The peripheral nerve tumor pictured here is best classified as a

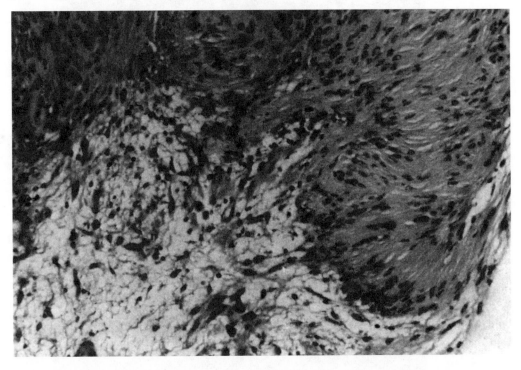

(A)   neurofibroma
(B)   traumatic neuroma
(C)   neurilemoma
(D)   triton tumor

40 Triglycerides are neutral fats of animals and food plants; they make up approximately 90% of the dietary intake of fats. An important step in their digestion in the gastrointestinal tract is

(A)   significant hydrolysis by gastric lipases
(B)   breakdown by biliary enzymes
(C)   formation of fatty acids and monoglyceride by pancreatic lipase
(D)   active transport of fatty acid products in the intestinal brush border

41 Which of these tracts, whose fibers traverse the spinal cord, brain stem, and higher structures, is thought to cross to the opposite side of the central nervous system (CNS) twice?

(A)   The anterior spinocerebellar tract, which conveys unconscious sensory information from joints, tendons, and muscles
(B)   The spinal thalamic tract, which conveys conscious sensory information of pain and temperature
(C)   The cuneocerebellar tract, which conveys conscious muscle and joint sensory information
(D)   The vestibulospinal tract, which conveys efferent fibers

42 A 62-year-old woman died of congestive heart failure due to severe mitral stenosis. At autopsy, sections of the heart revealed the lesions shown in the photomicrograph. This suggests a previous history of which one of the following conditions?

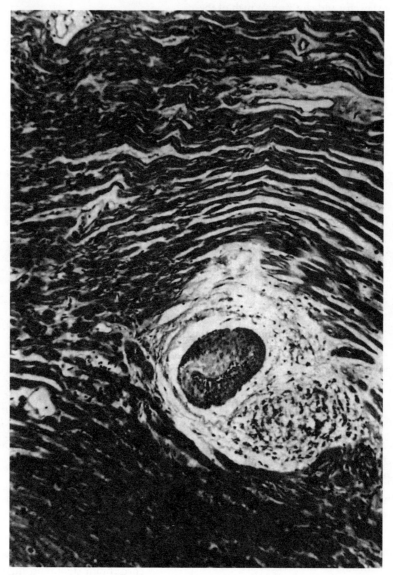

(A) Amyloidosis
(B) Rheumatic fever
(C) Polyarteritis nodosa
(D) Myocardial infarction

43 Which of the following tests is the major projective instrument of personality assessment?

(A) Rorschach inkblot test
(B) Minnesota Multiphasic Personality Inventory
(C) Thematic apperception test
(D) Sentence completion test
(E) Projective drawings

44 Proof of the presence of active disease caused by *Mycobacterium tuberculosis* is provided by which one of the following diagnostic measures?

(A) The tuberculin test
(B) Clinical findings (e.g., weight loss, night sweats, cough, low-grade fever)
(C) Finding acid-fast organisms in sputum
(D) Isolation of *M. tuberculosis*

45 Which of the following statements about the lesion depicted in Figure 55 of the color plate section is correct?

(A) It is associated with intravenous injection of heroin

(B) It is associated with peripheral basophilia (increased numbers of circulating basophils) and low serum fibrinogen levels in some patients

(C) Hypoxemia is a commonly associated problem in patients with this disorder

(D) Clefts do not contain cholesterol in the stained histologic section

46 Which of the following statements about the lesion in the muscularis propria of the colon (Figure 56 in the color plate section) is correct?

(A) It occurs with equal frequency in men and women

(B) It contains two distinctive cell types

(C) It is consistent with adenocarcinoma

(D) The lesion is primary to the colon

47 Several workers at a chemical manufacturing facility were referred to a physician for evaluation of connective tissue neoplasms. This physician could expect to find

(A) antigenic cross-reactivity between tumors

(B) distinct antigenic specificity for each tumor

(C) antigenic cross-reactivity between these tumors and those induced by ultraviolet light

(D) distinct antigenic specificity for different cells from the same tumor

48 A 29-year-old white woman comes to the physician's office stating that she recently discovered a 2-hour gap in her memory. Her friends informed her that she has been acting inappropriately. Suddenly the patient becomes confused but remains docile. She asks the physician from where the overwhelming smell of rotten food is emanating. The patient most likely suffers from

(A) Klüver–Bucy syndrome of the temporal lobes

(B) temporal lobe epilepsy

(C) jacksonian epileptic seizures

(D) petit mal seizures

49 A 5-year-old child in Bangladesh drinks untreated river water and develops cholera. Which of the following scenarios is most likely?

(A) Recovery following treatment is slow because *Vibrio cholerae* causes chronic intracellular infections

(B) Microscopic examination of stools reveals leukocytes

(C) Disease symptoms are due to cholera toxin–mediated elevation in cyclic adenosine monophosphate (cAMP) levels in intestinal cells

(D) *V. cholerae* attaches to the dental flora

50 Centrioles are replicated in which phase of the cell cycle?

(A) G_0 phase

(B) G_1 phase

(C) S phase

(D) G_2 phase

(E) M phase

Answer Key

1-E	11-C	21-B	31-E	41-A
2-B	12-D	22-E	32-D	42-B
3-B	13-B	23-C	33-C	43-A
4-B	14-E	24-D	34-C	44-D
5-B	15-B	25-D	35-C	45-D
6-D	16-C	26-B	36-E	46-B
7-D	17-C	27-B	37-D	47-B
8-D	18-C	28-D	38-E	48-B
9-D	19-C	29-C	39-C	49-C
10-A	20-B	30-C	40-C	50-C

Answers and Explanations

1 **The answer is E** *General principles / Microbiology / Bacterial pigment production*

P. aeruginosa, S. aureus, and *S. marcescens* are all pigment producers. Pigment production by bacteria is associated with both gram-positive and gram-negative organisms. *P. aeruginosa* and *S. marcescens* produce endotoxins, and only *S. aureus* produces enterotoxin and lipoteichoic acids. None of the organisms listed produces mycolic acids.

2 **The answer is B** *General principles / Microbiology / Mycobacteria*

Mycobacterium tuberculosis produces factors such as sulfatides, which inhibit the fusion of phagosomes with lysosomes. In addition to inhibiting phagosome–lysosome fusion, *M. tuberculosis* escapes engulfment by lysosomes. The organisms are also resistant to phagocytic killing because of their tough cell surface.

3 **The answer is B** *General principles / Pharmacology / Antimuscarinic agents*

Atropine may abolish the parasympathetic input that normally maintains a relatively slow heart rate. Indeed, atropine is often used intraoperatively and in emergencies to increase heart rate. Atropine inhibits secretions from salivary, lacrimal, bronchial, and sweat glands. It causes mydriasis and cycloplegia. It has no effect on skeletal muscle in which neuromuscular transmission involves acetylcholine (ACh) and nicotinic, not muscarinic, receptors.

4 **The answer is B** *General principles / Cell biology / G proteins and signal transduction*

GTP-binding proteins (G proteins) are involved with the process of signal transduction and are the target of toxins, such as pertussis and cholera toxins. G proteins are activated when bound to GTP and deactivate via the hydrolysis of GTP to form GDP.

5 **The answer is B** *General principles / Genetics / Cell division*

Down's syndrome is caused by trisomy 21. This syndrome affects approximately 1 in 800 live births and is marked by characteristic facial features including a low nasal root, up-slanting palpebral fissures, and epicanthal folds; congenital cardiac defects; and moderate to severe mental retardation. Ninety-five percent of the time, the extra copy of chromosome 21 is caused by meiotic nondisjunction (almost always maternal). This occurs when the two copies of chromosome 21 do not correctly separate during meiosis and yield an abnormal gamete with two copies of chromosome 21 instead of one. Down's syndrome is caused by unbalanced translocation in approximately 4% of cases, and mosaicism (the body is a mosaic with some somatic cells that are normal; some cells have three copies of chromosome 21—usually a milder phenotype) in approximately 1% to 3% of the cases. Trinucleotide repeat expansions cause diseases such as Huntington's chorea, myotonic dystrophy, fragile X syndrome, and spinocerebellar ataxia type 1, but not Down's syndrome.

6 **The answer is D** *General principles / Biochemistry / Protein synthesis, posttranslational modification, and targeting*

After the correct addition of the first 8 to 20 amino acids, a special signal is encountered in most of the proteins that are destined for secretion, lysosomes, or the plasma membrane. This signal peptide causes the ribosome to stop translating the transcript and move to the ER. ER with aggregations of ribosomes is often called the rough ER because of its dense, speckled appearance. Proteins that are ultimately destined for the cytoplasm (e.g., hexokinase) do not have a special signal, and their translation is finished on free ribosomes void of any ER interaction. Proteins are typically translocated across the ER membrane into the lumen co-translationally. *N*-linked glycosylation occurs in the ER. The ER plays a major role not only in protein synthesis but also in lipid biosynthesis. It may also function to sequester calcium from the cytoplasm by actively pumping calcium into the ER lumen (e.g., sarcoplasmic reticulum in skeletal muscle).

7 **The answer is D** *Respiratory system / Pathology / Bronchioloalveolar carcinoma*

Bronchioloalveolar carcinomas are well-differentiated adenocarcinomas, which grow in a nondestructive fashion over the matrix of the alveolar septa, replacing normal pneumocytes. This pattern has been called lepidic growth. Bronchioloalveolar carcinomas also have a propensity for aerogenous and lymphatic spread, and widespread intrapulmonary metastases may occur.

8 **The answer is D** *Hematopoietic and lymphoreticular system / Pathology / Therapeutic effects in neoplasia*

Paradoxically, patients with histologically unfavorable high-grade lymphomas show long-term survival if a complete clinical remission can be attained. However, it is rare to attain cure in histologically low-grade favorable non-Hodgkin's lymphomas—patients die gradually of bone marrow compromise or lymphoma over many years. Long-term survival after 5 years for diffuse large cell lymphomas is roughly 50%. Those who do not attain complete remission usually die within several years. Spontaneous remissions are rarely seen in aggressive lymphomas.

9 **The answer is D** *Endocrine system / Pathology; pathophysiology / Diabetes mellitus*

The β cells of the islets of Langerhans are the major site of insulin production in the pancreas. In IDDM, these cells are affected by genetic, autoimmune, viral, or other environmental factors so that they produce inadequate or no insulin.

10 **The answer is A** *General principles / Pathology / Amyloid biology*

Amyloid is composed of nonbranching fibrils (paired fibers) of indefinite length (95%) and nonprotein minor compounds (5%), including component P, proteoglycans, and sulfated glycosaminoglycans. All types of amyloid have an identical EM structure and are found as β-pleated sheets.

11 **The answer is C** *Endocrine system / Endocrinology / Blood glucose*

The α cells of the endocrine pancreas secrete glucagons, which increases blood glucose by increasing glycogenolysis and gluconeogenesis in the liver. GH opposes the action of insulin by interfering with the body's ability to use glucose. Somatostatin suppresses glucagons secretion and therefore tends to decrease blood glucose.

12 **The answer is D** *Renal/urinary system / Pathology / Amyloidosis involving kidney stained with Congo red, and without polarized light*

Amyloid is a pathologic proteinaceous substance composed of a primary fibril protein (95%) and amyloid P protein (5%), organized in β-pleated sheets. Two β-pleated sheets form an amyloid fibril 7.5 to 10 nm in diameter. Ultrastructurally, amyloid deposits consist of numerous haphazardly arranged fibrils. Amyloid fibrils bind Congo red dye and produce apple-green birefringence under polarized light. There are approximately 15 biochemically distinctive forms of amyloid, each with a unique primary fibrillary protein. The most common and clinically important forms involving the kidney are AL (i.e., light chain) and AA (i.e., amyloid A). Light-chain amyloid occurs in patients with plasma cell dyscrasias (e.g., multiple myeloma, monoclonal gammopathy of undetermined significance); the primary protein is a modified immunoglobulin light chain, usually a λ-light chain. Amyloid A protein is produced by the liver in chronic inflammatory disorders (e.g., rheumatoid arthritis, inflammatory bowel disease, chronic osteomyelitis, tuberculosis). The wild-type protein is nonamyloidogenic, but in some patients this protein is converted into an amyloidogenic protein by reticuloendothelial cells, including glomerular mesangial cells. Patients with a familial form of the disease (e.g., familial Mediterranean fever) have a mutant form of amyloid A, which is amyloidogenic in its de novo form. Amyloid is immunologically inert but causes injury by depositing in vessel walls. The result is vascular narrowing and increased serum protein permeability and deposition in the interstitium of organs, resulting in progressive ischemic injury, pressure atrophy, and organ dysfunction.

13 The answer is B *Respiratory system / Physiology / Surfactant*

Surfactant is a mixture of approximately 90% lipids (about half being dipalmitoyl phosphatidylcholine) and approximately 10% proteins. It increases pulmonary compliance by decreasing alveolar surface tension. Surfactant is synthesized by the alveolar type II epithelial cells. Reduced or excessive production by these cells can lead to conditions such as respiratory distress syndrome (RDS) of the newborn and pulmonary alveolar proteinosis, respectively. Decreases in the production of surfactant are involved in the pathogenesis of ARDS. Surfactant is secreted in a multilamellar form, and then it transforms into a lattice-like tubular myelin on top of which a lipid monolayer forms. The dipalmitoyl phosphatidylcholine within this monolayer is oriented so that the hydrophobic tails point toward the air-filled alveoli. Surfactant replacement therapy is recommended in both neonatal RDS and prophylactically in premature infants who are at high risk for RDS.

14 The answer is E *General principles / Pharmacology / Characteristics of volatile anesthetics*

Halothane and methoxyflurane are typical inhalational drugs that tend to depress both the cardiovascular and respiratory systems. Methoxyflurane is more potent (i.e., has a lower minimal alveolar concentration) than halothane, as predicted from its higher oil:gas partition coefficient. Both result in considerably slower induction than nitrous oxide because their respective blood:gas partition coefficients are greater than that of nitrous oxide. Similarly, recovery from methoxyflurane is slower than from halothane because its oil:gas partition coefficient is greater than that of halothane. An increase in ventilatory rate hastens the onset of anesthesia for all inhalational anesthetics.

15 The answer is B *General principles / Cell biology / DNA and restriction enzymes*

Restriction enzymes recognize specific base sequences in double-helical DNA and cleave both strands of the duplex at specific sites. Most of the cleavage sites contain a twofold rotational symmetry (the recognized sequence is palindromic). The cuts resulting from these enzymes may be either staggered or blunt. Restriction enzymes can cleave DNA molecules into a number of specific fragments. These enzymes are specific for DNA; they do not cleave RNA.

16 The answer is C *General principles / Behavioral science / Physician–patient interactions*

Regular structured visits by the nurses can help to reassure a dependent and frightened patient and keep the nurses from feeling resentful. The patient's disease and disability have made him feel angry and out of control, and he is acting out his feelings by bothering the nurses. Punitive actions and indirect warfare with the patient will not remedy the situation.

17 The answer is C *General principles / Behavioral science / Suicide risk*

Elderly men have the highest suicide rate of any group, especially with the additional risk factors of widowerhood, alcohol abuse, chronic medical problems, and living alone. Although renal insufficiency, silent myocardial infarction, peripheral neuropathy, and pneumonia are valid concerns, suicide has the highest lethal potential and need for active monitoring.

18 The answer is C *General principles / Pharmacology / Antibiotic action*

Chloramphenicol is bacteriostatic and therefore is responsible for the leveling off of *curve A*. All of the agents listed, except chloramphenicol, are bactericidal. Cephalothin, methicillin, and vancomycin all interfere with cell wall synthesis, leading to bursting and cell death. Polymyxin affects cell membrane function, causing irreversible loss of small molecules from the cell. Chloramphenicol inhibits protein synthesis and is bacteriostatic. Therefore, the cell number in the culture with chloramphenicol does not decrease, and the organisms are viable. Removal of chloramphenicol will result in growth.

19 **The answer is C** *General principles / Physiology / Acid–base balance*

According to the Henderson–Hasselbalch equation, the patient's pH is approximately 7.4 (normal), and his P_{CO_2} and $[HCO_3^-]$ are elevated. The elevation in P_{CO_2} (respiratory acidosis) has been compensated (i.e., normal pH) by a rise in $[HCO_3^-]$. This latter phenomenon is brought about by the kidneys excreting more acid and reabsorbing more HCO_3^-. Full compensation as in this example is most likely to be associated with chronic perturbations in acid–base balance. Such changes may be common in COPD.

20 **The answer is B** *General principles / Physiology / Na + transport; ATP production*

The ability of erythrocytes to pump Na + from the cytoplasm depends on a source of ATP. All of the erythrocyte's ATP is generated by glycolysis. The compound 1,3-diphosphoglycerate is a high-energy glycolytic intermediate that is converted to 3-phosphoglycerate with the concomitant phosphorylation of ADP to ATP. Phosphoglycerate kinase catalyzes this reaction. Pyruvate carboxylase and glucose 6-phosphatase are gluconeogenic enzymes and are not present in the erythrocyte. Malate dehydrogenase is a mitochondrial enzyme and is not present in the erythrocyte. Stearoyl CoA desaturase is an enzyme in β-oxidation and is not present in the erythrocyte.

21 **The answer is B** *General principles / Biostatistics / Paired t-test*

A paired *t*-test allows a comparison of mean K + values before and after treatment by comparing each patient's initial serum level with his or her repeat value.

22 **The answer is E** *Reproductive system / Biochemistry / Testosterone function*

Testosterone is produced by Leydig cells; it cannot be manufactured by Sertoli cells, which it reaches by diffusion from adjacent Leydig cells. Although essential for spermatogenesis, testosterone alone is not sufficient, and full maturation of the spermatids requires follicle-stimulating hormone. Because many major steps in steroid hormone synthesis are common to men and women, both produce testosterone. In women, however, it is mainly converted to estradiol by aromatase. LH tightly controls testosterone production via a negative feedback loop. Hypothalamic LH-releasing hormone (LHRH) stimulates LH release from the pituitary. In turn, LH stimulates testosterone production in Leydig cells. As testosterone levels rise, they inhibit both LH and LHRH release, acting at the levels of both hypothalamus and pituitary. High-plasma testosterone affects LH release by decreasing its sensitivity to LHRH. It decreases LHRH release by inhibiting LHRH synthesis and secretion. Because LHRH is normally released in a pulsatile manner, testosterone levels fluctuate diurnally such that highest testosterone levels are observed in the morning.

23 **The answer is C** *General principles / Genetics / Single-strand conformational polymorphism analysis; PCR*

SSCP analysis can be used as a screening test for mutations within a region of DNA. It uses the differences in intrastrand binding to separate DNA strands of different sequences. Because complementary strands take different conformations when using this technique, the physician sees two bands, one for each of the complementary strands, in a homozygote. If the patient is a heterozygote, the physician sees four bands. However, the physician cannot tell whether a point mutation within the examined region is responsible for the disease by analyzing the patient's DNA alone. It is necessary either to sequence the region or to compare the banding patterns to those of both normal and mutant controls. Otherwise, the physician may misdiagnose someone who merely has a silent point mutation or rule out a disease for which the patient is actually homozygous. In addition, errors may occur during PCR amplification.

24 **The answer is D** *Endocrine system / Pathology / Pheochromocytoma*

The paroxysmal symptoms and detection of an abdominal mass within the adrenal gland are consistent with a diagnosis of pheochromocytoma, a relatively rare tumor of the chromaffin cells of the adrenal medulla. The cells of the adrenal cortex are generally not affected, although extra-adrenal chromaffin cells are often involved.

25 **The answer is D** *Endocrine system / Pharmacology / Pheochromocytoma*

Pheochromocytoma is a relatively rare tumor of the chromaffin cells of the adrenal medulla. Pharmacotherapy to manage the clinical symptoms of pheochromocytoma includes the use of an α-adrenergic receptor blocker (phenoxybenzamine) either alone or in combination with a β-blocker. β-Blockers alone are contraindicated, as they may leave the α-adrenoreceptor-mediated effects of the disorder unopposed. Clonidine is a useful test for the disorder; peripheral catecholamine levels are not depressed after patients with pheochromocytoma take clonidine, whereas normal subjects show a prompt decline. Methyldopa is likely to be converted in significant amounts to the weak vasoconstrictor α-methyl norepinephrine, which may exacerbate the symptoms.

26 **The answer is B** *General principles / Pathology / Helicobacter pylori gastritis*

Helicobacter pylori is a corkscrew-shaped gram-negative rod that is a major cause of chronic gastritis throughout the world. The disease is transmitted through ingestion of contaminated material. The organism lives in the mucous layer overlying gastric fundal and antral mucosa. It is a urease producer and generates ammonia to neutralize gastric acid locally. Although *H. pylori* does not invade the gastric mucosa, it produces protease and elicits an inflammatory response characterized by active (i.e., neutrophils) and chronic (i.e., lymphocytes, plasma cells) inflammation. Patients with concurrent hyperacidity and *H. pylori* infection are predisposed to peptic ulcer disease. Patients with duodenal gastric surface cell metaplasia infected by *H. pylori* may also develop duodenal ulcers. *H. pylori* gastritis has been associated with an increased risk of gastric adenocarcinoma and lymphoma.

27 **The answer is B** *General principles / Pharmacology / Insecticide poisoning*

Treatment of cholinesterase inhibitor poisoning includes pralidoxime and atropine. Chlorinated hydrocarbons block the inactivation of Na channels on nerve membranes. Organophosphates and carbamate inhibit cholinesterase. Symptoms of anticholinesterase poisoning include salivation, bronchoconstriction, vomiting, diarrhea, and pupil constriction. Cholinesterase inhibitors have a much shorter half-life than do chlorinated hydrocarbons, which have environmental half-lives of years.

28 **The answer is D** *Cardiovascular system / Microbiology / Differential diagnosis of infectious mononucleosis*

This patient presents the classic picture of infectious mononucleosis caused by EBV infection. Extreme fatigue, difficulty concentrating, and fever are systemic symptoms. Pharyngitis reflects the local immunologic response by T cells reactive against viral antigens on infected tonsillar B cells. Splenomegaly is also a consequence of immunologic response to EBV. Morphologic examination of lymphocytosis in the peripheral blood should reveal atypical lymphocytes, which are activated T cells with increased cytoplasm and less mature nuclear chromatin. Lymphocytes of infectious lymphocytosis and pertussis are morphologically normal, albeit increased in number; also pertussis is a disease of young children. Serum from this patient should yield a positive test for heterophile antibodies. The combination of pharyngitis and lymphadenopathy is characteristic of EBV-associated mononucleosis. CMV mononucleosis lacks both of these features. Toxoplasmosis, a rare cause of mononucleosis, may have lymphadenopathy but not pharyngitis.

29 **The answer is C** *Central and peripheral nervous system / Anatomy / Nutrition*

A bitemporal loss of vision is caused by impingement on the optic nerves as they cross over near the seat of the pituitary. A defect in the optic nerve (cranial nerve II) would cause a complete loss of vision in one eye. An oculomotor nerve (cranial nerve III) defect will not affect visual fields but could affect the stability of vision because of the control of eye movements may be lost. A defect near the right lateral geniculate body would cause a left homonymous hemianopia, while a left occipital cortex defect could cause anything from a right homonymous quadrantopia to right homonomous hemianopia depending on the size of the defect.

30 **The answer is C** *General principles / Microbiology / Replication cycle of viruses*

During the eclipse phase, it is impossible to recover virus particles from infected cells. The eclipse phase of the virus replication cycle is the final stage of adsorption (during which the virus invades the cell, multiplies, kills, and lyses the cell) and penetration and uncoating (during which the virus particles become engulfed by the cytoplasm of the host cell where virus particles are broken down and released).

31 **The answer is E** *General principles / Histology / Cell function; organelles*

Catalase is an enzyme that catalyzes the synthesis and degradation of hydrogen peroxide. Peroxisomes, also called microsomes, contain large amounts of catalase and therefore can be visualized after staining for catalase. Peroxisomes function in the metabolism of hydrogen peroxide, cholesterol, and lipids.

32 **The answer is D** *General principles / Immunology / Delayed-type hypersensitivity reactions*

The reaction observed was most likely caused by CD4+ T cells. It is a delayed reaction, demonstrating that the T cells are working fine; therefore, the patient could neither lack all T cell–mediated immune function nor suffer from DiGeorge's syndrome. Sensitization has already occurred; therefore, the secondary exposure shows symptoms faster than the primary reaction.

33 **The answer is C** *Central and peripheral nervous system / Pathology / Open-angle glaucoma*

Primary open-angle glaucoma is a genetically determined disorder that is the most common form of glaucoma in the general population. In the patient described in the question, decreased outflow facility resulted in an imbalance between aqueous humor inflow and outflow. Outflow of aqueous humor is accomplished primarily by filtration through the trabecular network to the canal of Schlemm and to a lesser extent via absorption into iris blood vessels (uveoscleral outflow).

34 **The answer is C** *Central and peripheral nervous system / Pharmacology / Open-angle glaucoma*

Cholinomimetics contract the ciliary muscle, thereby reducing resistance of aqueous humor outflow through the trabecular mesh of canal of Schlemm. Accordingly, topical administration of pilocarpine is the agent of choice for this patient. Atropine is a muscarinic antagonist and may exacerbate this problem. Succinylcholine is a depolarizing muscle relaxant and may exacerbate this condition by acutely contracting the accessory striated muscles of the eye before its paralyzing effects. Dexamethasone is a glucocorticoid that may exacerbate primary open-angle glaucoma by further reducing aqueous outflow via the trabecular meshwork. Tubocurarine is a nondepolarizing muscle relaxant that has relatively little effect on muscarinic receptors of the ciliary muscle.

35 **The answer is C** *Respiratory system / Physiology / Mechanical ventilation*

Hypoxemic or hypercarbic respiratory failure or both can be an indication for mechanical ventilation. Both the assist–control and synchronized intermittent mandatory ventilation modes involve a backup respiratory rate. The difference is that only the assist–control mode provides mechanical support (providing a preset volume) to each breath that the patient takes (including breaths above the backup rate). Frequently, assist–control is the mode used initially for acute respiratory failure. Pressure support ventilation (PSV) is more frequently used to help wean patients off of a ventilator. One reason for this difference is that PSV does not initiate breaths for the patient but controls only the airway pressure for breaths initiated by the patient. Positive end-expiratory pressure can often decrease the number of collapsed alveoli and increase the arterial partial pressure of oxygen Po_2, but it may cause decreased oxygen delivery to the tissues because of a decrease in cardiac output. This lowering of cardiac output is due to the increased intrathoracic pressure, which reduces venous return to the heart. In any of the methods of mechanical ventilation, it is possible to set the oxygen concentration anywhere between room air and 100%. Tight control of this parameter is not possible with other methods, including a nasal cannula or a face mask, because they do not completely shut off access to room air as is done in mechanical ventilation.

36 The answer is E *General principles / Cell biology / Cell cycle*

Cellular proteins involved in regulating the cell cycle are often mutated in human cancers. The resultant dysregulation of cell cycle caused by activation of proto-oncogenes and/or loss of tumor suppressor proteins leads to unregulated cell growth (cancer). Mutations in p53 are the most common genetic abnormalities in human cancers. Li-Fraumeni syndrome is caused by germline mutations in the p53 gene. It is characterized by multiple primary tumor development, usually at an early age. Tumors include breast and colon carcinomas, leukemia, osteosarcomas, and soft tissue sarcomas. Neurofibromatosis (NF) type I, characterized by café au lait spots and neurofibromas, is caused by a mutation in neurofibromin, a tumor suppressor gene. NF type II, characterized by acoustic neuromas bilaterally, is caused by a genetic defect on chromosome 22. Familial adenomatous polyposis coli, characterized by large numbers of precancerous polyps in the colon, is caused by mutations in the APC gene, a tumor suppressor gene. Disease states caused by mutations in mismatch repair genes include hereditary nonpolyposis colorectal cancer and xeroderma pigmentosum.

37 The answer is D *Endocrine system / Biochemistry / Glycogen metabolism*

Glucagon functions to increase plasma glucose, primarily by two mechanisms. First, it stimulates conversion of glycogen to glucose in the liver (glycogenolysis). The signal transduction mechanism involves activation of adenyl cyclase, which eventually activates phosphorylase *a*. Phosphorylase *a* stimulates debranching and conversion of glycogen to glucose-1-phosphate (G-1-P). G-1-P is then dephosphorylated to yield glucose. The effect of glucagon on hepatic phosphorylase is similar to that exerted by epinephrine, which raises available plasma glucose during periods of stress. The second mechanism by which glucagon increases plasma glucose is stimulation of de novo glucose synthesis from amino acids (gluconeogenesis) in hepatocytes.

38 The answer is E *Central and peripheral nervous system / Behavioral science / Personality disorders*

Spending sprees and grandiosity that extend to energetic dysfunctional actions are characteristic of manic episodes, which are seen in bipolar I disorder. Although acute states such as these can be present in patients with narcissistic personality disorder, they are usually brief. A histrionic personality disorder is characterized by extroverted, emotional, dramatic, and possibly sexually provocative behavior, whereas a borderline personality disorder is characterized by chronic feelings of emptiness and loneliness. Finally, a person suffering from major depression exhibits seven major signs: decreased sleep, decreased interest, increased guilt, decreased energy, decreased concentration, decreased psychomotor activity, and suicidal ideation. Such depression is devoid of periods of mania. Obsessive-compulsive disorder is typified by perfectionistic, orderly, and indecisive behavior.

39 The answer is C *Central and peripheral nervous system / Histology; pathology / Peripheral nerve tumors*

Schwannomas, such as neurilemomas, are solitary encapsulated tumors that form eccentric masses derived from peripheral nerves. The histologic appearance in the photomicrograph reveals Antoni A areas (*right*), cellular regions with spindle cells that have elongated tapered nuclei. These nuclei may palisade to form a picket fence-like array called a Verocay body. The looser edematous zones with hyalinized blood vessels are called Antoni B areas. In contrast, neurofibromas form unencapsulated onion-like, bulbous expansions of the nerve and are composed of loose interlacing bands of spindle cells with wavy nuclei.

40 The answer is C *General principles / Physiology / Gastrointestinal transport of fats*

The formation of fatty acids and monoglyceride by pancreatic lipase is an important step in the digestive fate of triglycerides. Although there are gastric lipases, they have a relatively insignificant effect on ingested neutral fats. This is in contrast to a critical role for pancreatic lipase in the pancreatic juice. Neutral fats are emulsified by bile salts, and further agitation within the intestine makes their surface available for significant hydrolysis by the water-soluble pancreatic lipase. The products, fatty acids and 2-monoglyceride, would quickly convert back to fat if they were not made into micelles by bile salts. These bile salts ferry the micelles to the intestinal brush border, where the hydrophobic fatty acid (and monoglyceride) rapidly diffuse passively through the lipid membrane.

41 **The answer is A** *Central and peripheral nervous system / Neuroanatomy / Anterior spinocerebellar tract*

The anterior spinocerebellar tract is thought to cross the spinal cord and ascend to the cerebellum, where it crosses the spinal cord again. The spinal thalamic tract crosses the cord only once. The cuneocerebellar tract contains fibers that run from the nucleus gracilis and nucleus cuneatus to the ipsilateral cerebellar hemisphere. The vestibulospinal tract also remains ipsilateral.

42 **The answer is B** *Cardiovascular system / Histology; pathology / Rheumatic fever*

The photomicrograph of the heart shows an Aschoff body (*lower right*), which is pathognomonic of a history of rheumatic fever, and the mitral stenosis is also probably a consequence. Aschoff bodies constitute foci of fibrinoid necrosis surrounded by histiocytes, giant cells, and specialized histiocytes with linear chromatin called caterpillar cells, which are seen with acute rheumatic fever and are eventually replaced by scar tissue. Tissue affected by rheumatic heart disease usually shows pericardial adhesions, valvular deformities, and fusion and shortening of the chordae tendineae.

43 **The answer is A** *General principles / Behavioral science / Personality assessment*

The major projective instrument of personality assessment is the Rorschach test. The thematic apperception test, sentence completion test, and projective drawings all are projective tests, but they are less well studied and yield more limited information. The Minnesota Multiphasic Personality Inventory, which is the most frequently used personality test, is an objective instrument, not a projective test.

44 **The answer is D** *General principles / Microbiology / Tuberculosis culture; diagnostic tests*

Isolation of *Mycobacterium tuberculosis* is diagnostic of active tuberculosis. The tuberculin test can be positive in the absence of active disease. The clinical findings are not specifically pathognomonic for tuberculosis, nor is demonstration of acid-fast organisms.

45 **The answer is D** *Cardiovascular system / Pathology / Occlusive cholesterol atheroembolus in an intrarenal artery*

Cholesterol atheroemboli arise from dislodged atherosclerotic plaque material occurring in medium-sized and large arteries, most frequently the aorta. Atheroembolization commonly follows an intravascular procedure (e.g., cardiac catheterization) in patients with complicated atherosclerosis. Clinical presentation depends on the specific vascular distribution of embolization, resulting in ischemic toes, renal dysfunction, gastrointestinal tract ulcers, CNS and visual alterations, and so forth. Because the embolic material arises in the large arteries of the systemic circulation, the pulmonary circulation is typically spared (i.e., patients do not develop pulmonary thromboemboli). Some affected patients have peripheral eosinophilia and hypocomplementemia. Owing to tissue processing in organic solvents, the cholesterol is dissolved and removed from the atheroemboli, leaving empty clefts in the actual stained tissue section. Patients using illicit drugs (e.g., heroin) sometimes have emboli containing foreign material, most frequently talc.

46 **The answer is B** *Reproductive system / Pathology / Endometriosis*

Endometriosis is a disorder characterized by the ectopic growth of benign endometrial glands and associated stroma outside of the uterus. Sites of involvement in descending order of frequency include ovary, uterine ligaments, rectovaginal septum, pelvic peritoneum, laparotomy scars, umbilicus, vagina, vulva, and appendix and/or intestines. Clinical presentation includes dysmenorrhea, pelvic pain, infertility, dyspareunia, dysuria, and rectal pain with defecation. Peak age is in the third and fourth decades. Individual endometriotic foci undergo hormonal menstrual cyclic changes with intermittent bleeding, resulting in scarring. Typical lesions are red-blue to yellow-brown subserosal nodules and chocolate cysts.

Theories of pathogenesis include (1) retrograde regurgitation of endometrial tissue through the fallopian tubes into the peritoneal cavity, (2) angiolymphatic dissemination, and (3) endometrial metaplasia of coelomic mesothelium. Extensive endometriosis throughout the pelvic cavity may result in ovarian and intraperitoneal adhesions. The photomicrograph shows an endometriotic focus within the wall of the intestine.

47 **The answer is B** *General principles / Immunology / Tumor*

Antigens of physically induced tumors, such as those induced by chemical carcinogens, ultraviolet light, or x-rays, exhibit little or no antigenic cross reactivity. Because random mutations are the most likely explanation for these types of tumors, each tumor displays distinct antigenic specificity. The cells of a given tumor arise from a single cell and are therefore antigenically similar.

48 **The answer is B** *Central and peripheral nervous system / Neuroanatomy / Epilepsy*

The patient most likely has temporal lobe epilepsy, in which seizures are sometimes preceded by acoustic or olfactory hallucinations. Patients are also confused or anxious and sometimes perform complex and bizarre behaviors with no recall of events after the attack. Klüver–Bucy syndrome results from bilateral destruction of the temporal lobes and manifests as loss of fear and anger along with docility, increased appetite, and hypersexuality. Jacksonian seizures are the classic tonic-clonic convulsions due to focal activity in the primary motor cortex. Petit mal (or absence) seizures usually occur in children and involve brief myoclonic jerks, sudden loss in body tone with rapid recovery, or brief losses of consciousness during which the patient stares into space.

49 **The answer is C** *General principles / Microbiology / Enteric infection by enterotoxic bacteria*

The symptoms of cholera result from the attachment of *Vibrio cholerae* to the intestinal mucosa and production of cholera toxin. The infection is acute, and the bacteria remain extracellular. The action of cholera toxin involves elevation of intestinal cAMP levels, which results in massive fluid loss (diarrhea).

50 **The answer is C** *General principles / Histology / Cell cycle; organelles*

Centrioles are made of nine tubular triplets, and they function in mitotic spindle formation and in the production of cilia and flagella. Centrioles are self-duplicated in the S (synthesis) phase of the cell cycle.

test **13**

Questions

Directions: Single best answer questions consist of numbered items or incomplete statements followed by answers or by completions of the statement. Select the ONE lettered answer or completion that is BEST in each case.

1. A patient consults his physician because he is concerned about a recent growth on his right testicle. This has occurred rather suddenly, and although alarming, it has been completely painless. Assuming this growth represents a cancerous lesion, which of the following diagnoses is most likely?

   (A) Embryonal carcinoma
   (B) Yolk sac tumor
   (C) Sertoli cell tumor
   (D) Choriocarcinoma
   (E) Seminoma

2. Which of the following is true about fetal hematopoiesis?

   (A) It begins in the liver and moves to the spleen around the seventh week of gestation
   (B) It begins in the liver and moves to the bone marrow around the seventh week of gestation
   (C) It begins in the yolk sac and starts in the spleen around the seventh week of gestation
   (D) It begins in the yolk sac and starts in the liver around the sixth week of gestation

3. The extraction of β-hydroxybutyrate from blood and its oxidation to CO_2 and water requires the participation of

   (A) β-hydroxybutyrate dehydrogenase and 3-hydroxy-3-methylglutaryl (HMG) coenzyme A (CoA) lyase
   (B) acetoacetate thiokinase and β-hydroxybutyrate dehydrogenase
   (C) HMG CoA synthase and thiolase
   (D) short-chain fatty acetyl CoA dehydrogenase and thiolase
   (E) succinyl CoA:acetoacetate acyltransferase and HMG CoA lyase

4. What is the primary site of action of hydrochlorothiazide?

   (A) Proximal tubules
   (B) Early distal tubules
   (C) Late distal tubules
   (D) Thick ascending limb of the loop of Henle
   (E) Collecting ducts

5. A 43-year-old man who is being treated with hydrochlorothiazide for control of mild edema complains to the physician of malaise, fatigue, muscular weakness, and muscle cramps. Blood tests reveal elevated creatinine with an even greater elevation in blood urea nitrogen, high blood urate, and altered blood electrolytes. The patient's complaints most likely reflect the most serious adverse effect of diuretic therapy, which is

   (A) hyperglycemia
   (B) hyperuricemia
   (C) drug hypersensitivity
   (D) hyperkalemia
   (E) hypokalemia

6. A 21-year-old woman presents to the emergency department complaining of a loss of vision in the center of her visual field. What test should be performed in order to confirm her diagnosis?

   (A) Head computed tomography (CT)
   (B) Magnetic resonamce imaging (MRI) of head
   (C) Lumbar cerebrospinal fluid (CSF) tap
   (D) Corneal examination
   (E) Serological testing for toxoplasmosis

7 Which of the following statements about X chromosome inactivation is true?

(A) Female patients with Turner's syndrome have multiple Barr bodies

(B) The methylated X chromosome in cells is primarily transcriptionally inactive

(C) XIST, the gene responsible for X-inactivation, is transcribed only from the active X chromosome

(D) Depending on the cellular environment, cells shut down either the paternal or the maternal X chromosome

8 A mother takes her 7-year-old son for evaluation. The mother says her son makes funny, repetitive flapping movements with his hands. He does not make eye contact; he has never displayed any interest in playing with other children; he plays with objects in an idiosyncratic fashion; and he does not seem to respond appropriately to social or emotional cues. The child has

(A) Tourette's syndrome

(B) attention deficit hyperactivity disorder (ADHD)

(C) pica

(D) autism

(E) Rett's syndrome

9 Which of the following is a recently approved non-steroidal anti-inflammatory drug that has fewer gastrointestinal side effects than its predecessors?

(A) Ibuprofen

(B) Rofecoxib

(C) Ketorolac

(D) Prednisone

(E) Indomethacin

10 A 34-year-old woman has muscular weakness of 3 months' duration and says she tires easily when she is trying to work. After she rests for a while, some of her strength returns. She reports having some trouble with her vision, particularly diplopia; her speech appears to be dysarthric. During the physical examination, the physician notes bilateral facial weakness and a somewhat asymmetric distribution of proximal limb weakness. The woman's tendon reflexes are normal. Which of the following diagnoses is most likely to account for the patient's findings?

(A) Cerebrovascular accident in the motor cortex

(B) Guillain–Barré syndrome

(C) Myasthenia gravis

(D) Neurosyphilis

(E) Friedreich's ataxia

11 An investigator has isolated a bacterium that, in the absence of glucose, constitutively produces the proteins coded for by the lac operon. Which of the following statements explains this observation?

(A) The promoter has a mutation that prevents RNA polymerase from binding

(B) There is a missense mutation in the gene for β-galactosidase

(C) The gene for the catabolite activator protein is mutated and inactive

(D) There is a mutation in the attenuator sequence

(E) The gene for the repressor protein is mutated and inactive

12 An adolescent patient attends weekly individual psychodynamic psychotherapy sessions. When he begins to feel too close to and dependent on the psychiatrist, he often misses a scheduled appointment. This behavior is an example of

(A) acting out

(B) antisocial personality

(C) repression

(D) suppression

(E) identification with the aggressor

13 Which of the statements concerning the pictured disaccharide is most accurate?

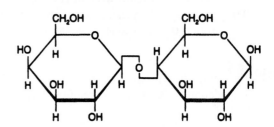

(A) It yields a negative result in the Fehling–Benedict reducing sugar test

(B) It is cleaved by isomaltose

(C) It is a β-galactoside

(D) It is digested and absorbed by a lactase-deficient child

(E) It is a good source of calories for a 2-week-old child with galactosemia

14 A 42-year-old woman with breast cancer was treated with radiation and is receiving chemotherapy. She complains of some left-sided chest pain, which is determined not to be cardiac. On the fourth day, several vesicles appear on her left thorax, following a rib in distribution; she also has several smaller vesicles at other sites (scalp, leg, forearm). Her physician diagnoses varicella zoster virus (VZV) infection and starts treatment with acyclovir. Which one of the following statements best describes the VZV in this case?

(A) Thymidine kinase-negative VZV mutants are likely to render the treatment ineffective

(B) The initial exposure to VZV in childhood could not have led to viral latency in the dorsal ganglia

(C) The lesions outside the dermatomal distribution are likely explained by depressed cell-mediated immunity

(D) The VZV is the most likely causal factor in the patient's breast cancer

(E) The acyclovir will alkylate the VZV DNA

15 Hodgkin's lymphoma can be distinguished from other forms of lymphoma by the presence of

(A) Reed–Sternberg cells

(B) the Philadelphia chromosome

(C) Auer rods

(D) decreased quantities of leukocyte alkaline phosphatase

16 An 86-year-old man has diminished vibratory sensation at the knees and toes, although his reflexes are intact, temperature sensation is normal, and he feels well, aside from having headaches. What is the most likely explanation?

(A) Peripheral neuropathy

(B) Normal age-related change

(C) Spinal cord lesion

(D) Small strokes

(E) Brain or brainstem tumor

17 The pressor response to an indirect-acting sympathomimetic agent, such as amphetamine, is

(A) associated with marked tolerance (tachyphylaxis)

(B) decreased in the presence of a monoamine oxidase (MAO) inhibitor

(C) potentiated by an uptake 1 inhibitor, such as imipramine

(D) potentiated by pretreatment with reserpine

(E) related to its direct effects on postsynaptic receptors

18 The introduction of foreign DNA into bacteria is an important tool in molecular biology. Which of the following statements concerning nucleic acid transfer is true?

(A) Transformation is the technique whereby a bacteriophage is used to introduce DNA into a bacterium

(B) Transduction is the technique whereby competent bacterial cells are suspended in a solution of calcium chloride and DNA

(C) The most common DNA used in transformation is plasmid DNA

(D) Conjugation is the technique whereby a bacteriophage is used to introduce DNA into a bacterium

19 The photomicrograph in Figure 57 from the color plate section is from a first-toe phalanx bone and soft tissue mass that was painful and warm. Which of the following statements about the disorder depicted is correct?

(A) It is associated with secondary nephropathy in a subset of patients

(B) Precipitated material is calcium pyrophosphate

(C) Deposition of material is pH- and temperature-independent

(D) Precipitated material is a product of nucleic acid pyrimidine metabolism

20 A 55-year-old man is seen in your office for a work-related checkup. Upon your questioning, the man gives you answers that don't really make much sense and seem to be made up. Upon physical examination an enlarged liver is discovered. Which diagnosis is most likely?

(A) Stroke-induced dementia

(B) Alzheimer's disease

(C) Pick's disease

(D) Wernicke's encephalopathy

(E) Korsakoff's psychosis

21 A 27-year-old man who has torn his anterior cruciate ligament (ACL) while skiing is sent to the operating room for ACL replacement and reconstruction. The anesthesiologist selects halothane. Induction of anesthesia is smooth, and the operation begins. Before any incision is made, the surgical resident informs the surgeon that this surgery is to be performed on the

(A) ankle
(B) knee
(C) hip
(D) elbow
(E) shoulder

22 A 32-year-old HIV-positive man is seen in his local emergency department for speech difficulties and asymmetric extremity weakness. He is admitted to the hospital and suffers a continuous decline in his condition, resulting in aphasia, blindness, and paralysis. A lumbar spinal tap is performed and JC virus presence is verified by polymerase chain reaction. What is the best diagnosis for this patient?

(A) AIDS-related dementia
(B) Toxoplasmosis infection
(C) Central nervous system (CNS) pheumocystis infection
(D) Subacute sclerosing pan-encephalitis
(E) Progressive multifocal leukoencephalopathy

23 A 60-year-old woman presents to her primary care physician with widespread dermatitis and her daughter says she also has suffered from persistent diarrhea and seems demented. What nutritional deficiency is most likely the cause of these symptoms in this patient?

(A) Thiamine
(B) Riboflavin
(C) Niacin
(D) Pyridoxine
(E) Folate

24 The primary site of long bone growth occurs at the

(A) epiphysis
(B) diaphysis
(C) epiphyseal plate
(D) medullary cavity
(E) primary ossification center

25 Which one of the following bones is a tarsal bone?

(A) Capitate
(B) Cuboid
(C) Trapezium
(D) Hamate
(E) Trapezoid

26 Which of the following descriptions is a characteristic of cancellous bone?

(A) Composed of parallel bony columns
(B) Thin and flat
(C) Composed of a network of trabeculae
(D) Contains haversian canals
(E) Found primarily in the shaft of long bones

27 Which of the following tests is contraindicated in patients with intracranial neoplasm?

(A) Computed tomography (CT) of the head because of the use of contrast dye
(B) Nuclear magnetic resonance (NMR) because of the length of time a patient must remain supine during testing
(C) Lumbar puncture to examine cerebrospinal proteins and relieve hydrocephalus
(D) Radiography of the skull because the radiation may shrink the tumor and cause hemorrhaging

28 A 3-year-old boy is febrile and breathing slowly, and he has a bark-like cough and inspiratory stridor. These symptoms have developed during the past 36 hours. He has been vaccinated against *Haemophilus influenzae* type B. Which one of the following statements is correct?

(A) The boy has epiglottitis and should be intubated immediately
(B) Cold air and quick temperature changes will make this boy appear much worse
(C) The organism causing this illness is respiratory syncytial virus
(D) The boy should be placed in a humidified room, and supplemental oxygen and racemic epinephrine should be considered if his condition continues to worsen
(E) The etiology of this disease is most commonly bacterial
(F) Croup can be eliminated from the differential diagnosis because he has inspiratory stridor and abnormal lung sounds are heard only during expiration in patients with croup

29 This figure is a stylized diagram of the juxtaglomerular apparatus of the kidney. A decrease in the flow of glomerular filtrate into the tubules might cause which one of the following actions?

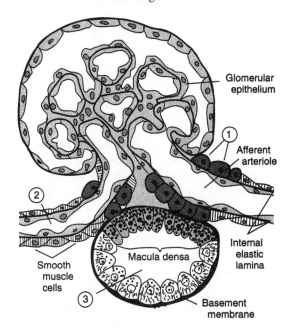

(A) Renin released from (1)
(B) Vasodilation of (2)
(C) An increase in Na+ concentration at (3)
(D) A reflexive vasoconstriction of the afferent arteriole

30 A quantitative Gram stain revealed many fewer cells than expected from the turbidity of a bacterial culture. The decrease in cells was most likely due to
(A) inactivation of the cytochromes
(B) digestion of the bacterial cell wall by autolytic processes
(C) presence of gram-negative organisms in the culture
(D) presence of bacterial spores in the culture

31 According to Fick's law, oxygen consumption is equal to the product of blood flow and arteriovenous oxygen difference. If the lungs absorb 300 mL/min of oxygen, arterial oxygen content is 20 mL/100 mL blood, pulmonary arterial oxygen content is 15 mL/100 mL blood, and heart rate is 60/min, stroke volume is
(A) 50 mL
(B) 60 mL
(C) 100 mL
(D) 5 L/min
(E) 6 L/min

32 Capsule production is essential for the virulence of many pathogenic bacteria. Which of the following statements best describes bacterial capsules?
(A) The most important function of the *Streptococcus pneumoniae* capsule is adhesion
(B) The capsule of *Haemophilus influenzae* type B stimulates a T cell-dependent immune response
(C) Opsonizing antibodies are often directed against *S. pneumoniae* capsules
(D) The capsule of group B *Neisseria meningitidis* is protein
(E) The licensed DTP (diphtheria–tetanus–pertussis) vaccine contains purified *Bordetella pertussis* capsules

33 True statements about the side chains of amino acids that are found in proteins include which one of the following?
(A) Serine provides strong buffering capacity at pH = 7
(B) Alanine absorbs ultraviolet light
(C) Glutamic acid and aspartic acid differ significantly in their isoelectric pH (pI)
(D) Proline often produces a bend in the protein chain
(E) Only D-amino acids are incorporated into protein

34 A 56-year-old woman with a history of ovarian cancer treated with chemotherapy several years ago visits a clinic with complaints of fatigue and the recent development of small hemorrhages on her arms. She has the following laboratory values: hemoglobin, 9.6 g/dL; white blood cells, 2,900/μL; platelets, 56,000/μL. A bone marrow aspirate is hypercellular and contains approximately 10% blasts (normal < 5%), with megaloblastic morphologic changes in the red cell precursors and megakaryocytes with abnormal nuclei. Cytogenetic analysis reveals a clone with a deletion of the long arm of chromosome 7. Which of the following diagnoses best fits this woman's condition?
(A) Preleukemia (myelodysplastic syndrome)
(B) Megaloblastic anemia
(C) Acute lymphocytic leukemia
(D) Acute nonlymphocytic (myeloid) leukemia
(E) Chronic myelogenous leukemia

35 Of these drugs, which one is thought to function through a receptor?

(A) Mannitol
(B) Dimercaprol
(C) Cimetidine
(D) Ethylenediaminetetraacetic acid (EDTA)

36 According to this figure, which one of the following conditions would result in a shift of the oxygen saturation curve from *a* to *b*?

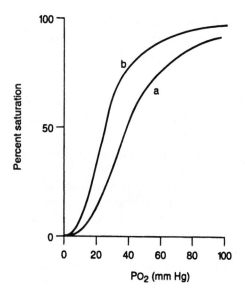

(A) A change in pH from 7.6 to 7.4
(B) A change in P_{CO_2} from 30 to 40 torr
(C) An increase in the concentration of 2,3-diphosphoglycerate (DPG)
(D) Fetal hemoglobin ($\alpha_2\gamma_2$)
(E) Oxidation of the heme iron from Fe^{2+} to Fe^{3+}

37 Which one of the following muscles raises the soft palate during swallowing?

(A) Levator veli palatini
(B) Palatoglossus
(C) Palatopharyngeus
(D) Superior constrictor

38 Which of the following is true about cell membranes?

(A) The cell membrane contains DNA
(B) The cell membrane is a cholesterol bilayer
(C) The lipid composition of the two halves of the membrane bilayer is the same
(D) Glycolipids in the bilayer are found in the noncytoplasmic leaflet
(E) Polypeptides usually cross the bilayer as a β-sheet

39 A previously healthy 27-year-old woman consults her physician about a petechial rash. She denies recent bleeding and has had no recent illnesses. Hemoglobin, hematocrit, and white blood cell counts are normal. Examination of the peripheral blood smear reveals normal red and white blood cells and is remarkable only for a paucity of platelets. The most likely diagnosis in this patient is

(A) aleukemic leukemia
(B) idiopathic thrombocytopenic purpura (ITP)
(C) Glanzmann's thrombasthenia
(D) amegakaryocytic thrombocytopenia
(E) drug-induced thrombocytopenia

40 Multiple mechanisms in the body maintain oxygen and carbon dioxide levels within a normal range. Which of the following statements about those mechanisms is correct?

(A) The aortic bodies are the primary sensors of decreases in arterial oxygen tension
(B) The Hering–Breuer reflex functions to terminate respiration and involves pulmonary stretch receptors and vagal afferents; however, this system is not important during normal resting
(C) Central chemoreceptors on the ventral medullary surface are the major mediators of the response to hypoxia
(D) During metabolic alkalosis, peripheral chemoreceptors cause hyperventilation to compensate with respiratory acidosis
(E) A person who has an increased resistive load will attempt to compensate by taking small breaths at a high rate
(F) The responsiveness to ventilatory stimuli is increased during sleep

41 This micrograph is a portion of the liver biopsy of a 42-year-old man. The microscopic features are most likely due to

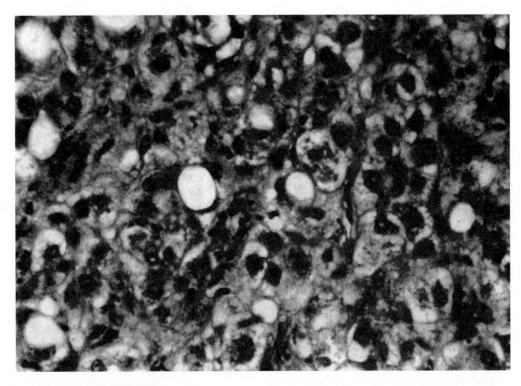

(A) exposure to carbon tetrachloride
(B) acetaminophen toxicity
(C) ethanol use
(D) acute rejection of a liver allograft

42 Which of the following statements correctly describes a tissue's germ layer origin?

(A) Adrenal cortex is derived from neuroectoderm
(B) Melanocytes are derived from neuroectoderm
(C) Liver is derived from mesoderm
(D) Thyroid gland is derived from ectoderm
(E) Gonads are derived from endoderm

43 A patient with familial lipoprotein lipase deficiency consults her physician for a checkup. Elevation of which of the following plasma components would support the patient's diagnosis?

(A) Low-density lipoprotein (LDL)
(B) Chylomicron remnants and intermediate-density lipoprotein
(C) Very-low-density lipoprotein
(D) Albumin
(E) Chylomicrons

44 Neuropathic pain syndromes often result from peripheral nerve injury and are characterized by increased sensitivity to pain. Which of the following neurotransmitters is likely to be involved in the primary synapse of sensory neurons in the spinal cord?

(A) Serotonin
(B) Dopamine
(C) Substance P
(D) Acetylcholine
(E) Norepinephrine

45 Which of the following is an accurate description of the pathologic event responsible for the symptoms of myasthenia gravis?

(A) An infectious agent resides in the neurons of the dorsal root ganglion and reactivates in times of stress or immunocompromise

(B) Large motor neurons of the ventral horn degenerate, causing muscle wasting

(C) An autoimmune attack is initiated against voltage-gated Ca^{2+} channels in the presynaptic membrane at the neuromuscular junction, resulting in interrupted neurotransmission and decreased ability to contract muscles

(D) An autoimmune attack against acetylcholine receptors at the neuromuscular junction results in interrupted neurotransmission and decreased ability to contract muscles

(E) An autoimmune attack against muscle cells results in muscle wasting

46 Oncogenesis, the production of tumors, occurs because of a dysregulation of cellular signaling, which is often caused by a protein that functions as an uncontrolled growth factor receptor. Which of the following normal physiologic receptors is correctly paired with the oncogene that it most closely resembles functionally and structurally?

(A) Insulin receptor—*ras*

(B) Nerve growth factor (NGF) receptor—*kit*

(C) Epidermal growth factor (EGF) receptor—*sis*

(D) Platelet-derived growth factor (PDGF) receptor—*trk*

(E) Glial cell line-derived neurotrophic factor (GDNF) receptor—*erbB*

47 The causative virus of the lesion depicted in Figure 58 in the color plate section is

(A) Human papilloma virus (HPV)

(B) Herpes zoster virus

(C) Molluscum virus

(D) Parvovirus B19

48 A pathology report describes a biopsy of the cervix in the following manner: "Atypical cells appear in the lower layers of the squamous epithelium, but there still remains a persistent differentiation of cells up to the keratinizing cell layers. The atypical cells show changes in nucleocytoplasmic ratio, variation in nuclear size, loss of polarity, increased mitotic figures, and hyperchromasia." This statement is consistent with a diagnosis of which of the following?

(A) Cervical intraepithelial neoplasia (CIN) I

(B) CIN II

(C) CIN III

(D) Cervical squamous carcinoma

(E) This biopsy report is of a normal cervix

49 A 32-year-old man is unemployed and lives in a personal care boarding home. He has a 10-year history of undifferentiated schizophrenia and has been observed pacing around the house and fidgeting whenever seated. Recently he received his monthly injection of fluphenazine. The most likely cause of his agitation is

(A) anxiety

(B) restless legs syndrome

(C) akathisia

(D) undiagnosed hyperthyroidism

(E) worsening psychosis

50 Which one of the following statements best describes chondroblasts?

(A) They are endosteal cells capable of secreting proteoglycan

(B) They are perichondrial cells capable of secreting type II collagen

(C) They are periosteal cells capable of secreting type I collagen

(D) They show little mitotic activity

(E) They are filled with rough endoplasmic reticulum but lack a Golgi apparatus

Answer Key

1-E	11-E	21-B	31-C	41-C
2-D	12-A	22-E	32-C	42-B
3-B	13-C	23-C	33-D	43-E
4-B	14-C	24-C	34-A	44-C
5-E	15-A	25-B	35-C	45-D
6-C	16-B	26-C	36-D	46-A
7-B	17-A	27-C	37-A	47-C
8-D	18-C	28-D	38-D	48-B
9-B	19-A	29-A	39-B	49-C
10-C	20-E	30-D	40-B	50-B

Answers and Explanations

1 **The answer is E** *Reproductive system / Pathology / Testicular tumors*

In the United States, testicular tumors occur in approximately 6/100,000 males and are the most common cause of cancer death in males aged 15 to 34 years. The most common tumor of one single histologic pattern is seminoma, which is also one of the more curable tumors. Other germ cell-derived tumors include embryonal carcinomas, yolk sac tumors, choriocarcinomas, and teratomas, but these tumors occur less frequently as discrete entities and are found more often in combination. Sertoli cell, Leydig cell, and granulosa cell tumors, the so-called stromal tumors, are also less common.

2 **The answer is D** *Hematopoietic and lymphoreticular system / Embryology / Fetal hematopoiesis*

Fetal hematopoiesis begins in the yolk sac, where it can be detected at 3 to 12 weeks' gestation. The liver is hematopoietically active between 6 and 30 weeks of gestation. Hematopoiesis begins in the spleen around 9 weeks of gestation, and the bone marrow takes over by 28 weeks of gestation. Bone marrow incompetence caused by various factors may lead to extramedullary hematopoiesis in one of these fetal sites (i.e., the liver or spleen).

3 **The answer is B** *General principles / Biochemistry / Oxidative enzymes*

The extraction of β-hydroxybutyrate from blood and its oxidation to carbon dioxide and water require the participation of acetoacetate thiokinase and β-hydroxybutyrate dehydrogenase. All tissues except the liver use β-hydroxybutyrate as a metabolic fuel. The enzymes required for catabolism of the ketone bodies are in the mitochondria. These enzymes are β-hydroxybutyrate dehydrogenase, succinyl CoA, acetoacetate acyltransferase, and acetoacetate thiokinase. HMG CoA lyase catalyzes a step in fatty acid oxidation that takes place in the kidneys or liver. HMG CoA lyase breaks down (*S*)-3-hydroxy-3-methylglutaryl CoA into acetyl CoA and acetoacetate.

4 **The answer is B** *General principles / Pharmacology / Thiazide diuretic therapy*

The thiazide diuretics, such as hydrochlorothiazide, primarily act in the early distal tubules by binding to a membrane protein that is a Na + and Cl − cotransporter. Thus, both Na + and the more important Cl − reabsorption in the early distal tubules are blocked. The thiazide diuretics also have a small effect in the late proximal tubules.

5 **The answer is E** *Renal/urinary system / Pharmacology / Diuretic therapy*

Although most diuretics can cause all of the untoward effects listed in the question, the patient's neuromuscular dysfunction is most likely the result of hypokalemia, the most important and most serious side effect listed. Hypokalemia is produced because the diuretics cause a large amount of Na + to collect in the distal tubules, which leads to Na + reabsorption (sodium avidity) and a concomitant depletion of K + . This Na + /K + exchange site is a primary mechanism for renal control of K + homeostasis.

6 **The answer is C** *Central and peripheral nervous system / Neuroscience / Multiple sclerosis*

A unilateral loss of vision in a young woman is likely optic neuritis in the absence of other retinal findings. Ten percent to 50% of these patients go on to develop multiple sclerosis (MS). Whereas an MRI of the head can be used to diagnose the development of CNS plaques in the MS, it is not useful for the diagnosis of optic neuritis. A better diagnostic test would be a spinal tap that is positive for oligoclonal gamma globulin bands. A head CT could show a cerebral hemorrhage but such a lesion is unlikely to cause a central scotoma (loss of vision from the central portion of the retina).

7 **The answer is B** *General principles / Genetics / Cell division*

Female cells normally have two X chromosomes, whereas male cells have only one X chromosome. Dosage compensation between males and females is achieved by a process called X-inactivation, whereby one X in every female cell is inactivated. This process occurs very early in development (at approximately the 50 to 100 cell stage) and is random; that is, each cell has a 50% chance of shutting down the paternal X or the maternal X chromosome. Although much of the process remains unclear, XIST is known to be an important gene involved in X-inactivation and is transcribed only from the inactive X chromosome. In addition, the inactive X chromosome is heavily methylated, which may be responsible for its transcriptional silence. Inactive X chromosomes are visible as densely stained chromatin in female somatic cells and are called Barr bodies. Female patients with Turner's syndrome are typically 45,X (i.e., they have only a single X chromosome) and therefore have no Barr bodies.

8 **The answer is D** *Central and peripheral nervous system / Behavioral science / Childhood development*

This is a classic description of an autistic child. ADHD is marked by inability to focus or sustain attention (concentration) in a developmentally appropriate manner. ADHD, although sometimes manifesting itself in impaired relationships and cognitive abilities, is not primarily characterized by an inability to acquire these communication and learning skills, as autism is; rather, children with ADHD are unable to apply these skills consistently in an age-appropriate manner. Although Tourette's syndrome, like autism, can manifest itself secondarily in impaired social functioning, Tourette's is characterized primarily by verbal and motor tics. The essential feature of pica is the persistent eating of nonnutritive substances such as paint, clay, and dirt. Although Rett's syndrome has some of the same signs as autism, including impaired social and emotional interactions and ritualized hand movements, it is unlikely here because this child is a boy. To date, Rett's syndrome has been seen only in girls, never in boys.

9 **The answer is B** *General principles / Pharmacology / Cyclo-oxygenase inhibitors*

Ibuprofen, ketorolac, and indomethacin are nonsteroidal anti-inflammatory drugs (NSAIDs) that inhibit both cyclo-oxygenase (COX) 1 and 2 enzymes, which are necessary for prostaglandin production. Because they are nonselective in inhibiting COX enzymes, they often have several gastrointestinal side effects. Rofec-oxib is a new, selective COX-2 inhibitor that is specifically useful because it has relatively few gastrointestinal side effects. Prednisone is a steroidal anti-inflammatory drug.

10 **The answer is C** *Central and peripheral nervous system / Pathology; neurobiology / Differential diagnosis of neuromuscular disease*

Myasthenia gravis, which occurs more commonly in women than in men, is an autoimmune disorder with antibodies directed against nicotinic cholinergic receptors of the neuromuscular junction. Treatment is somewhat effective, so that early diagnosis of this disease is critical. The features described, particularly weakness that subsides after rest, are cardinal symptoms of the disease. The characteristic distribution of fatigue that affects facial musculature earlier is a hallmark of the myasthenia pathology. Because this is not an upper-motor neuron disease, reflexes are maintained. Also, there are no sensory deficits.

11 **The answer is E** *General principles / Microbiology / Lac operon*

A gene that is expressed at a constant, unregulated, and often low rate is said to be constitutively expressed. A mutation in either the operator sequence or the lac I gene that produces an inactive repressor results in an operon that cannot be regulated by the presence or absence of lactose and is therefore inactive. With an inactive repressor, the lac operon can still be regulated by catabolite repression. With a mutated repressor and no glucose, the expression of the lac operon is high because there is no catabolite repression by glucose. In the presence of glucose, it is expressed, but at a low level. A mutated promoter that prevents RNA polymerase from binding leads to a complete inhibition of expression under all growth conditions. A missense mutation in the β-galactosidase gene is likely to reduce the activity of the enzyme but is not likely to affect its cellular levels. A mutated β-galactosidase has no effect on either of the other two enzyme products of the operon. A mutation in the catabolite activator protein (CAP) affects the lac operon's ability to be regulated by catabolite repression. The lac operon is not regulated by attenuation.

12 **The answer is A** *Central and peripheral nervous system / Behavioral science / Psychotherapy management*

The patient physically and nonverbally expresses (acts out) his conflicted feelings and anxiety about the closeness he feels toward his psychiatrist by avoiding a scheduled appointment. There is some degree of repression of these feelings, but the motor behavior indicates that the patient is acting out. Suppression is a *conscious* decision to postpone something, but missing these appointments was not done consciously.

13 **The answer is C** *General principles / Biochemistry / Disaccharide structure and function*

The structure is the milk disaccharide lactose. Lactose is composed of 1 mol of galactose and 1 mol of glucose, which are joined by a β-galactosidic linkage. Lactose is the substrate for the intestinal enzyme lactase, which hydrolyzes the disaccharide. Therefore, lactose is not digested or absorbed by a lactase-deficient child. Because galactosemia arises from an impaired ability to metabolize galactose, lactose is not a good source of calories for a child with galactosemia; additional galactose would augment the problem. Because the only requirement for a reducing sugar is an unsubstituted carbonyl group, the disaccharide gives a positive result in the Fehling–Benedict reducing sugar test. The anomeric carbon of the glucose residue is in equilibrium with the open chain structure, which provides an unsubstituted carbonyl group.

14 **The answer is C** *General principles / Microbiology / VZV*

The lesions outside the dermatomal distribution are explained by depressed cell-mediated immunity. When VZV goes outside a dermatomal distribution, it is because the affected person is immunosuppressed either from old age (>65 years) or medication (in this case, chemotherapy). Thymidine kinase-negative mutations rarely occur except in human immunodeficiency virus (HIV) patients receiving prolonged prophylaxis with acyclovir. Acyclovir blocks VZV thymidine kinase and does not alkylate DNA. Initial exposure to the infection always leads to viral latency of the dorsal ganglia. There is no evidence that VZV is oncogenic in breast cancer.

15 **The answer is A** *Hematopoietic and lymphoreticular system / Pathology / Hematopoietic and lymphoreticular system*

Reed–Sternberg cells are diagnostic for Hodgkin's lymphoma. The Philadelphia chromosome and decreased quantities of leukocyte alkaline phosphatase are commonly observed in chronic myelogenous leukemia. Auer rods are most often seen in increased numbers in acute myelogenous or myelomonocytic leukemia.

16 **The answer is B** *Central and peripheral nervous system / Neuroanatomy / Normal age-related change*

The selectivity of the deficit rules out a supraforaminal lesion and peripheral neuropathy. Whether position sense is impaired has not been determined. If it is impaired, the posterior column of the spinal cord becomes a possibility, but an isolated vibratory deficit can occur as a normal aging change. When diminished vibratory sensation is encountered, position sense must be tested carefully to make the branch point.

17 **The answer is A** *General principles / Pharmacology / Autonomic pharmacology*

Indirect-acting sympathomimetic agents, such as amphetamine, are transported by the uptake 1 mechanism into nerve terminals, where they displace norepinephrine to account for the pressor response. Because these agents lack hydroxyl groups on the catechol ring, they are without significant direct effects on synaptic receptors. Thus, their action is affected by the presence of other agents that modify adrenergic transmission. Reserpine depletes norepinephrine stores, and MAO inhibitors may potentiate norepinephrine levels. Therefore, the pressor response to amphetamine is potentiated by an MAO inhibitor and decreased by reserpine. Imipramine interferes with uptake of amphetamine and reduces its effect in this and other ways. A hallmark of indirect-acting sympathomimetics is tolerance, or tachyphylaxis. This is presumably secondary to depletion of endogenous norepinephrine pools after repetitive application of amphetamine.

18 **The answer is C** *General principles / Microbiology / Nucleic acid transfer*

Transduction is the technique whereby a virus, known as a bacteriophage, is used to introduce DNA into bacteria. Transformation uses high concentrations of calcium chloride to help DNA cross the bacterial plasma membrane. Conjugation refers to direct transfer of DNA between bacteria. Circular, or plasmid, DNA is the form of DNA most commonly used to transfer genes into bacteria via transformation.

19 **The answer is A** *Musculoskeletal system / Pathology / Tophaceous gout*

Gout is one of several crystal arthropathies; the other major endogenous crystal arthropathy (calcium pyrophosphate crystal deposition disease) is known as pseudogout. Hyperuricemia (>7 mg/dL) is a common feature in all patients with gout, which is caused by either overproduction or underexcretion of uric acid. Most (90%) affected patients have disease limited to one or several joints (primary gout); a few (10%) have concurrent extra-articular disease related to increased nucleic acid turnover (e.g., malignancies with high cell turnover), chronic renal disease (impaired uric acid excretion), or specific severe inborn purine metabolic disorders (e.g., Lesch–Nyhan syndrome, due to complete deficiency of hypoxanthine-guanine phosphoribo-syl transferase (HGPRT), a critical purine metabolism salvage enzyme that promotes nucleic acid synthesis from hypoxanthine preventing its conversion to uric acid). Monosodium urate precipitates when its concentration exceeds its solubility product, which is lower in synovial fluid than in serum, and is pH- and temperature-dependent. Urate microprecipitates form in synovial lining cells and articular cartilage, which are released into the synovial fluid following trauma. Sodium urate crystals activate complement and elicit acute inflammatory arthritis. Recurrent episodes of acute arthritis result in chronic arthritis, associated with an erosive pannus that destroys the articular cartilage. Large tophi form in the synovium and periarticular tissues, characterized by large aggregates of urate crystals surrounded by lymphocytes, macrophages, and multinucleate giant cells. A subset of patients develop urate precipitation in the interstitium and tubules of the kidney, leading to interstitial nephritis and urate nephrolithiasis (urate nephropathy).

20 **The answer is E** *Central and peripheral nervous system / Neuroscience / Korsakoff's psychosis*

The enlarged liver in this patient may suggest alcohol abuse. With the information given and the inability of the patient to answer questions, a diagnosis of Korsakoff's psychosis should be considered. This inability to answer questions is due to a loss of short-term memory acuity and patients normally try to conceal this difficulty by making up answers to question, a phenomenon known as confabulation.

21 **The answer is B** *Musculoskeletal system / Anatomy / Properties of halothane; skeletal muscles*

The ACL is important to the proper functioning of the knee joint. The ACL attaches the femur to the tibia. Damage to this ligament is usually sports-related and caused by rapid deceleration or torque. The ligament is essential to the stability of the knee joint, and surgery is necessary to prevent further damage.

22 **The answer is E** *Central and peripheral nervous system / Pathology / Progressive multifocal leu-koencephalopathy*

Progressive multifocal leukoencephalopathy (PML) is a severe demyelinating disease that occurs in the setting of immune suppression. It is caused by replication of the JC polyoma virus within oligodendrocytes and can be verified by JC virus amplification by PCR and evidence of multiple sites of demyelination on brain MRI.

23 **The answer is C** *General principles / Molecular biology / Vitamin deficiency*

This patient is suffering from niacin deficiency. Niacin is incorporated into nicotinamide adenine dinucleo-tide (NAD) and NAD phosphate which are utilized in many redox reactions. The classic symptoms of niacin deficiency are the three D's: dermatitis, dementia, and diarrhea.

24 **The answer is C** *Musculoskeletal system / Anatomy / Bone growth*

The epiphysyseal plate lies between the epiphysis and the diaphysis of the long bones, and is the area of highest mitotic activity. During bone growth, the epiphyseal plates migrate distally, finally becoming epiphyseal lines when growth is complete.

25 The answer is B *Musculoskeletal system / Anatomy / Tarsal bones*

The cuboid is a tarsal bone. All of the other bones listed (i.e., capitate, trapezium, trapezoid) are carpal bones.

26 The answer is C *Musculoskeletal system / Anatomy / Cancellous bone*

Trabeculae are characteristic features of cancellous (spongy) bone.

27 The answer is C *Central and peripheral nervous system / Pathology / Diagnostic tests*

Lumbar puncture is absolutely contraindicated in patients with intracranial neoplasm because it may cause a rapid extrusion of brain tissue of the cerebral hemisphere through the tentorial notch or of the medulla and cerebellum through the foramen magnum. These tumors usually cause CSF pressure buildup, and lumbar puncture causes rapid depressurization of the fluid. CT with contrast medium, MRI, and radiography are all useful tools in imaging brain tumors and do not cause these complications.

28 The answer is D *Respiratory system / Microbiology / Croup and other respiratory infections*

The age, timing of symptoms, fever, cough, and inspiratory stridor are typical of croup rather than bronchiolitis or epiglottitis. The etiology of croup is frequently parainfluenza virus type 1 or 2. Less likely causes are respiratory syncytial virus (RSV), other viral agents, and bacteria. However, RSV is the most common cause of bronchiolitis, which is more common in infants younger than 6 months old. Epiglottitis is frequently misdiagnosed as croup, but in this case the lack of drooling, slower onset (more than 1 day), and *Haemophilus influenzae* type B vaccination make epiglottitis less likely. However, intubation is the correct action in severe cases of epiglottitis. Temperature changes and cold air often improve the symptoms of croup for a brief period. Thus, they may not appear so severe when the patient arrives at the office. Children with croup should be put in a humidified room, although the benefit of this has not been proved. Oxygen, racemic epinephrine, and steroids are sometimes used in the treatment of croup.

29 The answer is A *Renal/urinary system / Physiology / Renal physiology*

If glomerular filtration decreases, excessive reabsorption of Na+ (and Cl−) occurs in the ascending limb of the loop of Henle. The decrease in ion concentration within the distal tubules causes the release of renin from the juxtaglomerular cells (*1*), with subsequent formation of angiotensin II and vasoconstriction of the efferent arteriole (*2*) to help return filtration to normal values. In addition, afferent arteriolar vasodilation will support glomerular filtration.

30 The answer is D *General principles / Microbiology / Gram stain; bacterial growth*

Bacterial spores probably caused the decrease in the number of cells expected from the turbidity of the culture. Spores contribute to turbidity, but they do not stain in Gram's procedure.

31 The answer is C *Cardiovascular system / Physiology / Hemodynamics*

Under the circumstances described in the question, the stroke volume is 100 mL. Cardiac output is the ratio of oxygen consumption to the arteriovenous difference. In this case, it is

$$\frac{300 \text{ mL/min}}{20 \text{ mL/100 mL} - 15 \text{ mL/100 mL}} = 6,000 \text{ mL/min}$$

Stroke volume is the ratio of cardiac output to heart rate:

$$\frac{6,000 \text{ mL/min}}{60/\text{min}} = 100 \text{ mL}$$

32 **The answer is C** *General principles / Microbiology / Antiphagocytic virulence factors*

Opsonizing antibodies promote phagocytosis and are often directed against the capsules of pathogens, including *S. pneumoniae*. The most important function of the *S. pneumoniae* capsule is to inhibit phagocytosis (until opsonizing antibodies are produced). The capsules of both *H. influenzae* type B and *N. meningitidis* are polysaccharides that elicit a poor T cell-dependent immune response. The existing DTP vaccine contains killed whole *B. pertussis* cells, not purified capsules.

33 **The answer is D** *General principles / Biochemistry / Structure and function of proteins*

The chemical properties of proteins are determined by the nature of the constituent amino acid side chains. There are no ionizing groups, physiologically speaking, on the side chain of serine to provide buffering capacity. Only amino acids with aromatic side chains absorb significantly in the ultraviolet range. Both glutamic acid and aspartic acid have a pI of approximately 4.5, and only L-amino acids are incorporated into protein. The side chain of proline contains a cyclic ring that cannot bond hydrogen and therefore disrupts the α-helical structure.

34 **The answer is A** *Hematopoietic and lymphoreticular system / Immunology / Diagnosis of myelodysplastic syndrome*

Clinically persistent and unexplained cytopenias associated with morphologically abnormal differentiation in bone marrow precursors define preleukemia, often referred to as myelodysplastic syndrome. Many of these individuals have bone marrow blast percentages of less than 5%, and patients suffer from complications of bone marrow failure, such as bleeding, infection, and anemia. Others show an increase in bone marrow blasts of 5% to 30% and have a propensity to develop frank, acute myeloid leukemia, particularly at the higher levels. Bone marrow blasts greater than 30% define acute leukemia. If present in myelodysplastic syndrome, cytogenetic changes, such as an extra chromosome 8, loss of chromosome 5 or 7, or loss of the long arm of chromosome 5 or 7, are similar to those observed with acute myeloid leukemia. Despite megaloblastoid morphologic changes, these patients do not resolve with treatment for megaloblastic anemia. It is rare for chronic myelogenous leukemia to present with a low white cell and platelet count and bone marrow dyspoiesis.

35 **The answer is C** *General principles / Pharmacology; toxicology / Histamine (H_2) receptor agonists*

Cimetidine, like most drugs, interacts with a specific receptor, the H_2 receptor. Mannitol is the osmotic diuretic used most frequently in the prevention and treatment of acute renal failure in conditions such as cardiovascular surgery, trauma, and hemolytic transfusion reactions. EDTA and dimercaprol chelate heavy metals but need not interact directly with any receptor for their pharmacologic actions.

36 **The answer is D** *Hematopoietic and lymphoreticular system / Physiology / Hemoglobin–oxygen interaction*

The affinity of hemoglobin A_1 ($\alpha_2\beta_2$) for oxygen is decreased by an increase in H+ concentration (a decrease in pH), by an increase in the PCO_2, or by an increase in the concentration of DPG. All of these conditions result in a shift of the oxygen saturation curve to the right. Fetal hemoglobin ($\alpha_2\gamma_2$) has a higher affinity for oxygen than does adult hemoglobin ($\alpha_2\beta_2$) and consequently becomes saturated at a lower PO_2.

37 **The answer is A** *Musculoskeletal system / Anatomy / Musculature of the oral cavity*

During deglutition, the levator veli palatini muscle raises the soft palate to seal the nasopharynx. Contraction of the palatoglossus elevates the base of the tongue and with help from the palatopharyngeus muscle, closes the oropharyngeal isthmus behind the food bolus. The superior constrictor muscle helps raise the posterior portion of the pharynx over the bolus.

38 The answer is D *General principles / Cell biology / Cell membranes*

Biomembranes are made up of an enclosed phospholipid bilayer. The hydrocarbon side chains of the phospholipids pack together to minimize exposure to water. This allows the hydrophilic side chains to associate with the aqueous surroundings. The lipid composition of the two leaflets is asymmetric. The large hydrophobic side chains of cholesterol insert themselves within the membrane, orienting the hydrophilic head toward the water to make the membranes more fluid. Carbohydrate chains that are covalently bonded to lipids form glycolipids in cell membranes. These glycolipids are found almost exclusively in the noncytoplasmic leaflet, where they can engage in important cell–cell and cell–extracellular matrix interactions. They also serve as antigens for recognition of specific antibodies. Proteins that contain stretches of hydrophobic amino acids associate with membranes as integral membrane proteins to form cellular components (e.g., channels and transporters). The bilayer-spanning portion of the proteins is usually an α-helix. DNA is confined to the nucleus of cells because of the nuclear membrane; it is not associated with cell membranes.

39 The answer is B *Hematopoietic and lymphoreticular system / Pathology; physiology / Idiopathic thrombocytopenic purpura*

Idiopathic thrombocytopenic purpura (ITP) is most common in young women, and the usual presentation is isolated thrombocytopenia without associated illness. Amegakaryocytic thrombocytopenia can occur, but it is much less common, especially in this age group. Drug-induced thrombocytopenia is also possible but is unlikely in a healthy woman who has no reason to take medications. Patients with thrombasthenia are not thrombocytopenic, and aleukemic leukemia is unlikely to occur without other cytopenias.

40 The answer is B *Respiratory system / Physiology / Control of respiration*

The carotid bodies are the major sensors of hypoxia (the aortic bodies being much less sensitive), and the central chemoreceptors are the major sensors of hypercapnia. However, there is a synergistic effect of hypoxia and hypercapnia on respiratory rate. The level of response to ventilatory stimuli is reduced during sleep because of decreased neural output and increased upper airway resistance (caused by the relaxation of dilator muscles). The Hering–Breuer reflex acts to terminate inspiration at tidal volumes greater than 1 L, and it is mediated through stretch receptors and vagal afferents. Peripheral chemoreceptors are the major mediator of the compensatory hyperventilation that occurs during metabolic acidosis. Individuals with increased elastic loads compensate with short, rapid breaths, whereas people with increased resistive loads generally take deeper breaths and decrease breathing frequency.

41 The answer is C *Gastrointestinal system / Histology; pathology / Alcohol-induced acute liver damage*

The liver biopsy shows the typical features of alcohol-induced acute liver injury, which include steatorrhea, acute inflammation, and Mallory bodies. Mallory bodies are intracellular filamentous material believed to be related to prekeratin, which is normally produced by the liver. This injury to the liver is a direct effect of alcohol.

42 The answer is B *General principles / Embryology / Germ layer origin*

Melanocytes in the dermis arise from neuroectoderm. Ectoderm gives rise to the nervous system, sensory epithelia, epidermis, mammary glands, and pituitary gland. Mesoderm gives rise to cartilage, bone, connective tissue, muscles, the cardiovascular system, kidneys, gonads, spleen, and the adrenal cortex. Endoderm gives rise to gastrointestinal and respiratory mucosa and the parenchyma of the tonsils, thyroid gland, parathyroid glands, thymus, liver, and pancreas.

43 The answer is E *General principles / Genetics; biochemistry / Lipoproteins and genetic disorders*

Lipoprotein lipase is an enzyme normally found within the capillary endothelium; it is involved in converting chylomicrons to chylomicron remnants. A deficiency in lipoprotein lipase leads to elevated circulating levels of chylomicrons. Chylomicron levels may also be elevated in systemic lupus erythematosus.

44 **The answer is C** *Central and peripheral nervous system / Neuroanatomy / Neurotransmitters*

Substance P is a peptide neurotransmitter that is specific to the dorsal horn of the spinal cord. It is often associated with sensory neurons that encode painful stimuli, such as extreme temperature, intense mechanical stimuli, or chemical irritation.

45 **The answer is D** *Central and peripheral nervous system / Pathology; neuroscience / Myasthenia gravis*

Myasthenia gravis is caused by an autoimmune attack against acetylcholine receptors at the neuromuscular junction. It can be treated by giving acetylcholinesterase inhibitors that prolong the action of acetylcholine at the synapse, partially compensating for the lack of postsynaptic receptors. An autoimmune attack against muscle is a feature of polymyositis. Herpes viruses, such as herpesvirus or VZV, remain latent in the neurons of dorsal root ganglia or the trigeminal ganglion, but these agents have nothing to do with the etiology of myasthenia gravis. Amyotrophic lateral sclerosis is characterized by progressive muscle weakness owing to the destruction of motor neurons in the ventral horn. Lambert–Eaton syndrome is caused by an autoimmune attack against presynaptic Ca^2+ channels at the neuromuscular junction. Lambert–Eaton syndrome can be distinguished from myasthenia gravis because in myasthenia gravis there is a lack of enhanced neurotransmission with repetitive stimulation.

46 **The answer is A** *General principles / Biochemistry / Oncogenes*

Alteration of almost any cellular signaling system has the potential to cause oncogenesis. The *ras* oncogene product is an activated insulin receptor. The homologue of one of the two subunits of the NGF receptor is *trk*. The oncogene *erbB* has activated tyrosine kinase, which is also activated when EGF binds to the EGF receptor. The oncogenic homologue of the PDGF receptor is *kit*, whereas *sis* binds to the PDGF receptor. The nuclear oncogene *jun* is involved in the control of gene transcription. GDNF signals through its receptor, which consists of *ret* subunits. The oncogene *ret* has been implicated in the genesis of multiple endocrine neoplasia (MEN) types 2A and 2B.

47 **The answer is C** *Skin and other related connective tissue / Pathology / Molluscum virus*

Molluscum contagiosum is a warty lesion of the skin and mucous membranes caused by a double-stranded DNA poxvirus and is acquired through direct contact with a lesion. It manifests as one or more small, pruritic, umbilicated, skin-colored papules, most commonly on the trunk and anogenital areas. Histologically, the lesion shows cup-like verrucous epidermal hyperplasia, and the squamous cells of the stratum granulosum and stratum corneum contain pathognomonic molluscum bodies (i.e., large, homogeneous, eosinophilic, cytoplasmic viral inclusions). HPV is a double-stranded DNA papovavirus that causes cutaneous and anogenital warts, papillomas of oral and respiratory mucosa, and squamous neoplasms. Infected squamous cells containing replicated virions are referred to as koilocytes and are characterized by cytoplasmic clearing and cavitation. Herpes zoster is a double-stranded DNA herpesvirus that causes chickenpox and shingles. The virus is spread by direct contact with an infectious lesion. The virus infects keratinocytes and causes an intraepidermal vesicular lesion that may ulcerate. Infected cells are often multinucleate, with nuclear molding, and individual nuclei have eosinophilic, glassy intranuclear inclusions with peripheral margination of host chromatin (Cowdry type A inclusions). The virus develops latency in dermatomal neurons, with reactivation manifested as a vesicular skin rash in a dermatomal distribution (i.e., shingles). Parvovirus B19 is a single-stranded DNA virus that causes transient bone marrow (predominantly erythroid) suppression in immunocompetent patients and aplastic anemia in immunocompromised patients. It is a cause of nonimmune gestational hydrops fetalis. Infected erythroid precursor cells contain intranuclear gelatinous inclusions. Primary infection is often subclinical or associated with a flu-like illness, followed 1 or 2 weeks later by an immune complex-mediated rash ("slapped cheek"), that is, Fifth disease.

48 **The correct answer is B** *Reproductive system / Pathology / Cervical intraepithelial neoplasia*

Normal cervical epithelium should be nonkeratinized stratified squamous epithelium with no atypical cells. CIN I is the earliest stage of neoplasia on a path to cervical carcinoma. It is distinguished by the presence of koilocytes, large vacuolated cells within a mainly normal epithelium. CIN II is characterized by atypical cells showing changes in nucleocytoplasmic ratio, nuclear size, loss of polarity, increased mitoses, abnormal mitoses (i.e., two nuclei), and hyperchromasia. These are all distinctly precancerous changes. However, CIN II differs from CIN III in that the atypical cells are restricted to subsurface levels and do not penetrate to the top strata of the epithelium. A somewhat differentiated surface epithelial layer remains in CIN II, whereas in CIN III, the atypia occurs throughout the entire epithelium. Cervical carcinoma is diagnosed if there is any evidence of invasion through the basal layers into the underlying stroma.

49 **The answer is C** *Central and peripheral nervous system / Pharmacology / Side effects of neuroleptics*

Akathisia, an extrapyramidal side effect of neuroleptics, causes restlessness and an urge to keep moving. The agitation seems more motoric than psychic, making worsening psychosis relatively unlikely. Although hyperthyroidism causes hyperactivity, this patient has no other symptoms of thyroid disease. Restless legs syndrome is a sleep-related disorder generally associated with nocturnal myoclonus. It is described as a creepy, crawly feeling in the legs at rest, especially when supine, that is relieved by walking.

50 **The answer is B** *General principles / Histology / Extracellular matrix production and chondroblasts*

Chondroblasts are cartilage cells deep in the perichondrium, the dense connective capsule that surrounds cartilage. As chondroblasts secrete an extracellular matrix rich in type II collagen and cartilage proteoglycan, they become surrounded by their own extracellular matrix and differentiate into chondrocytes. Both chondroblasts and chondrocytes are capable of cell division by mitosis. The endosteum is a layer of osteoblasts in bone. The periosteum is the outer connective tissue covering of bone.

test 14

Questions

Directions: *Single best answer questions consist of numbered items or incomplete statements followed by answers or by completions of the statement. Select the ONE lettered answer or completion that is BEST in each case.*

1 A 50-year-old man goes to the emergency department with severe epigastric pain, low-grade fever, tachycardia, and mild hypotension. The patient relates a history of moderate to heavy social drinking. The chief resident suspects acute pancreatitis. The single most important laboratory finding to confirm the diagnosis of pancreatitis would be

(A) hyperlipidemia
(B) hyperbilirubinemia
(C) elevated serum amylase
(D) elevated serum phospholipase A
(E) elevated serum alkaline phosphatase

2 An abnormally small child from a migrant community is seen in a local clinic. The child's mother complains that the child has little interest in eating and suffers from chronic diarrhea. Upon physical examination the child also presents with a hemorrhagic dermatitis around the eyes, nose, and mouth. What type of a deficiency would you suspect?

(A) Folate
(B) Zinc
(C) Selenium
(D) Vitamin D
(E) Vitamin C

3 A 7-year-old child presents to a local clinic with a beefy red tongue, a widespread dermatitis, numbness and tingling in his hands and feet, and severe cracking around the corners of the mouth. What type of deficiency do you suspect?

(A) Thiamine
(B) Riboflavin
(C) Niacin
(D) Pyridoxine
(E) Folate

4 Which of the following activation pathways are used by leukocytes to respond to chemotactic agents?

(A) Tyrosine–kinase activation
(B) Phospholipase C
(C) Src–kinases
(D) Potassium–sodium fluxes across cell membrane
(E) Serine–threonine kinase

5 Which of the following statements about secretin, a polypeptide that has a significant effect on pancreatic secretion, is correct?

(A) It is synthesized in the pancreatic acinar cells
(B) It causes the pancreas to secrete large amounts of enzyme
(C) Its release is caused by fats and amino acids in the upper small intestine
(D) It causes the pancreas to secrete large amounts of bicarbonate ion (HCO_3^-)
(E) It is stored in an active form within S cells of the duodenum

6 A 1-year-old boy is brought to his pediatrician by his mother. She says that he had a fever of 39°C for three days that she treated with acetaminophen. Yesterday the fever subsided and the boy developed a fine, erythematous rash over his entire body. What is the best diagnosis for this condition?

(A) Rubella
(B) Chicken pox
(C) Rubeola
(D) Exanthem subitem
(E) Measles

7 A complement fixation test is performed on a patient's serum by first adding influenza type A virus antigen and then adding complement, followed by antibody-coated sheep red blood cells (SRBC), which are then lysed. A possible explanation for this is that

(A) the patient has no immunoglobulin (Ig) E or IgA anti-influenza type A antibodies
(B) the patient's serum contains an antibody that crossreacts with SRBC
(C) the patient has no complement-fixable anti-influenza type A antibodies
(D) the patient's serum contains high levels of IgM, which cause SRBC lysis

8 Volume and pressure (alveolar; pleural) for a normal respiratory cycle are shown in the figure. Which one of the following statements about respiration is correct?

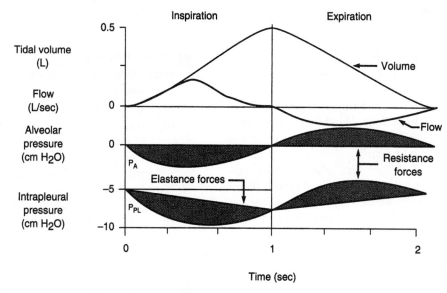

(A) Inspiration is the result of a passive process
(B) Gas flow is greatest at the end of inspiration
(C) Elastic recoil of the lung is identical at the beginning and end of inspiration
(D) During expiration, alveolar pressure becomes greater than atmospheric pressure

9 Which one of the following areas in a eukaryotic cell is a site of RNA processing?

(A) Mitochondria
(B) Golgi complex
(C) Rough endoplasmic reticulum
(D) Endosome

10 In humans, the major route of nitrogen metabolism from amino acids to urea involves which one of the following sets of enzymes?

(A) Amino acid oxidases and arginase
(B) Glutaminase and amino acid oxidases
(C) Glutamate dehydrogenase and transaminases
(D) Transaminase and glutaminase
(E) Glutamine synthetase and urease

11 A reading disability is best characterized by which of the following?

(A) Comprehension of written material when someone else reads it aloud but difficulty in forming symbol–sound relationships when reading independently

(B) Slow development in all conceptual areas

(C) Poor development of social skills

(D) Problems with maintaining attention and concentration in school

12 Which one of the following central nervous system stimulants is a hallucinogen?

(A) Caffeine

(B) Amphetamine

(C) Theobromine

(D) Nicotine

(E) Doxapram

(F) Tetrahydrocannabinol (THC)

(G) Nikethamide

13 A couple asks you for advice concerning their second pregnancy. The father is Rh+, and the mother is Rh−. Their first child is Rh−; however, they have heard of risks to subsequent offspring if the mother and father are opposite Rh factors. What advice would you give to the parents?

(A) Inform the parents that the risk of developing antibodies to the red blood cells of subsequent children is high, so the mother should receive an injection of Rh immunoglobulin (Rho-GAM) to prevent hemolytic anemia in the new fetus.

(B) Inform the parents that there is no risk of developing antibodies to the red blood cells of subsequent children; however, the mother should still receive an injection of RhoGAM to minimize any risks to a new fetus.

(C) Inform the parents that because the first child was Rh−, no antibodies were generated in the mother and so no RhoGAM is needed to protect a new fetus. Normal pregnancy precautions will be sufficient.

(D) Inform the parents that the risk to subsequent pregnancies is very high and advise against subsequent pregnancies.

14 Which of the following statements about the lesion depicted in Figure 59 of the color plate section is true?

(A) It may be confused with pneumonia on a chest radiograph

(B) Multifocal character is uncommon

(C) Regional lymph node metastasis is frequent at presentation

(D) Invasive carcinoma is demonstrated in the photomicrograph

15 A patient who is receiving cyclophosphamide for breast cancer begins to have nausea, vomiting, weakness, and inability to think clearly. No evidence of infection is found, but her serum sodium has dropped to 115 mEq/L (normal = 134 to 146 mEq/L). Although there are no signs of edema, a urinalysis reveals a urinary sodium level of 500 mEq/L. Which one of the following statements is most likely correct?

(A) Because the patient is hyponatremic, she must also be volume-depleted

(B) Diuretics should not be given to this patient

(C) Administration of normal saline is the only form of treatment required

(D) No treatment is required, because this patient should recover rapidly on her own

(E) This case is consistent with a diagnosis of syndrome of inappropriate secretion of antidiuretic hormone (SIADH)

16 A 35-year-old man contracts something resembling influenza, receives no treatment, and is sick for a few days. Then, 25 days later, he develops a feeling of pins and needles in his fingers and toes; 3 days after that, he has trouble speaking and eating, and he keeps cutting the right side of his face while shaving because it is numb. The next day, upon waking, he has trouble walking. He goes to the hospital and tells the physician that he has never been ill before in his life. He is barely able to lift his arms to a horizontal position, and he cannot walk well. All of his tendon reflexes are absent. Which one of the following diseases is the patient most likely to have?

(A) Myasthenia gravis

(B) Polio

(C) Guillain–Barré syndrome

(D) Raynaud's phenomenon

17 Which of the following disease is an example of the deleterious effects of improper protein folding following polypeptide translation?

(A)   Duchenne's muscular dystrophy
(B)   Tay–Sachs disease
(C)   Alpha-1 antitrypsin deficiency
(D)   Hemophilia A
(E)   Hemophilia B

18 Which of the following inherited cancer syndromes is caused by autosomal recessive syndromes of defective DNA repair?

(A)   Familial retinoblastoma
(B)   Multiple endocrine neoplasia syndromes
(C)   Von Hippel–Lindau syndrome
(D)   Familial adenomatous polyps of the colon
(E)   Xeroderma pigmentosum

19 Angiotensin-converting enzyme (ACE) hydrolyzes angiotensin I to angiotensin II. Which of the following statements correctly explains why inhibition of this enzyme with an agent such as captopril reduces blood pressure in some subjects?

(A)   Increased Na + absorption by the renal tubules owing to increased renin levels
(B)   Increased synthesis and release of aldosterone
(C)   Centrally mediated increase in water intake
(D)   Decreased production of a vasoconstrictor (angiotensin II)
(E)   Inhibition of synaptic transmission in the peripheral sympathetic nervous system

20 Which one of the following statements regarding pulmonary emboli is true?

(A)   Pulmonary emboli can usually be diagnosed by the clinical presentation
(B)   The most common source of pulmonary emboli is the internal jugular vein
(C)   Risk factors for pulmonary emboli include indwelling catheters, sickle cell disease, and hypocoagulable states
(D)   Pulmonary angiography is the gold standard test for the diagnosis of pulmonary emboli
(E)   Pulmonary emboli lead to a decrease in pulmonary vascular resistance
(F)   All pulmonary emboli share a characteristic abnormality on chest radiograph

21 Which of the following gives rise to the right ventricle of the heart?

(A)   Right horn of the sinus venosus
(B)   Bulbus cordis
(C)   Truncus arteriosus
(D)   Primitive ventricle
(E)   Wolffian duct

22 Which of the following is true about Meckel's diverticulum?

(A)   It is usually in the duodenum
(B)   It lies on the mesenteric side of the intestinal wall
(C)   It is due to the persistence of the Müllerian duct
(D)   It is usually asymptomatic
(E)   It is present in more than 30% of the population

23 Which of the following is true about liver tissue?

(A)   Many hepatocytes are binucleate
(B)   Hematoxylin and eosin (H&E)-stained hepatocytes appear smooth by light microscopy owing to the abundance of smooth endoplasmic reticulum
(C)   Kupffer cells are specialized neutrophils that line the liver sinusoids
(D)   The tough collagenous capsule surrounding the liver is called Bowman's capsule

24 A 47-year-old man with cardiac insufficiency is diagnosed with familial hypercholesterolemia. Which of the following serum components is most likely to be elevated?

(A)   Ig against apoprotein E
(B)   Chylomicron remnants and intermediate-density lipoproteins (IDLs)
(C)   Very-low-density lipoproteins
(D)   Low-density lipoproteins (LDLs)
(E)   Chylomicrons

25 Which one of the following statements concerning the effects of diuretics on the kidney is correct?

(A) Diuretics that affect the proximal tubule are the most efficacious class of diuretics because the majority of reabsorption occurs in the proximal tubules

(B) Loop diuretics may cause kidney stone formation because of the reduction of the electrical potential that normally enhances the reabsorption of calcium

(C) Thiazide-type diuretics, which act in the distal tubule, can cause metabolic acidosis

(D) Because only approximately 20% of sodium reabsorption occurs in the loop of Henle, loop diuretics are suitable only for cases of very mild edema

(E) Aldosterone antagonists act mainly in the proximal tubule

(F) Osmotic diuretics are frequently useful as oral agents in patients with severe edema

26 A 22-year-old woman has orange discolorations on her palms and bulbous, cutaneous xanthomas. An analysis of her serum indicates elevated levels of chylomicron remnants and IDLs. Which of the following is the most likely diagnosis?

(A) Combined hyperlipidemia

(B) Hypertriglyceridemia

(C) Type III hyperlipoproteinemia

(D) Hypercholesterolemia

(E) Lipoprotein lipase deficiency

27 Ablation of the medial forebrain bundle results in the depletion of which neurotransmitters in the cerebral cortex?

(A) Acetylcholine (ACh) and dopamine

(B) γ-Aminobutyric acid (GABA) and glycine

(C) Nitric oxide

(D) Serotonin and catecholamines

(E) GABA and dopamine

28 A patient with atrial fibrillation who is not maintained on anticoagulant therapy has an embolic stroke. Given that the patient cannot move his right leg or feel any sensation on the right leg, which of the following arteries is most likely to have the embolism?

(A) The left middle cerebral artery

(B) The right posterior cerebral artery

(C) The left anterior cerebral artery

(D) The right middle cerebral artery

(E) The left vertebral artery

29 Patients with persistent, chronic gastroesophageal reflux can eventually develop changes in the epithelium of the esophagus called Barrett's esophagus. Which of the following cancers is 30 to 40 times as likely to occur in these patients as in the general population?

(A) Squamous cell carcinoma of the upper esophagus

(B) Adenocarcinoma of the esophagus

(C) Adenocarcinoma of the stomach

(D) Squamous cell carcinoma of the lower esophagus

(E) Lymphoma

30 Three days after returning from a camping trip in Texas, an 18-year-old man develops a high fever, muscle and joint pain, weakness, and anorexia. Five days after the onset of these symptoms, he has a brief period of shaking chills; then his symptoms resolve. Seven days later, the initial symptoms reappear. The patient is diagnosed with relapsing fever. Which of the following is the etiologic agent?

(A) *Treponema pallidum*

(B) *Treponema pertenue*

(C) *Treponema carateum*

(D) *Leptospira interrogans*

(E) *Borrelia recurrentis*

31 Bejel, or nonvenereal endemic syphilis, is usually seen in children of the Middle East or Africa. Which of the following is the causative agent?

(A) *Treponema pallidum*

(B) *Treponema carateum*

(C) *Borrelia recurrentis*

(D) *Leptospira interrogans*

(E) *Treponema pertenue*

32 An 80-year-old man has congestive heart failure, angina pectoris, and exertional syncope. Physical examination reveals left ventricular hypertrophy and a delayed upstroke of the carotid arteries. Which of the following findings are you also most likely to observe in this patient?

(A) A midsystolic click

(B) A coarse crescendo–decrescendo systolic ejection murmur

(C) An apical pansystolic murmur

(D) A diastolic sharp opening snap

(E) A mid- to late-diastolic murmur

33 Extracts of glycosides from the foxglove plant *Digitalis purpurea* provide an important family of drugs in the treatment of heart failure. In high concentrations, however, cardiac glycosides can have severe toxic effects. Which of the following statements about digitalis toxicity is correct?

(A) High levels of digitalis activate Na+/K+-adenosine triphosphatase (ATPase)

(B) High levels of digitalis lower the resting potential in cardiac myocytes

(C) High levels of digitalis can result in third-degree atrioventricular block

(D) High levels of digitalis increase the action potential duration in cardiac myocytes

34 Which one of the following statements correctly describes the mechanism of action of mast cells in people with allergies?

(A) Fc receptors on the surface of mast cells bind to IgE. When antigen crosslinks the bound IgE antibodies, the mast cell is triggered to release secretory granules that contain inflammatory mediators (e.g., leukotrienes and histamine).

(B) Mast cells are triggered by the release of cytokines during the allergic response. Interleukin (IL) 4 and IL-5 cause the mast cell to release secretory granules containing more IL-4 and IL-5 in a positive-feedback loop.

(C) Receptors on the surface of mast cells can specifically bind to foreign antigen. Upon binding, mast cells begin to secrete and release inflammatory mediators.

(D) The IgD antibody binds to mast cells via Fab receptors. When antigen crosslinks the bound antibodies, the mast cell is triggered to release its secretory granules, which contain inflammatory mediators such as leukotrienes and histamine.

(E) Mast cells phagocytose foreign antigen and process it for presentation to other mast cells. These cells will then begin secreting IL-8 and tumor necrosis factor-α.

35 Which of the following hematologic malignancies is properly matched with the most common oncogenic translocations?

(A) Chronic myeloid leukemia (9:22)

(B) Acute myelogenous leukemia (11:22)

(C) Follicular lymphoma (8:14)

(D) Burkitt lymphoma (11:14)

(E) Mantle cell lymphoma (14:18)

36 Which of the following statements regarding contraction in skeletal and smooth muscles is correct?

(A) The same tension of contraction requires more energy in smooth muscle than in skeletal muscle

(B) The maximum force of contraction is greater in smooth muscle than in skeletal muscle

(C) The contractions are faster in smooth muscle than in skeletal muscle

(D) The smooth muscle can shorten a smaller percentage of its length while maintaining the full force of contraction than can skeletal muscle

37 A 10-year-old child has exertional dyspnea, cyanosis, and clubbing of the fingers and toes. Tetralogy of Fallot is diagnosed by echocardiography. Which of the following abnormalities would an electrocardiogram of this patient indicate?

(A) Left ventricular hypertrophy

(B) Right ventricular hypertrophy

(C) Third-degree atrioventricular conduction block

(D) Left atrial hypertrophy

(E) Sick sinus syndrome

38 What is the most common cause of cirrhosis in industrialized countries?

(A) Hepatitis A

(B) Hepatitis B

(C) Hepatitis C

(D) Hepatitis B and E

(E) Alcohol abuse

39 Which of the following is true about the control of cell proliferation?

(A) Uncontrolled cell proliferation can result from inactivation of proto-oncogenes

(B) Loss of one tumor suppressor allele in a cell leads directly to uncontrolled cell proliferation

(C) The retinoblastoma gene is an important proto-oncogene

(D) p53 is elevated in cells exposed to ultraviolet light and is important in blocking cellular proliferation

40 Which one of the following fatty acids found in a normal diet is metabolized by the α-hydroxylase pathway?

(A) Linoleic acid
(B) Phytanic acid
(C) Arachidonic acid
(D) Palmitic acid
(E) Decanoic acid

41 Low levels of cellular 3-hydroxy-3-methylglutaryl (HMG) coenzyme A (CoA) reductase activity in humans is most likely to result from

(A) a vegetarian diet
(B) the administration of a bile acid-sequestering resin
(C) familial hypercholesterolemia
(D) a long-term high-cholesterol diet

42 A particular recessive trait (e.g., purple fingers) is found in 4.5% of a population, and the penetrance of the trait is 50% in the homozygous recessive state (0% in heterozygotes and dominant homozygotes). What is the percentage of the population that is heterozygous for the purple finger allele, assuming only two possible alleles (dominant and recessive), random mating, no selection bias for the trait, and no new mutations?

(A) 5.82%
(B) 9%
(C) 30%
(D) 42%
(E) 49%

43 Deficiency in absorption of which of the following vitamins may result in prolonged prothrombin times in a patient who is noted to have pancreatic achylia (no secretion of pancreatic digestive enzymes)?

(A) Vitamin A
(B) Vitamin B_6
(C) Vitamin C
(D) Vitamin D
(E) Vitamin K

44 A teenager who is below average in both weight and height is seen because of vomiting of bile-stained material, abdominal distention, and pain. Further questioning reveals a periodic history of respiratory infections. Cystic fibrosis is suspected, and the diagnosis is confirmed when pilocarpine iontophoresis produces an abnormally high sweat chloride concentration (>60 mEq/L). The patient has a history of frequent respiratory infections. A recent sputum analysis indicates the presence of *Staphylococcus aureus, Haemophilus influenzae,* and *Pseudomonas aeruginosa.* Although the value of antibiotic therapy in cystic fibrosis remains unclear, a conventional approach to such therapy based on sputum culture might include

(A) gentamicin and ceftazidime
(B) nalidixic acid and kanamycin
(C) nitrofurantoin
(D) pentamidine
(E) rifampin and isoniazid

45 Which of the following glomerular diseases is strongly responsive to steroid treatments?

(A) IgA nephropathy
(B) Nephrotic syndrome
(C) Rapidly progressive glomerulonephritis
(D) Membranous glomerulonephritis
(E) Minimal change disease

46 Before it was banned in 1971, the estrogen analogue diethylstilbestrol (DES) was commonly prescribed to prevent miscarriages in pregnant women. Daughters of DES-treated mothers have been found to have a host of health problems. Which of the following cancers has an increased frequency in women exposed to DES in utero?

(A) Uterine carcinoma
(B) Clear cell carcinoma of the vagina
(C) Transitional cell carcinoma of the bladder
(D) Cervical carcinoma
(E) Ovarian carcinoma

47 Which of the following statements about generalized tonic–clonic seizures is correct?

(A) They do not cause a general increase in muscle tone
(B) They rarely cause a loss of consciousness
(C) They result in postictal lethargy and confusion
(D) They are also called petit mal seizures
(E) They are preceded by an aura of abnormal smells, tastes, or visual sensations

48 Which of the following findings is most consistent with the diagnosis of Parkinson's disease?

(A) Seizures
(B) Postural dizziness and syncope
(C) Rigidity
(D) Isolated tics and involuntary vocalizations
(E) Diminished strength

49 Which of the following descriptions are consistent with a diagnosis of nonfluent aphasia?

(A) It is produced by lesions in the basal ganglia
(B) Naming and repetition are preserved
(C) Comprehension is fairly well preserved
(D) It is produced by lesions in the angular gyrus
(E) Speech is polysyllabic and repetitious

50 Which of the following teratogens is correctly paired with its associated toxicity?

(A) Sulfonamides—gray baby syndrome
(B) Tetracycline—tooth enamel dysplasia and bone growth inhibition
(C) Chloramphenicol—kernicterus
(D) Valproic acid—ototoxicity
(E) Streptomycin—neural tube defects

Answer Key

1-C	11-A	21-B	31-A	41-D
2-B	12-F	22-D	32-B	42-D
3-D	13-C	23-A	33-C	43-E
4-B	14-A	24-D	34-A	44-A
5-D	15-E	25-B	35-A	45-E
6-D	16-C	26-C	36-B	46-B
7-C	17-C	27-D	37-B	47-C
8-D	18-E	28-C	38-E	48-C
9-A	19-D	29-B	39-D	49-C
10-C	20-D	30-E	40-B	50-B

Answers and Explanations

1 The answer is C *Endocrine system / Physiology / Exocrine pancreatic function*

Elevated serum amylase is the single most important diagnostic finding for confirmation of acute pancreatitis. A serum amylase level three times as high as normal virtually confirms the diagnosis.

2 The answer is B *General principles / Pathology / Nutrition*

The symptoms described in this patient are pathonomonic for zinc deficiency. The common findings are growth retardation, anorexia, diarrhea, poor wound healing, and acrodermatitis enteropathica (a hemorrhagic dermatitis around the eyes, nose, mouth, anus, and other distal parts.

3 The answer is D *General principles / Pathology / Nutrition*

The symptoms found in this patient are consistent with the diagnosis of pyridoxine deficiency (vitamin B_6). The symptoms of pyridoxine deficiency are glossitis (beefy red tongue), cheilosis (cracking of the corners of the mouth), dermatitis, and peripheral neuropathy.

4 The answer is B *General principles / Immunology / Leukocyte activation*

The binding of chemotactic agents to receptors on the surface of leukocytes results in the activation of phospholipase C. Phospholipase C mediates the hydrolysis of PIP2 to IP3, diacylglycerol (DAG), and the influx of extracellular calcium. The increased calcium concentration triggers the assembly of contractile elements that results in the movement of leukocytes.

5 The answer is D *Endocrine system / Physiology / Exocrine pancreatic function*

The mucosa of the small intestine secretes cholecystokinin and secretin into the bloodstream. They exert their effects after entering the pancreatic circulation. Secretin is stored in an inactive form in the S cells of the duodenum and is released and activated in response to acid. It causes the pancreas to secrete copious amounts of HCO_3^-; but unlike cholecystokinin, which is secreted in response to food, secretin does not significantly affect pancreatic enzyme secretion. The proteolytic enzymes are synthesized as proenzymes, inactive precursors that must be processed before they are active. Many proenzymes, including chymotrypsinogen, procarboxypeptidase, and prophospholipase, are activated by trypsin. Trypsinogen is activated by enterokinase.

6 The answer is D *General principles / Pathology / Infectious disease*

Exanthem subitem (roseola infantum) is a common malady of young children that normally begins with 3 to 4 days of fever followed by the cessation of the fever followed by the development of fine, erythematous maculopapular rash over a large portion of the body. The rash is normally self-limited and resolves within 24 to 48 hours. Treatment of exanthem subitem is usually supportive except for the use of acetaminophen as an antipyretic.

7 The answer is C *General principles / Immunology / Complement fixation*

The complement fixation test is composed of SRBC, antibodies to SRBC, and complement. The concentration of complement is limiting, and any loss of complement is reflected by a decrease in the extent of SRBC lysis. This loss of complement may occur during preincubation of the complement with an antigen–antibody complex not related to the SRBC, which would cause fixation and activation of the cascade. All or most of the complement would be consumed, so that the introduction of SRBC does not result in lysis. In this case, because lysis did occur, the patient's serum possesses no complement-fixable (IgG) anti-influenza type A antibodies. A crossreactive antibody has no bearing on the complement fixation test.

8 **The answer is D** *Respiratory system / Physiology / Pulmonary mechanics*

Inspiration is an active process brought about by contraction of the diaphragm. This contraction increases chest volume, lowering pleural and alveolar pressure and creating a gradient for the movement of air. At the end of inspiration, flow is zero and alveolar pressure equals atmospheric pressure. The difference between alveolar and pleural pressure is the recoil pressure of the lung, which is always greatest at higher lung volumes, hence is greater at the end of inspiration. During expiration, inspiratory muscles relax, and the elastic forces of the lungs compress alveolar gas, which raises alveolar pressure to values greater than atmospheric pressure and creates a pressure gradient to expel gas from the lung.

9 **The answer is A** *General principles / Cell biology / RNA processing*

RNA processing occurs in two locations within cells. The most common site is the cell nucleoplasm, where most RNA transcribed in the nucleus is spliced, capped, and polyadenylated. The other site is the mitochondria, each of which contains a ring of DNA that codes for two ribosomal RNA (rRNA) molecules, proteins, and all the transfer RNA (tRNA) required to synthesize the encoded proteins.

10 **The answer is C** *General principles / Biochemistry / Urea metabolism; amino acid enzymes*

The pathway by which the α-amino groups of the amino acids are incorporated into urea involves a number of transaminases that transfer the amino group from the amino acids to α-ketoglutarate, with the concomitant formation of glutamate. The mitochondrial enzyme glutamate dehydrogenase converts the glutamate back to α-ketoglutarate and ammonium. The ammonium produced in the reaction is the substrate for carbamoyl phosphate synthesis. This reaction constitutes the first step in urea biosynthesis.

11 **The answer is A** *Central and peripheral nervous system / Behavioral science / Childhood development*

Children with reading disabilities are characterized by average or above-average intelligence. They have difficulty forming sound–symbol relationships of written material, but otherwise they follow normal developmental patterns. Although slow development in all concept areas, poor development of social skills, and difficulty maintaining attention and concentration may occur in children with a reading disability, these problems are not directly attributable to the reading disability.

12 **The answer is F** *Central and peripheral nervous system / Pharmacology / Central nervous system stimulants*

Tetrahydrocannabinol (THC) is a hallucinogen found in marijuana that produces euphoria followed by drowsiness and relaxation, depending on the social situation. Caffeine, amphetamine, theobromine, and nicotine are psychomotor stimulants; they cause excitement and euphoria, decrease feelings of fatigue, and increase motor activity. Doxapram and nikethamide are convulsants and respiratory stimulants, which have minimal effect on mental function but produce exaggerated reflex responses, increase activity in the respiratory and vasomotor centers, and cause convulsions at high doses.

13 **The answer is C** *General principles / Hematology / Rh factor incompatibility*

If a fetus has the Rhesus antibody and the mother does not, fetal Rh + blood exposure to maternal Rh − blood may result in the development of antibodies to fetal red blood cells with the Rhesus factor. As a result, a subsequent fetus is at risk of *hydrops fetalis,* a condition of high-output cardiac failure owing to hemolytic anemia, which occurs as a result of maternal antibody formation to fetal red blood cells and the subsequent hemolytic destruction of those fetal cells and ensuing anemia.

14 The answer is A *Respiratory system / Pathology / Bronchioloalveolar carcinoma*

This pulmonary neoplasm arises peripherally in the lung in the distribution of terminal bronchioles and alveoli. Patients have cough, pain, hemoptysis, and/or asymptomatic radiographic abnormalities on a chest radiograph. There is no obstructive bronchial component, in contrast to primary bronchogenic neoplasms. Neoplastic cells spread in a contiguous fashion on the surfaces of alveolar septa (lepidic growth), replacing the normal type II pneumocytes. The abnormal cells show type II pneumocyte, Clara cell, or mucinous bronchiolar cell differentiation. The carcinoma remains in situ; invasion and metastasis occur in a few patients late in the course of the disease. Lesions may be single but are frequently multifocal; these lesions are represented radiographically as nodules or diffuse infiltrates, with the latter mimicking pneumonia. Intrapulmonary dissemination is common and is typically due to aerosols resulting in multifocal lesions. Invasive pulmonary carcinomas may show a bronchioloalveolar growth pattern at the periphery of the tumor, mimicking bronchioloalveolar carcinoma.

15 The answer is E *Renal/urinary system / Physiology / Syndrome of inappropriate secretion of anti-diuretic hormone*

Syndrome of inappropriate secretion of antidiuretic hormone (SIADH) is characterized by urine osmolality that is too concentrated relative to serum tonicity. In the case of hyponatremia, the urine should be maximally diluted to limit further sodium losses. Diagnosis entails ruling out other causes of water retention (e.g., volume depletion and congestive heart failure). Total body sodium must also be normal. Although water restriction may be sufficient therapy for mild cases, symptoms of the central nervous system and a serum sodium level lower than 120 mEq/L require treatment with both saline and diuretics. Correction of the hyponatremia must be done slowly to avoid causing brain damage.

16 The answer is C *Central and peripheral nervous system / Pathology / Neurologic disease topography*

Guillain–Barré syndrome causes peripheral sensory defects and motor defects that progress from distal areas of the body to involve more proximal regions. It usually follows a viral illness of unknown origin and affects mostly young people. Loss of deep tendon reflexes is also present. Guillain–Barré syndrome is thought to involve antimyelin autoantibodies against motor neurons that evolve after viral illness or influenza vaccine. There is a progressive mixed motor and sensory loss, even though motor neurons are the target of these antibodies, due to the inflammation of spinal nerves in which both motor and sensory fibers travel together. Myasthenia gravis is a disease of the neuromuscular junction and most commonly causes ocular symptoms, such as ptosis, diplopia, and dysarthria. It manifests as muscle fatigue without sensory symptoms. Deep tendon reflexes are diminished but not lost. Myasthenia gravis is an autoimmune disease that involves ACh receptors in the postsynaptic neuromuscular junction.

Poliovirus is a picornavirus that usually causes an intestinal disease that can progress to viremia and cause the destruction of anterior horn cells of the spinal cord, resulting in paralysis of the innervated muscles. It usually manifests as a purely muscular disorder, and deep tendon reflexes are absent only if the muscles involved in the reflex lose their motor innervation.

Raynaud's phenomenon is a peripheral vascular syndrome manifested by sensitivity to cold, livedo reticularis, and acrocyanosis. It occurs primarily in women in their late teens. The cause is unknown, but the condition is associated with vasospasms.

17 The answer is C *General principles / Molecular biology / Alpha-1 antitrypsin deficiency*

Alpha-1 antitrypsin deficiency is caused by improper folding of the mutated protein. The genetic mutation causes slow folding of the protein resulting in the accumulation of nonfolded proteins within the endoplasmic reticulum of hepatocytes and an inability to release the protein into the bloodstream.

18 The answer is E *General principles / Pathology / Neoplasia*

Except for xeroderma pigmentosum, the neoplastic conditions listed are all caused by mutations that are inherited in an autosomal dominant manner. The genetic mutation that causes xeroderma pigmentosum are mutations in one of the seven xeroderma DNA repair genes named XPA through XPG.

19 **The answer is D** *Endocrine system / Physiology / Blood pressure regulation*

ACE hydrolyzes the decapeptide angiotensin I to the vasoconstrictor octapeptide angiotensin II. Inhibition of this enzyme by a number of competitive antagonists is a useful way to lower blood pressure in some individuals. In addition to reducing circulating levels of the endogenous angiotensin II peptide, inhibition of ACE may have central effects, including a decrease in the dipsogenic effect of angiotensin II. Furthermore, angiotensin II appears to facilitate neurotransmission in the central and peripheral sympathetic nervous systems. Angiotensin II is a potent stimulator of aldosterone secretion in the zona glomerulosa of the adrenal cortex and inhibition of this effect may be expected to reduce blood pressure by enhancing Na + excretion by the kidneys. However, there is usually little change in aldosterone levels because other endogenous secretagogues, including steroids, K +, and minimal levels of angiotensin II, can maintain aldosterone secretion. Nonetheless, there is little indication to suggest that the aldosterone level would actually increase, and if it did, this would result in Na + reabsorption, water retention, and an increase in arterial blood pressure.

20 **The answer is D** *Respiratory system / Physiology / Pulmonary emboli*

Diagnosis of pulmonary emboli is difficult but critical because pulmonary emboli may be life-threatening. Pulmonary emboli cause a wide array of symptoms and are often asymptomatic. In addition, patients with pulmonary emboli may have a normal chest radiograph. Thus, other diagnostic tests are often required. Among these tests are ventilation–perfusion lung scan, venous ultrasonography, spiral computed tomography, and the gold standard—pulmonary angiography. The most common source of the thromboemboli are the deep veins of the leg (popliteal and femoral). Risk factors include indwelling catheters, sickle cell disease, surgery, and hypercoagulable states, including factor V Leiden mutation. Pulmonary emboli may affect both gas exchange and hemodynamics. These disruptions include an increase in pulmonary vascular resistance.

21 **The answer is B** *Cardiovascular system / Embryology / Myocardial development*

The bulbus cordis gives rise to the right ventricle of the heart. The right horn of the sinus venosus gives rise to the smooth part of the right atrium. The truncus arteriosus gives rise to the pulmonary trunk and ascending aorta. The primitive ventricle gives rise to most of the left ventricle. The Wolffian duct, which is not involved in the development of the heart, develops into the ductus deferens, seminal vesicles, and epididymis.

22 **The answer is D** *Gastrointestinal system / Embryology / Meckel's diverticulum*

Meckel's diverticulum is one of the most common congenital anomalies of the gastrointestinal tract. It is caused by the persistence of the vitelline duct or yolk sac and is present in approximately 2% of the population. It is found approximately 1 to 2 feet from the ileocecal valve and lies on the antimesenteric side of the intestine wall. Although it can cause complications such as bleeding or obstruction, it is usually asymptomatic.

23 **The answer is A** *Gastrointestinal system / Histology / Hepatic histology*

Many hepatocytes are binucleate, and many hepatocyte nuclei contain twice the normal amount of DNA (i.e., they are tetraploid). Although hepatocytes do have a large amount of smooth endoplasmic reticulum, which is important for drug detoxification and steroid synthesis, they also have enormous amounts of ribosomes and rough endoplasmic reticulum. This gives the cytoplasm a fine, granular appearance on light microscopy after H&E staining. The tough capsule surrounding the liver is called Glisson's capsule (Bowman's capsule is in the kidney). Kupffer cells are specialized macrophages that line the liver sinusoids.

24 **The answer is D** *General principles / Genetics; biochemistry / Lipoproteins and genetic disorders*

Familial hypercholesterolemia, caused by mutation within a single gene, is one of the most common human Mendelian disorders. LDL levels are elevated in the serum because this disorder greatly decreases the number of high-affinity LDL receptors within the liver. LDL levels may also be elevated in nephrotic syndrome and hyperthyroidism. Abnormalities in apoprotein E have been associated with an increased risk of Alzheimer's disease.

25 **The answer is B** *Renal/urinary system / Pharmacology / Diuretics*

Most reabsorption takes place in the proximal tubule, but diuretics that act in this segment are not very efficacious because their effects may be compensated for by increased reabsorption in the loop of Henle. Conversely, although only approximately 20% of sodium reabsorption occurs in the loop of Henle, drugs that act in this segment make up the most efficacious class of diuretics. Thus, loop diuretics are often used for rapid diuresis in severe cases of edema. Kidney stones are a possible side effect of loop diuretics because they decrease the electrical potential that increases the reabsorption of calcium and magnesium. Thus, the calcium concentration increases in the tubular lumen, and kidney stones may form. Loop diuretics and thiazide-type diuretics may cause metabolic alkalosis because of the increased proton secretion in the collecting duct. This excess secretion of hydrogen ions is caused by increased sodium delivery to the collecting duct. Aldosterone antagonists act in the collecting duct, and they may cause metabolic acidosis because of the reduction in sodium reabsorption and proton secretion. Almost all osmotic diuretics are ineffective orally and are not efficacious for severe edema.

26 **The answer is C** *General principles / Genetics; biochemistry / Lipoproteins and genetic disorders*

Familial (type III) hyperlipoproteinemia has been traced to a single amino acid substitution within the receptor for apoprotein E. Because the apoprotein E receptor is required for the normal metabolism of both chylomicron remnants and IDLs, both of these molecules accumulate in the blood.

27 **The answer is D** *Central and peripheral nervous system / Anatomy / Neuroscience; neurotransmitters*

Sectioning of the medial forebrain bundle would destroy many of the axons that connect the catecholaminergic and serotoninergic nuclei of the brainstem with the cerebral cortex. Destruction of the medullary raphe would destroy the serotoninergic neurons of the medulla that project to the spinal cord.

28 **The answer is C** *Central and peripheral nervous system / Anatomy; neuroscience / Cerebral ischemia; embolism*

Given that the patient's symptoms are on the right side, the lesion is likely to be on the left hemisphere of the brain. Because the symptoms are localized to the leg, not the arms or head, it is likely that the most medial areas of primary motor and somatosensory cortex are ischemic, because the representation of the body is mapped from the feet to the head in a medial to lateral direction. Therefore, the anterior cerebral artery is the artery with the thromboembolism, because this artery supplies the medial portion of the cortex.

29 **The answer is B** *Gastrointestinal system / Pathology / Barrett's esophagus*

Barrett's esophagus, a metaplasia of normal esophageal squamous epithelium to columnar epithelium in response to chronic acidic irritation from gastroesophageal reflux, is a distinctly precancerous condition. These patients have a 30- to 40-fold increased risk of developing adenocarcinoma of the lower third of the esophagus.

30 **The answer is E** *General principles / Microbiology / Etiology of spirochetal diseases*

Borrelia recurrentis is the etiologic agent of relapsing fever in humans. The disease is worldwide and is characterized by febrile bacteremia. The disease name is derived from the fact that there can be 3 to 10 recurrences, apparently from the original infection. The disease is transmitted to humans from infected animals by ticks and from human to human by lice.

31 **The answer is A** *General principles / Microbiology / Etiology of spirochetal diseases*

Bejel is nonvenereal endemic syphilis that is caused by a variant of *Treponema pallidum*. It is most commonly seen in children in the Middle East and Africa. Transmission appears to be through the shared use of drinking and eating utensils; bejel is not transmitted sexually. It develops in primary, secondary, and tertiary stages.

32 **The answer is B** *Cardiovascular system / Pathology / Aortic stenosis*

The patient most likely has idiopathic calcific aortic stenosis. These patients commonly have the triad of congestive heart failure, angina pectoris, and exertional dyspnea or syncope. Left ventricular hypertrophy arises from the increased pressure gradient necessary to push blood through the stenotic aortic valve. Aortic stenosis produces a coarse crescendo–decrescendo systolic ejection murmur that is best heard in the second right intercostal space. A midsystolic click is usually the result of mitral valve prolapse. An apical holosystolic or pansystolic murmur most commonly results from mitral or tricuspid regurgitation in adults or from ventricular septal defect in children. Although the murmur of aortic stenosis is present throughout systole, it is not considered pansystolic. For a murmur to be called pansystolic, it must be homogeneous throughout systole. A diastolic sharp opening snap and mid- to late-diastolic murmur indicate mitral or tricuspid valve stenosis.

33 **The answer is C** *Cardiovascular system / Pharmacology / Mechanism of action and toxicity of cardiac glycosides*

Digitalis glycosides improve cardiac contractility by inhibiting the sarcolemmal $Na+/K+$-ATPase pump. This causes intracellular $Na+$ to rise, leading to increased $Na+/Ca^2+$ exchange and increased intracellular Ca^2+. Sarcoplasmic reticulum thus accumulates higher than normal levels of Ca^2+, which are released during an action potential. Because contraction strength directly depends on the amount of Ca^2+ released during an action potential, digitalis improves cardiac contractility. Digitalis also produces electrical effects on the heart, the most important of which is slowed conduction and increased refractoriness at the atrioventricular node. This property makes it useful in the treatment of atrial fibrillation. Digitalis toxicity results directly from magnification of its therapeutic effects on the heart. Inhibition of $Na+/K+$-ATPase raises the membrane resting potential, which has two important effects. First, it leads to voltage-dependent inactivation of fast $Na+$ channels, which are responsible for the upstroke of the action potential. The resultant decrease in conduction velocity can lead to re-entrant arrhythmias if several myocyte populations are affected heterogeneously. Second, it further raises intracellular Ca^2+ levels, which activates a Ca^2+-dependent $K+$ channel. Increased $K+$ efflux promotes rapid repolarization, shortening the action potential. A shortened action potential allows myocytes to spend more time in an excitable state, promoting development of arrhythmias. Exaggeration of the therapeutic effect of digitalis on the AV node can lead to a complete AV block such that the electrical system in the ventricles is uncoupled from that in the atria.

34 **The answer is A** *General principles / Immunology / Mast cells and allergies*

Upon first encounter between an allergic individual and the allergen, IgE antibodies are produced. These antibodies bind to high-affinity Fc receptors on the surface of mast cells and basophils. The antigen-binding portion of the antibodies are unbound and can bind to allergens during the next encounter. When enough IgE coats the mast cell so that antibodies are close to one another, the allergen crosslinks the adjacent IgE, triggering the release of granules containing inflammatory mediators (i.e., leukotrienes, histamine, and serotonin).

35 **The answer is A** *General principles / Pathology / Neoplasia*

The most common oncogenic translocation associated with chronic myeloid leukemia is a 9:22 (q34:q11) translocation that results in the fusion of the Abl and bcr sequences. The proper combinations for the other listed neoplasia are AML (4:11) or (6:11), Burkitt lymphoma (8:14), Mantle cell lymphoma (11:14), and follicular lymphoma (14:18).

36 **The answer is B** *Musculoskeletal system / Physiology / Smooth and skeletal muscle contraction*

Although the general contraction mechanism is similar between smooth and skeletal muscle, some important features differentiate the two muscle types. The major reason for some of these differences is that the process of myosin cross-bridge attachment, detachment, and reattachment to actin is much slower in smooth muscle than in the skeletal muscle. Because one cross bridge uses one adenosine triphosphate (ATP) molecule per cycle, the energy required to sustain a contraction of a given force in smooth muscle is less than in skeletal muscle. The slow cycle also explains why contractions tend to be much longer in smooth muscle than in skeletal muscle. However, despite a slow cycling time in smooth muscle, the fraction of the cycle that cross-bridges spend attached to actin is greater in smooth muscle than in skeletal muscle. This allows smooth muscle to generate a greater force of contraction per unit area than skeletal muscle. In addition, smooth muscle can contract a much greater percentage of its length while maintaining contraction force than can skeletal muscle. The exact reason for this is unknown, but it is believed that longer actin filaments in smooth muscle permit myosin chains to slide a greater distance in smooth versus skeletal muscle.

37 **The answer is B** *Cardiovascular system / Pathology / Tetralogy of Fallot*

Tetralogy of Fallot is characterized by four components: ventricular septal defect, obstruction of the right ventricular outflow, aortic override of the septal defect (straddle), and right ventricular hypertrophy. An electrocardiogram shows right ventricular hypertrophy, which worsens with age because of the increased load on the right ventricle. Cardiac angiography would show a ventricular septal defect, obstruction to flow into the pulmonary arteries, and flow of blood from the right ventricle directly into the aorta.

38 **The answer is E** *General principles / Pathology / Alcohol abuse*

Alcohol abuse is the most common cause of cirrhosis in industrialized countries. Hepatitis A infection is usually self-limited and does not result in chronic infections that can cause cirrhosis. Hepatitis B infection results in chronic infection capable of generating cirrhosis in about 10% of cases. The risk for chronic hepatitis C infection is about 40% but is much less common than alcohol abuse.

39 **The answer is D** *General principles / Cell biology / Cell cycle*

The cell cycle is tightly regulated by cellular proteins. Two important classes of cell cycle regulators are cellular proto-oncogenes and tumor suppressor genes. Proto-oncogenes favor entry into the cell cycle and therefore cellular proliferation. Thus, uncontrolled cell proliferation can result from activation of a proto-oncogene. Tumor suppressor proteins keep the cell from entering the cell cycle. Loss of one tumor suppressor allele does not directly lead to uncontrolled cellular proliferation, because there is still another copy to carry out the tumor suppressor function. Thus, within a cell, both copies of the tumor suppressor allele must be lost or mutated to ablate the tumor suppressor function, and this results in uncontrolled cellular proliferation. An important cell cycle regulator is p53. One of its functions is to block cellular proliferation in the face of DNA damage. It is elevated in cells exposed to DNA-damaging agents, including ultraviolet light and radiation. The retinoblastoma gene is an important tumor suppressor gene.

40 **The answer is B** *General principles / Biochemistry / Fatty acid metabolism*

Because of a methyl group on the third carbon, phytanic acid cannot be metabolized through β-oxidation. Phytanic acid is converted to pristanic acid in peroxisomes by the decarboxylation of the hydroxylated intermediate. Pristanic acid can then be used as a substrate for β-oxidation, as can linoleic acid, arachidonic acid, palmitic acid, and decanoic acid. Phytanic acid is toxic if it is not metabolized.

41 **The answer is D** *General principles / Biochemistry / Cholesterol biosynthesis*

The rate-limiting and regulated step of cholesterol biosynthesis is the formation of mevalonate from HMG CoA catalyzed by HMG CoA reductase. This enzyme is inhibited by dietary cholesterol and endogenously synthesized cholesterol. A vegetarian diet, a diet low in cholesterol, and the administration of a bile acid-sequestering resin all result in a reduced intake of cholesterol, which will not inhibit HMG CoA reductase activity. Familial hypercholesterolemia is a result of a deficiency of LDL receptors.

42 **The answer is D** *General principles / Genetics / Hardy–Weinberg equilibrium*

The Hardy–Weinberg equilibrium equation ($p-$ + 2pq + $q-$ = 1) includes random mating and no selection or mutations. If the penetrance of the trait is only 50%, the percentage of people who are homozygous recessive is twice the percentage with the trait (4.5% × 2 = 9%). Thus, q may be calculated by taking the square root of 0.09 (= 0.3), and p may be determined by subtracting 1 − q (= 0.7). Thus, the percentage of heterozygotes in the population should be 2pq, or 2 × 0.3 × 0.7 = 0.42 = 42%.

43 **The answer is E** *Hematopoietic and lymphoreticular system / Biochemistry / Clotting factors; pancreatic achylia*

A deficiency in pancreatic lipases reduces the absorption of fat-soluble vitamins (A, D, and K). Vitamin K is critically important in the synthesis of clotting factors II, VII, IX and a deficiency in vitamin K leads to bleeding diatheses manifested by a prolonged prothrombin time. Vitamin B_6 and C are water-soluble and are less likely to be affected by pancreatic lipase deficiency.

44 **The answer is A** *General principles / Microbiology / Cystic fibrosis*

An aminoglycoside antibiotic like gentamicin is needed for *Pseudomonas* infections with a late generation cephalosporin added for *Staphylococcus* and *Haemophilus* infections.

45 **The answer is E** *Renal/urinary system / Pathology / Minimal change disease*

Minimal change disease is the most common cause of nephrotic syndrome in children. It is characterized by loss of foot processes of epithelial cells as visualized by electron microscopy. It is strongly responsive to steroid treatment and usually results in a complete recovery.

46 **The answer is B** *Reproductive system / Pathology / Diethylstilbestrol*

Although adenocarcinomas of the vagina are quite rare in the general population, between 1 and 2 in 1,000 DES-exposed women develop this condition, usually between the ages of 15 and 20. The cells are often vacuolated, contain glycogen, and appear clear, hence the term clear cell carcinoma.

47 **The answer is C** *Central and peripheral nervous system / Pathology / Generalized seizures*

Generalized tonic–clonic (grand mal) seizures consist of the sudden onset, often without any preceding aura, of jerky tonic and clonic activity of both arms and legs with a general increase in muscle tone and loss of consciousness. Tongue-biting and incoherence may also be involved. Seizures usually last 1 to 2 minutes and often resolve with postictal lethargy and confusion.

48 **The answer is C** *Central and peripheral nervous system / Pathology / Parkinson's disease*

Parkinson's disease is a gradually progressive degenerative disease of the basal ganglia (extrapyramidal) motor system. Seizures are not a feature of Parkinson's disease. Parkinson's disease consists of four cardinal features: (1) a to-and-fro pronation–supination resting tremor that diminishes with voluntary movement; (2) rigidity with diffuse increase in muscular tone and sometimes a cogwheel property to joints when passively moved; (3) Bradykinesia (slowness of movement); and (4) postural instability. Although fine or alternating movements may be impaired, power is preserved in Parkinson's disease. Isolated tics and involuntary vocalizations are not found in Parkinson's disease; however, if they begin in childhood, they may suggest Tourette's syndrome. Postural dizziness, syncope, decreased sweating, and bladder dysfunction are not cardinal symptoms of Parkinson's disease; however, they are typical findings in Shy's syndrome and Drager's syndrome (which in later stages may exhibit extrapyramidal signs and symptoms similar to those of Parkinson's disease).

49 **The answer is C** *Central and peripheral nervous system / Pathology / Aphasia*

The two main types of aphasia are fluent and nonfluent. Nonfluent aphasia is generally produced by lesions in the cortex in the anterior part of the dominant hemisphere around the sylvian fissure and is often referred to by other names (e.g., Broca's aphasia). Patients with nonfluent aphasia have difficulty producing language and either cannot speak or do so only in monosyllabic and short telegraphic phrases. Naming and repetition are also impaired, but comprehension is fairly well preserved. Fluent aphasia results in speech that is fluent and even loquacious but nonsensical.

50 **The answer is B** *General principles / Pharmacology / Toxicological effects of drugs*

Tetracyclines may cause tooth enamel dysplasia and bone growth inhibition. Sulfonamides can displace bilirubin from serum albumin, leading to kernicterus in neonates. Chloramphenicol can cause gray baby syndrome. Neonates can neither efficiently glucuronidate chloramphenicol nor efficiently excrete the conjugated metabolite. Toxic levels can accumulate and inhibit normal mitochondrial function, leading to cardiovascular compromise, depressed breathing, cyanosis, and death. Streptomycin can cause ototoxicity, whereas valproic acid is associated with neural tube defects.

test **15**

Questions

Directions: Single best answer questions consist of numbered items or incomplete statements followed by answers or by completions of the statement. Select the ONE lettered answer or completion that is BEST in each case.

1 One week after boot camp, an 18-year-old recruit goes to the infirmary with a fever, headache, stiff neck, and visual sensitivity to light. A lumbar puncture is performed, and meningitis is diagnosed. Several other recruits have since reported similar symptoms. The most likely cause of this outbreak of meningitis is

(A) *Haemophilus influenzae* type B
(B) *Streptococcus pneumoniae*
(C) *Neisseria meningitidis*
(D) *Escherichia coli*
(E) *Streptococcus agalactiae*

2 Which of the following statements describes the mechanism of action of amphetamine?

(A) It is mediated through the cellular release of stored catecholamines
(B) It blocks the reuptake of norepinephrine, serotonin, and dopamine by presynaptic fibers
(C) It blocks the ability of adrenergic neurons to transport norepinephrine from the cytoplasm into storage vesicles
(D) It blocks the release of stored norepinephrine
(E) It acts directly on α- or β-adrenergic receptors

3 Which of the following infectious diseases is caused by a spirochete?

(A) Lyme disease
(B) Yellow fever
(C) Typhus
(D) Dengue fever

4 The most common malignant childhood brain tumor is

(A) schwannoma
(B) medulloblastoma
(C) meningioma
(D) squamous cell carcinoma

5 Bell's palsy is the most common ailment of which of the following cranial nerves (CN)?

(A) CN III (oculomotor)
(B) CN VII (facial)
(C) CN VI (abducens)
(D) CN VIII (acoustic)
(E) CN X (vagus)

6 An α-helix protein conformation is an example of which one of the following structures?

(A) Primary structure
(B) Secondary structure
(C) Tertiary structure
(D) Quaternary structure

7 Which of the following statements pertains to the gross autopsy photograph in Figure 60 of the color plate section?

(A) Complication in 20% of patients sustaining the cardiac event
(B) Association with acute hemopericardium in this patient
(C) Peak incidence occurring 2 weeks after the onset of the initiating cardiac event
(D) Association with development of acute initial regurgitation and pulmonary congestion in this patient

8 People often have difficulty changing their behavior, even when change would benefit their health. Which one of the following is the most effective way to help someone modify his or her behavior?

(A) Continually give positive reinforcement, whether or not the person is achieving the goal
(B) Give positive reinforcement for coming close to the goal and gradually become stringent
(C) Do not give positive reinforcement until the person has completely reached the goal
(D) Give negative reinforcement to make a person's old behavior less likely to occur
(E) Punish the person's undesired behavior

9 In tropical areas, a form of endemic syphilis, yaws, is found in children and is transmitted orally. Which of the following agents is most closely associated with yaws?

(A) *Borrelia recurrentis*
(B) *Treponema pertenue*
(C) *Treponema pallidum*
(D) *Leptospira interrogans*
(E) *Treponema carateum*

10 Which of the following neurotransmitters is correctly paired with its primary source in the brain?

(A) Dopamine—pontine nuclei
(B) Norepinephrine—locus ceruleus
(C) Acetylcholine—substantia nigra
(D) Serotonin—nucleus basalis
(E) γ-Aminobutyric acid (GABA)—dorsal raphe

11 The most common agent in narcotic endocarditis is

(A) *Streptococcus pneumoniae*
(B) *Staphylococcus aureus*
(C) gram-negative bacilli
(D) *Neisseria gonorrhoeae*

12 Which human herpes virus is implicated in the etiology of AIDS-associated non-Hodgkin's lymphoma?

(A) Herpes simplex virus type 1
(B) Herpes simplex virus type 2
(C) Epstein–Barr virus (EBV)
(D) Cytomegalovirus

13 To withdraw cerebrospinal fluid (CSF) (i.,e., perform a spinal tap), a needle tip must pass successively through the

(A) pia mater, dura mater, epidural space, and arachnoid membrane
(B) arachnoid membrane, epidural space, dura mater, and subdural space
(C) subdural space, dura mater, epidural space, and arachnoid membrane
(D) arachnoid membrane, subdural space, dura mater, and epidural space
(E) epidural space, dura mater, subdural space, and arachnoid membrane

14 Which of the following organisms extrude sulfur granules from a draining wound?

(A) *Francisella tularensis*
(B) *Pasteurella multocida*
(C) *Actinomyces israelii*
(D) *Yersinia pestis*

15 The accompanying graph shows the tubular loss of glucose (excretion rate) plotted against the rate at which glucose is filtered at the glomerulus (filtered load). Which lettered point on the curve corresponds to the tubular maximal (Tm) for glucose?

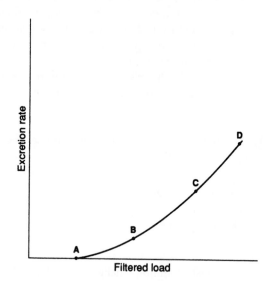

16 The most common type of primary brain tumor is

(A) meningioma
(B) glioma
(C) neural sheath tumor
(D) squamous cell carcinoma
(E) osteosarcoma

17 The accompanying micrograph depicts a section of distal lung. Which lettered structure is a cell that secretes surfactant?

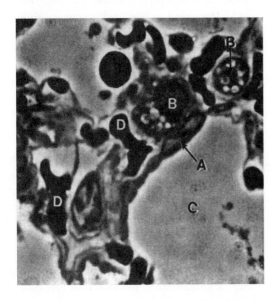

18 The gross photograph in Figure 61 of the color plate section is from an autopsy of a 35-year-old woman. The photograph shows multinodular thickenings of the vagal nerves. Which of the following is this patient also likely to have?

(A) Cutaneous angiofibromas
(B) Café au lait spots
(C) Renal angiomyolipomas
(D) Cerebral cortical tubers
(E) Cutaneous ash leaf patches

19 The most common cause of posttransfusion hepatitis is

(A) hepatitis A virus
(B) hepatitis B virus
(C) hepatitis C virus
(D) hepatitis D virus
(E) hepatitis E virus

20 In intravenous drug abusers, the valves most commonly affected in narcotic endocarditis are

(A) right-sided valves
(B) left-sided valves
(C) both right-sided and left-sided valves
(D) neither right- nor left-sided valves

21 Drugs used in multiple-drug therapies of choice for tuberculosis include

(A) isoniazid, rifampin, pyrazinamide, penicillin
(B) penicillin, rifampin, pyrazinamide, ethambutol
(C) isoniazid, penicillin, pyrazinamide, ethambutol
(D) isoniazid, rifampin, pyrazinamide, ethambutol
(E) isoniazid, rifampin, penicillin, ethambutol

22 A 34-year-old woman has intermittent dysesthesia, paresthesia, and hypesthesia in the middle digits of her right hand. History, physical findings, and decreased nerve conduction velocity indicate that she has carpal tunnel syndrome. In the accompanying diagram of the brachial plexus, identify the nerve that is compressed in this syndrome.

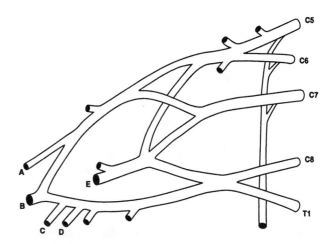

23 A 6-month-old child is seen by his pediatrician for a routine check up. The pediatrician suspects that the child has a distended abdomen that seems to be worsening upon repeat examination 2 weeks later. An abdominal computed tomography (CT) scan is performed and a mass is discovered. What is the most likely tumor type seen in a child of this age?

(A) Hepatocellular carcinoma
(B) Renal cell carcinoma
(C) Small intestinal carcinoid
(D) Small round cell tumor
(E) Neuroblastoma

24 In the accompanying diagram, which lettered point provides the best point for auscultation of mitral stenosis?

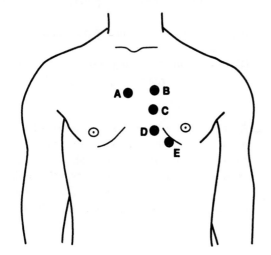

25 Which statement below is correct about the enzyme it describes?

(A) Aldolase cleaves a carbon–carbon bond to create a carboxyl group

(B) Dehydrogenase adds water to a carbon–carbon bond without either breaking the bond or removing water to create a double bond

(C) Hydrolase adds water to break a bond

(D) Isomerase hydrolyzes ester linkages to form an acid and an alcohol

26 Which of the following congenital immunodeficiencies involves only a T cell deficiency?

(A) Thymic aplasia (DiGeorge's syndrome)

(B) Ataxia–telangiectasia

(C) X-linked hypogammaglobulinemia (Bruton's agammaglobulinemia)

(D) Chronic granulomatous disease

(E) Hereditary angioedema

27 Which of the following special maneuvers intensifies the murmur associated with aortic insufficiency?

(A) The patient rolls into the left lateral decubitus position

(B) While sitting, the patient leans forward, exhales, and holds his or her breath

(C) While sitting, the patient expires against a closed glottis (i.e., bears down)

(D) The patient stands

(E) The patient exercises briefly

28 Which of the following physical findings make up the classic triad in cardiac tamponade in patients with penetrating cardiac injuries, aortic dissection, or intrapericardial rupture of aortic or cardiac aneurysms?

(A) Hypotension, elevated systemic venous pressure, and small, quiet heart

(B) Hypotension, elevated systemic venous pressure, and enlarged heart

(C) Hypotension, decreased systemic venous pressure, and small, quiet heart

(D) Hypertension, elevated systemic venous pressure, and small, quiet heart

29 A 72-year-old asthmatic man comes in for management of stable exertional angina that he has had for 2 years. Which of the following treatments for managing angina is contraindicated in this patient?

(A) Calcium channel blockers

(B) Nitrates

(C) Noncardioselective β-blockers at low doses

(D) Cardioselective β-blockers at low doses

30 Which of the following congenital variable immunodeficiencies involves a combined B cell and T cell deficiency?

(A) Hyperimmunoglobulin M syndrome

(B) Wiskott–Aldrich syndrome

(C) Chronic mucocutaneous candidiasis

(D) Chediak–Higashi syndrome

(E) Leukocyte adhesion deficiency syndrome

31 Which of the following vitamins can be synthesized by intestinal bacteria?

(A) Vitamin E

(B) Vitamin C

(C) Vitamin A

(D) Vitamin K

(E) Niacin

32 Reciprocal innervation is most accurately described as

(A) inhibition of flexor muscles during an extension

(B) activation of contralateral extensors during a flexion

(C) reduction of Ia fiber activity during a contraction

(D) simultaneous stimulation of α- and γ-motor neurons

(E) inhibition of α-motor neurons during a contraction

33 Which of the following may be associated with the lesion depicted in Figure 62 of the color plate section?

(A) Addison's disease
(B) Conn's syndrome
(C) Elevated serum adrenocorticotropic hormone (ACTH) level
(D) Pituitary adenoma

34 A hyperventilating patient has untreated diabetes. Over the past several days, he has had thirst, frequent urination, weight loss, and fatigue. Analysis of his blood reveals subnormal pH, bicarbonate level, and partial pressure of carbon dioxide (P_{CO_2}) and above-normal glucose level. The acid–base abnormalities of this patient can best be described as

(A) compensated respiratory acidosis with metabolic alkalosis
(B) compensated respiratory alkalosis with metabolic acidosis
(C) compensated metabolic acidosis with respiratory alkalosis
(D) compensated metabolic alkalosis with respiratory acidosis
(E) compensated metabolic acidosis with respiratory acidosis

35 A renal allograft recipient develops fever and adenopathy 3 months after engraftment. Serum studies show markedly elevated anti-EBV titers. A biopsy of the allograft is most likely to show

(A) fibrinoid necrosis of the small vessels
(B) vascular sclerosis
(C) interstitial fibrosis
(D) a dense lymphoplasmacytic interstitial infiltrate with cytologic atypia
(E) isometric vacuolar change in the tubular epithelial cells

36 A 20-year-old disoriented woman goes to an emergency department with high fever, nausea, vomiting, watery diarrhea, hypotension, and diffuse erythema. A tentative diagnosis of toxic shock syndrome (TSS) is made. Which of the following organisms is the etiologic agent of TSS?

(A) *Staphylococcus aureus*
(B) *Staphylococcus epidermidis*
(C) *Staphylococcus saprophyticus*
(D) *Pseudomonas aeruginosa*
(E) *Clostridium perfringens*

37 Hereditary spherocytosis is a disorder of red blood cells that is characterized by a spheroid shape of erythrocytes that leads to splenic sequestration and an increased rate of red cell destruction. What is the molecular modification of red blood cells that causes this disorder?

(A) Spectrin deficiency
(B) Ankyrin deficiency
(C) Hemoglobin mutation
(D) Glucose-6-phosphate dehydrogenase deficiency
(E) Glycan anchor deficiency

38 Which of the following drugs is a monoamine oxidase inhibitor?

(A) Trazodone
(B) Amitriptyline
(C) Phenelzine
(D) Fluoxetine
(E) Nortriptyline

39 A 22-year-old man has shortness of breath and a cough. The accompanying chest radiographs show mediastinal lymphadenopathy and bilateral pulmonary infiltrates. After bronchoalveolar lavage failed to grow micro-organisms, a transbronchial biopsy was performed. The best diagnosis for this case is

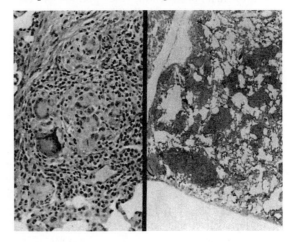

(A) sarcoidosis
(B) Hodgkin's disease
(C) aspiration pneumonia
(D) alveolar proteinosis

40 Trypsin cleaves peptide bonds on the carboxyl side of which of the following amino acids?

(A) Arginine only
(B) Lysine only
(C) Either arginine or lysine
(D) Phenylalanine only
(E) Either phenylalanine or lysine

41 Which of the following is the drug of first choice in the treatment of absence seizures?

(A) Primidone
(B) Valproic acid
(C) Ethosuximide
(D) Phenytoin
(E) Carbamazepine

42 The primary screening method in the detection of AIDS carriers is

(A) virus isolation
(B) Western blot followed by immunoassay
(C) immunoassay followed by Western blot
(D) immunoassay for viral antigen
(E) DNA hybridization for viral RNA

43 If an area of the lung is not ventilated because of bronchial obstruction, the pulmonary capillary blood serving that will have a P_{O_2} that is

(A) equal to atmospheric P_{O_2}
(B) equal to mixed venous P_{O_2}
(C) equal to normal systemic arterial P_{O_2}
(D) higher than inspired P_{O_2}
(E) lower than mixed venous P_{O_2}

44 In a study designed to test the effect of a new knee brace on running speed, eight college athletes who wore the brace turned in the following times in minutes in a 1,000-meter speed trial: 4, 2, 5, 2, 4, 5, 5, and 9. The mean finishing time for this group of subjects is

(A) 8 minutes
(B) 5 minutes
(C) 4 minutes
(D) 4.5 minutes

45 The figure below shows the DNA typing for a family that has Huntington's disease (HD). I-1 has HD, as does his son, II-2. Family members II-1, II-3, and II-4 want to know their risk of having the abnormal gene. The family members have had DNA analysis with a marker approximately 2 million base pairs from the mutation causing HD. The risk of HD in II-1 is

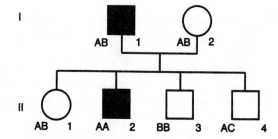

(A) significantly increased
(B) significantly decreased
(C) mildly increased
(D) not changed because the markers are uninformative
(E) nonexistent

46 A hematologist is asked to see a 52-year-old man who has been hospitalized for 6 weeks because of various complications beginning with a bowel obstruction. The patient has had several operative procedures, one of which required transfusion of three units of packed red cells. He has been unable to eat and has been receiving broad-spectrum antibiotics almost continuously. Recent tests show a prolonged prothrombin time (PT) and partial thromboplastin time (PTT) that were corrected when the patient's plasma was mixed with an equal volume of normal plasma. Quantitative fibrinogen, thrombin time, and platelet count all are normal. The most likely cause of the coagulation abnormality is

(A) an acquired inhibitor
(B) dilution of coagulation factors as a result of transfusions
(C) vitamin K deficiency
(D) folate deficiency
(E) von Willebrand's disease

47 The anamnestic response is defined as

(A) a gradual rise in antibody titers
(B) true immunologic paralysis
(C) prompt production of antibodies after a second exposure to antigen
(D) species-specific antibodies
(E) the lag in antibody production after initial antigen exposure

48 Which of the following drugs is a potassium-sparing diuretic?

(A) Furosemide
(B) Amiloride
(C) Acetazolamide
(D) Chlorothiazide
(E) Indapamide

49 Lung compliance in a 32-year-old woman is studied. Data collected under control and experimental conditions are listed in the accompanying table. This patient's lung compliance during control and experimental conditions was

TABLE 15-1

	Respiratory Rate (breaths/min)	Tidal Volume (ml)	Change in Interpleural Pressure during Inspiration (cm H_2O)
Control	15	600	4
Experimental	25	600	10

(A) unchanged
(B) 40 mL/breath and 24 mL/breath, respectively
(C) 150 mL/cm H_2O and 60 mL/cm H_2O, respectively
(D) 150 cm H_2O/mL and 60 cm H_2O/mL respectively

50 A pediatrician wanted to determine the relation between chronic otitis media in young children and parental history of such infections. From the records of a large pediatric practice, he identified 50 children aged 1 to 3 years who had had at least three middle-ear infections during the preceding year. He also identified 50 children in the same age group, treated by the same practice for other illnesses. The pediatrician interviewed the parents of subjects in both groups to determine their history of chronic otitis media as young children. Of the children with recurrent ear infections, 30 had a family history of chronic otitis media, compared with 20 of the children treated for other illnesses. This study is an example of

(A) a cross-sectional study
(B) a prospective cohort study
(C) a case-control study
(D) an experimental study
(E) a randomized controlled clinical trial

Answer Key

1-C	11-B	21-D	31-D	41-C
2-A	12-C	22-B	32-A	42-C
3-A	13-E	23-E	33-B	43-B
4-B	14-C	24-E	34-C	44-D
5-B	15-B	25-C	35-D	45-D
6-B	16-B	26-A	36-A	46-C
7-B	17-B	27-B	37-A	47-C
8-B	18-B	28-A	38-C	48-B
9-B	19-C	29-C	39-A	49-C
10-B	20-A	30-B	40-C	50-C

Answers and Explanations

1 **The answer is C** *General principles / Microbiology / Neisseria meningitidis*

Neisseria meningitidis is the most common cause of meningitis in adolescents and young adults and is the most likely cause of epidemics of meningitis. *Haemophilus influenzae* type B is responsible for 70% of cases of bacterial meningitis in children aged 2 months to 5 years. *Escherichia coli* and *Streptococcus agalactiae* cause meningitis in neonates who acquire the infection during passage through the birth canal. *S. pneumoniae* predominates in adults over 40 years of age, in the very young, and in trauma patients.

2 **The answer is A** *General principles / Pharmacology / Central nervous system stimulants*

Amphetamine's mechanism of action is mediated through the cellular release of stored catecholamines. Cocaine blocks the reuptake of norepinephrine, serotonin, and dopamine by presynaptic fibers. Reserpine blocks the ability of adrenergic neurons to transport norepinephrine from the cytoplasm to storage vesicles. Guanethidine blocks the release of stored norepinephrine. Isoproterenol acts directly on α- or β-adrenergic receptors, producing effects similar to those that follow stimulation of sympathetic nerves. Unlike isoproterenol, amphetamine's agonist activity is indirect.

3 **The answer is A** *General principles / Microbiology / Spirochete; Borrelia burgdorferi*

Three genera of spirochetes can cause human infections: *Treponema*, which causes syphilis; *Leptospira*, which causes leptospirosis; and *Borrelia*, which causes a number of tickborne diseases. Lyme disease is caused by the *B. burgdorferi* spirochete. Upon Giemsa stain, *B. burgdorferi* appear as large, loosely coiled organisms. Lyme disease is treated with tetracycline or amoxicillin for acute infections and penicillin for chronic infections. Dengue fever is caused by the dengue virus, and yellow fever is caused by the yellow fever virus; both are transmitted by the *Aedes aegypti* mosquito. Typhus is caused by the bacteria *Rickettsia typhi* and is transmitted by flea bites.

4 **The answer is B** *Central and peripheral nervous system / Pathology / Cancer; medulloblastoma*

Medulloblastoma is the most common malignant tumor of the brain in children. Its most frequent site of occurrence is the cerebellum. Meningioma is a primary brain tumor arising from the meninges. It is the second-most common primary intracranial neoplasm. Squamous cell carcinoma is a tumor composed of cells that resemble cells of the squamous layer of the epidermis. Schwannoma is a neural sheath tumor. Its most frequent site of occurrence is the CN VIII, and it is the third most common primary intracranial neoplasm.

5 **The answer is B** *Central and peripheral nervous system / Pathology; neuroanatomy / Bell's palsy*

Bell's palsy is a demyelinating viral inflammatory disease that is the most common ailment of CN VII. Onset usually is preceded by viral prodrome and is acute. Duration is approximately 5 days. Findings are unilateral; they can involve loss of facial expression, widened palpebral fissure, diminished taste, difficulty in chewing, hypesthesia in one or more branches of CN V, and hyperacusis.

6 **The answer is B** *General principles / Cell biology / Structure of polypeptides*

Polypeptides can be arranged in four structure types. Primary structure refers to the linear arrangement of a polypeptide chain along with the available corresponding cysteine side chains. Secondary structure consists of two forms, α-helix and β-pleated sheet. Tertiary structure combines secondary structures into complex and compact domains. The combination of several polypeptide chains into one molecule is an example of a quaternary structure.

7 **The answer is B** *Cardiovascular system / Pathology / Rupture of the left ventricular free wall in an acute myocardial infarct*

After the initial ischemic event, multiple complications may develop in 80% to 90% of patients with myocardial infarction. Lethal arrhythmias lead to sudden cardiac death in 10% to 20% of patients. Complications in patients admitted to hospitals include cardiac arrhythmias (75% to 95% of complicated cases); left ventricular congestive heart failure and pulmonary edema (60%); cardiogenic shock (10% to 15%); thromboembolism (15% to 40%); fibrinous pericarditis local to the area of infarct; and ventricular aneurysm (i.e., a late complication). Cardiac rupture syndromes occur in 1% to 5% of patients, with a peak incidence 4 to 7 days after the ischemic event, when the myocardium is structurally the weakest. Disintegration of dead myocytes by macrophages begins, and early fibrovascular development at the margin of the infarct leads to the formation of granulation tissue by day 10. Rupture of the free wall results in hemopericardium and tamponade. Rupture of the septum leads to left-to-right shunting. Rupture of a papillary muscle results in acute mitral or tricuspid valvular insufficiency. The probability of specific complications after a cardiac ischemic event depends on the size, location, and transmural extent of the myocardial ischemic injury.

8 **The answer is B** *General principles / Behavioral science / Modifying consequences to change behavior*

The most effective use of positive reinforcement is to give it frequently and easily and then gradually become stringent. This method is called shaping. It is more effective than giving continual praise regardless of the result or only giving praise when the final goal is reached. Using negative reinforcement makes a person's undesired behavior more likely to occur (i.e., the desired behavior becomes difficult). Punishment reduces the undesired behavior, but is ineffective if it is not directly related to the behavior.

9 **The answer is B** *General principles / Microbiology / Etiology of spirochetal diseases*

Treponema pertenue is the etiologic agent of yaws. The disease occurs primarily in children in tropical regions, where it appears to be transmitted by direct contact or by vectors such as flies. This potentially disfiguring disease has primary, secondary, and tertiary stages.

10 **The answer is B** *Central and peripheral nervous system / Neuroanatomy / Neuroscience; neurotransmitters*

Norepinephrine is produced by cells in the locus ceruleus. A major source of dopamine in the brain is the substantia nigra. Acetylcholine is made primarily in the nucleus basalis. Serotonin is made in neurons of the dorsal raphe. GABA is made primarily by the interneurons of the brain.

11 **The answer is B** *Cardiovascular system / Pathology; microbiology / Infective endocarditis*

Although *S. pneumoniae* is the most common cause of infective endocarditis in general (65% of cases), *S. aureus* is the most common agent in narcotic endocarditis (>50% of cases).

12 **The answer is C** *General principles / Microbiology / Herpes virus*

EBV is present in about half of AIDS-associated non-Hodgkin's lymphomas; tumor cells carry EBV DNA and express viral proteins. Herpes simplex virus type 1 can cause gingivostomatitis, recurrent herpes labialis, keratoconjunctivitis, and encephalitis. Herpes simplex virus type 2 causes genital herpes, neonatal herpes, and aseptic meningitis. Cytomegalovirus causes cytomegalic inclusion disease in neonates and can cause pneumonia in immunocompromised patients. Neither herpes simplex virus nor cytomegalovirus has been implicated in the etiology of AIDS-associated non-Hodgkin's lymphoma.

13 **The answer is E** *Central and peripheral nervous system / Neuroanatomy / Spinal tap*

The physician can insert a needle into the subarachnoid space to withdraw CSF for diagnostic analysis. The needle tip passes successively through the epidural space, the dura mater, the subdural space, and the arachnoid membrane. The CSF is between the arachnoid membrane and the pia mater, the innermost of the three meningeal sheaths.

14 The answer is C *General principles / Microbiology / A. israelii*

A. israelii is an anaerobe that is a part of the normal flora of the oral cavity. It may invade tissues after local trauma, forming filaments surrounded by areas of inflammation. Hard yellow granules, called sulfur granules, are formed in pus in the area of infection. *Y. pestis* causes plague. The most common form of plague is bubonic plague, also known as black plague. *P. multocida* causes wound infections associated with cat and dog bites. *F. tularensis* causes tularemia. None of these organisms is associated with the extrusion of sulfur granules from a draining wound.

15 The answer is B *Renal/urinary system / Biochemistry / Tubular loss of glucose*

When the filtered load of a substance exceeds the Tm for that substance, the excess is not reabsorbed, so proportionately more of the substance is excreted. In this example, the Tm for glucose (*B* on the curve) is determined by extrapolation of the linear portion of the curve from *C* to *D* to the abscissa (filtered load). The splay of the curve from *A* to *C* indicates that the tubules are not all uniform in length, number of glucose transporters, or renal threshold.

16 The answer is B *Central and peripheral nervous system / Pathology / Brain tumor*

Most primary brain tumors can be divided into three classes: gliomas, meningiomas, and neural sheath tumors. Gliomas, the most common type of primary brain tumor, include astrocytomas, ependymomas, oligodendrogliomas, and medulloblastomas. Meningiomas are the next most common type of primary brain tumor. Neural sheath tumors are less common. Squamous cell carcinoma is a tumor composed of cells that resemble cells of the squamous layer of the epidermis. It is the second-most common skin cancer. Osteosarcoma arises from primitive mesenchymal cells and is a malignant primary bone tumor. Neither osteosarcoma nor squamous cell carcinoma is a type of primary brain tumor.

17 The answer is B *Respiratory system / Histology / Distal lung components*

Alveoli (*C*) in the lungs are lined by an epithelium that contains type I and type II cells. Type I cells (*A*) are extremely attenuated squamous cells specialized for gas exchange. Type II cells (*B*) are rounded cells containing phospholipid-rich multilamellar bodies of secretion product (surfactant). Alveoli are adjacent to capillaries, which are filled with erythrocytes (*D*). Macrophages are abundant in alveoli, where they phagocytose and destroy inspired debris, such as bacteria.

18 The answer is B *Central and peripheral nervous system / Pathology / Plexiform neurofibromas of the vagus nerves*

Neurofibromatosis encompasses two distinct neurocutaneous syndromes (phakomatoses). Type I neurofibromatosis (NF-1) (von Recklinghausen's disease) is characterized by neurofibromas, unilateral acoustic nerve schwannomas, gliomas of the optic nerve, pheochromocytomas, meningiomas, cutaneous hyperpigmented macules (café au lait spots), and pigmented nodules of the iris (Lisch nodules). Multinodular neurofibromatous expansion of a peripheral nerve (i.e., plexiform neurofibroma) is the pathognomonic feature of NF-1. Some patients develop malignant peripheral nerve sheath tumors. The NF-1 gene, mapped to chromosome 17q11.2, encodes for neurofibromin, a protein with homology to a family of guanosine triphosphatase (GTPase) activating signal transduction proteins, which down-regulate the function of the p21 *ras* oncoprotein and act as a tumor suppressor gene. NF-2 (i.e., central neurofibromatosis), a disorder mapped to a gene on chromosome 22, is characterized by bilateral acoustic nerve schwannomas, meningiomas, and café au lait spots. The target protein is believed to link integral cell membrane proteins to the cytoskeleton. Cutaneous angiofibromas, ash leaf patches, and renal angiomyolipomas are extra-central nervous system (CNS) manifestations of tuberous sclerosis, an autosomal dominant phakomatosis characterized by CNS hamartomas (i.e., cortical tubers and subependymal giant cell astrocytomas). Affected patients are commonly mentally retarded and have a seizure disorder. Additional manifestations include visceral (e.g., liver, kidney, pancreas) cysts, pulmonary and cardiac myomas, subungual fibromas, and shagreen patches (e.g., cutaneous local thickenings). Tuberous sclerosis has been linked to genetic loci on chromosomes 9 and 16, the latter encoding the protein tuberin that exhibits homology to a GTPase-activating protein that is distinct from neurofibromin.

19 **The answer is C** *General principles / Microbiology / Hepatitis*

Hepatitis C virus is the most common cause of posttransfusion hepatitis. Hepatitis A is easily spread by the oral–fecal route and is often called infectious hepatitis. Hepatitis B is contracted by contact with blood or other bodily secretions from infected individuals and is often called serum hepatitis. Hepatitis D requires hepatitis B surface antigen (HBsAg) to become pathogenic, and transmission is closely linked with the transmission of the hepatitis B virus. Hepatitis E is a major enterically transmitted hepatitis. It is the most common cause of waterborne epidemics in Asia, Africa, India, and Mexico but is uncommon in the United States.

20 **The answer is A** *Cardiovascular system / Pathology; microbiology / Infective endocarditis*

Intravenous drug abuse-associated infective endocarditis usually has acute vegetation on right-sided valves. Most other cases of infective endocarditis are associated with left-sided valves.

21 **The answer is D** *Respiratory system / Pharmacology / Pulmonary tuberculosis*

Multiple-drug therapy is used to prevent the emergence of drug-resistant mutants during the 6 to 9 months of treatment. Isoniazid (a bactericidal drug), rifampin, and pyrazinamide are the drugs used to treat most patients with pulmonary tuberculosis. Ethambutol is added initially for those who have AIDS with CNS involvement, dissemination, or suspected isoniazid resistance. Penicillin is not effective against the tubercle bacillus.

22 **The answer is B** *Central and peripheral nervous system / Neuroanatomy / Carpal tunnel syndrome*

Carpal tunnel syndrome results from compression of the median nerve as it passes deep within tissue to the flexor retinaculum. The median nerve originates in the brachial plexus by the joining of the lateral and medial cords. The nerves labeled *A, C, D,* and *E* are the musculocutaneous nerve, medial cutaneous nerve of the forearm, ulnar nerve, and radial nerve, respectively.

23 **The answer is E** *Renal/urinary system / Oncology / Neuroblastoma*

Neuroblastoma is the most common malignancy of children of less than 1 year of age. Twenty-five percent to 35% of neuroblastomas develop in the adrenal medulla. Whereas most cases are sporadic, there are some rare cases of familial neuroblastoma.

24 **The answer is E** *Cardiovascular system / Anatomy / Auscultation of heart sounds*

When routinely auscultating the heart, one should listen in the second intercostal space along the right sternal border, in the second through the fifth intercostal spaces along the left sternal border, and at the apex. Locations for auscultations of heart valve sounds are aortic valve (*point A*), pulmonary valve (*point B*), tricuspid valve (*points C* and *D*), and mitral valve (*point E*).

25 **The answer is C** *General principles / Biochemistry / Enzymes*

Hydrolase adds water to break a bond. This is called hydrolysis. Aldolase cleaves a carbon–carbon bond to create an aldehyde group. Dehydrogenase removes hydrogen atoms from its substrate. Hydratase adds water to a carbon–carbon bond without breaking the bond or removing water to create a double bond. Isomerase converts between *cis* and *trans* isomers, D- and L-isomers, or aldose and ketose. Esterase hydrolyzes ester linkages to form an acid and an alcohol.

26 **The answer is A** *General principles / Immunology / Congenital immunodeficiencies*

Thymic aplasia (DiGeorge's syndrome) involves a T cell deficiency caused by failure of the thymus and parathyroids to develop properly because of a defect in the third and fourth pharyngeal pouches. Ataxia–telangiectasia is an autosomal recessive disease that appears by age 2 years and combines B cell and T cell deficiency. X-linked hypogammaglobulinemia (Bruton's agammaglobulinemia) is a B cell deficiency caused by a mutation in the gene encoding a tyrosine kinase. Hereditary angioedema is a complement deficiency caused by an uncommon autosomal dominant disease that results from a deficiency of C1 esterase inhibitor. Chronic granulomatous disease is a phagocyte deficiency caused by an X-linked disease in most cases (in some patients the disease is autosomal) that appears by age 2 years.

27 The answer is B *Cardiovascular system / Physiology / Aortic insufficiency*

Aortic insufficiency (regurgitation) is accentuated by leaning forward while seated, exhaling completely, and holding one's breath. The Valsalva maneuver, in which the patient expires against a closed glottis while seated, is useful for diagnosing mitral valve prolapse. Having the patient roll into the left lateral decubitus position aids diagnosis of mitral stenosis, as does brief exercise. Standing decreases ventricular filling and increases the murmurs associated with mitral valve prolapse and idiopathic hypertrophic subaortic stenosis (IHSS). Squatting increases the murmurs associated with mitral and aortic valve insufficiencies.

28 The answer is A *Cardiovascular system / Pathology / Cardiac tamponade*

Hypotension, elevated systemic venous pressure, and small, quiet heart make up the classic triad of physical findings in cardiac tamponade in patients with penetrating cardiac injuries, aortic dissection, or intrapericardial rupture of aortic or cardiac aneurysms. These are uncommon causes today. The most common causes of cardiac tamponade are neoplastic disease and idiopathic pericarditis, followed by acute myocardial infarction and uremia.

29 The answer is C *Cardiovascular system / Pharmacology / Antianginal drugs*

This patient has two medical problems: asthma and chronic stable angina. Available antianginal drugs are classified as (1) nitrates, (2) β-blockers, and (3) calcium channel blockers. The asthma constitutes a contraindication to the use of noncardioselective β-blockers. β-Adrenergic antagonists can induce acute episodes of asthma, and they regularly produce airway obstruction in asthmatics. Even the selective β-adrenergic antagonists do this, particularly at high doses. Low-dose cardioselective β-blockers may be used with caution. Calcium channel blockers and nitrates can also be used to treat this patient.

30 The answer is B *General principles / Immunology / Congenital immunodeficiencies*

Hyper-IgM syndrome and chronic mucocutaneous candidiasis also involve T cell deficiency. Hyper-IgM syndrome results from a defect in helper T cells in a surface protein that interacts with the CD40 antigen on the B cell surface. Chronic mucocutaneous candidiasis results from a T cell deficiency specifically for *Candida albicans;* other T cell and B cell functions are normal. Wiskott–Aldrich syndrome also involves a combined B cell and T cell deficiency in which B cell numbers are normal but antibody responses to polysaccharide antigens are absent and T cell deficiencies are variable. Chediak–Higashi syndrome and leukocyte adhesion deficiency syndrome are phagocyte deficiencies. Chediak–Higashi syndrome is an autosomal recessive disease, and leukocyte adhesion deficiency syndrome is caused by a defective adhesion (LFA-1) protein on the surface of their phagocytes.

31 The answer is D *Gastrointestinal system / Biochemistry / Vitamins*

Intestinal bacteria synthesize vitamin K. The main dietary source of vitamin K is green leafy vegetables. Vitamin E, vitamin A, vitamin C, and niacin are not synthesized by intestinal bacteria. The main dietary source for vitamin E is vegetable oils. The main dietary sources for vitamin C are fresh fruit and vegetables. The main dietary sources for vitamin A are liver, whole milk, fish oils, and eggs. The main dietary sources for niacin are meat and nuts.

32 The answer is A *Central and peripheral nervous system / Neuroanatomy / Reciprocal innervation*

Reciprocal innervation is most accurately described as inhibition of the antagonist muscle when the agonist muscle is activated. For example, flexor muscles are inhibited during an extension. Reciprocal innervation allows extensor contraction to occur without interference from the flexor muscles that are being stretched during the movement. Under normal circumstances, stretching the flexors elicits a stretch reflex leading to contraction of the flexor muscles. Inhibiting the α-motor neurons that innervate the flexor muscles prevents the stretch reflex from interfering with the extension. Reciprocal innervation characterizes all movements, not just extension.

33 The answer is B *Endocrine system / Pathology / Adrenal cortical adenoma*

Proliferative adrenal cortical disorders include diffuse and nodular cortical hyperplasia and cortical neoplasms (e.g., adenoma, carcinoma). Primary hyperadrenalism arises from adrenal cortical neoplasms, which are typically unilateral (in contrast to hyperplasia, which is bilateral); functioning neoplasms are yellow, produce steroid hormones, and often suppress pituitary secretion of ACTH. Carcinomas are distinguished from adenomas by their larger size (>100 g), necrosis, increased mitotic activity, local invasiveness, and metastatic potential. Secondary hyperadrenalism results from increased ACTH secretion from a basophilic pituitary microadenoma or ectopically from an extrapituitary neoplasm (e.g., paraneoplastic syndrome). Tertiary hyperadrenalism results from increased hypothalamic production of corticotropin-releasing hormone (CRH). Clinical disorders associated with adrenal cortical hyperfunction include Cushing's syndrome, Conn's syndrome, and various adrenogenital syndromes. Cushing's syndrome is caused by hypersecretion of cortisol and is manifested by central obesity, moon face, hirsutism, hypertension, glucose intolerance or diabetes, osteoporosis, neuropsychiatric disorders, menstrual abnormalities, abdominal skin striae, and impaired cell-mediated immunity. Conn's syndrome (i.e., primary hyperaldosteronism), a cause of hypertension in 0.05% to 0.2% of hypertensive patients, is characterized by elevated serum aldosterone and low renin levels, sodium retention, and hypokalemia. Adrenogenital syndromes (e.g., adrenal virilism) may be caused by an androgen-secreting adrenal cortical neoplasm or may be the congenital result of an enzyme deficiency in the synthesis of cortisol or aldosterone, which results in pituitary ACTH hypersecretion, bilateral adrenal cortical hyperplasia, and shunting of adrenal cortical steroidogenesis toward excessive androgen production. Adrenal cortical insufficiency may take any of three clinicopathologic forms: (1) primary acute adrenocortical insufficiency (adrenal crisis); (2) primary chronic adrenocortical insufficiency (Addison's disease); and (3) secondary adrenocortical insufficiency (i.e., low ACTH).

34 The answer is C *Respiratory system / Biochemistry / Acid–base disorders*

Metabolic acidosis is defined as a below-normal level of serum bicarbonate. Respiratory alkalosis is subnormal partial pressure of carbon dioxide (P_{CO_2}). The respiratory alkalosis represents an attempt by the lungs to compensate for the metabolic acidosis. If the lungs do not compensate, the blood pH is even lower.

35 The answer is D *General principles / Pathology / Renal transplant*

Transplant recipients are at risk for a variety of opportunistic infections. EBV infection with posttransplant lymphoproliferative disorder (PTLD) is one such complication. In PTLD, the immunosuppressed host has a primary or reactivated infection. EBV exerts a proliferative pressure on the B cells. In the absence of regulatory T cell control, B cells may expand and develop clonal populations (i.e., lymphoma).

36 The answer is A *Reproductive system / Microbiology / Toxic shock syndrome*

Toxic shock syndrome (TSS) is caused by TSS toxin-1 (TSST-1), produced by *S. aureus*. Although this disease is usually associated with tampon use in menstruating women, it can be associated with nonmenstruating women and men, most frequently as a postoperative wound infection. Recurrent episodes may occur in menstruating women with a frequency of up to 30%.

37 The answer is A *General principles / Molecular biology / Hereditary spherocytosis*

Hereditary spherocytosis is a disorder caused by a deficiency in the spectrin protein that, in concert with ankyrin, makes up the membrane cytoskeleton of the red blood cell. Although hereditary spherocytosis can also be caused by a deficiency in ankyrin, band 3, protein 4.1, or glycophorin A, the most common biochemical abnormality in these patients is a deficiency of spectrin.

38 The answer is C *General principles / Pharmacology / Antidepressants*

All clinically useful antidepressant drugs potentiate, either directly or indirectly, the actions of norepinephrine, dopamine, and serotonin in the brain. Phenelzine is a monoamine oxidase inhibitor. Trazodone and fluoxetine are serotonin uptake inhibitors. Amitriptyline and nortriptyline are tricyclic antidepressants that block norepinephrine, dopamine, and serotonin uptake into the neuron. All tricyclic antidepressants have similar therapeutic efficacy, and the choice of drug depends on the patient's tolerance of side effects and on the duration of action required.

39 The answer is A *Respiratory system / Pathology / Sarcoidosis*

The clinical presentation in this case is characteristic of sarcoidosis—a young person, often African American, with persistent symptoms and lymph node enlargement ("potato" nodes) with lung infiltrates. Fever, skin nodules, or iritis is often coexistent. The figure shows small nodules in the lung parenchyma (*left*) that at higher magnification are shown to be small, nonnecrotizing granulomas (*right*). The granulomas are composed of giant cells, epithelioid histocytes, and lymphocytes (usually T cells).

40 The answer is C *General principles / Biochemistry / Peptidases*

Trypsin cleaves peptide bonds on the carboxyl side of either arginine or lysine. The fragments are called tryptic peptides. Chymotrypsins can cleave peptide bonds on the carboxyl side of phenylalanine, tyrosine, tryptophan, and other bulky residues. Trypsin and chymotrypsin are both pancreatic enzymes.

41 The answer is C *Central and peripheral nervous system / Pharmacology / Antiepileptics*

Ethosuximide is the drug of first choice in the treatment of absence seizures. Primidone is used in the treatment of partial and tonic–clonic seizures. Although valproic acid diminishes absence seizures, it is the drug of second choice because of its hepatotoxic potential. Phenytoin is not effective for absence seizures; in fact, seizures may worsen if a patient with absence seizures is treated with this drug. Carbamazepine is highly effective for all partial seizures and is often the drug of first choice for partial seizures.

42 The answer is C *General principles / Microbiology / AIDS screening*

The current method of screening patients for evidence of infection by HIV is immunoassay of the serum to detect any antibodies to HIV. Immunoassay-positive sera are retested using a Western blot to confirm that the reactive antibodies are HIV-specific. Direct detection of the HIV virus itself, either by cultivation or by immunoassay, is not reliable. Detection of viral RNA in blood looks promising in some cases, but is still no more than a research tool.

43 The answer is B *Respiratory system / Physiology / Respiration*

If an area of lung is not ventilated, there can be no gas exchange in that region. The pulmonary capillary blood serving that region will not equilibrate with alveolar P_{O_2} but will have a P_{O_2} equal to that of mixed venous blood.

44 The answer is D *General principles / Biostatistics / Mean values*

The mean finishing time (Y) for this group of eight subjects is the arithmetic average of their individual times:

$$Y = \sum Y_i/n$$
$$= 36/8$$
$$= 4.5 \text{ minutes}$$

45 The answer is D *General principles / Genetics / DNA typing for Huntington's disease*

Evidently, the gene causing Huntington's disease (HD) in this family is inherited with the A marker. However, II-1 has AB markers, and it is impossible to know whether she inherited the A or the B marker from her father; therefore, her risk of having the HD gene has not changed.

46 **The answer is C** *Hematopoietic and lymphoreticular system / Hematology / Coagulation abnormality*

This patient's coagulation abnormality most likely is the result of vitamin K deficiency. Prolonged malnutrition with administration of broad-spectrum antibiotics commonly results in vitamin K deficiency. Correction of the PT and PTT in the mixing test excludes an acquired inhibitor. Coagulation factors would not have been diluted by the transfusion of three units of packed red cells; only massive transfusions might cause this effect. Folate deficiency is not associated with abnormalities of the coagulation cascade, and von Willebrand's disease does not affect the PT.

47 **The answer is C** *General principles / Immunology / Anamnestic response*

The anamnestic response, or anamnesis, is also called the booster response, memory response, or secondary immune response. It is characterized by the prompt production of high levels of antibody (i.e., a rapid rise in antibody titers) following a second exposure to antigen. Anamnesis is caused by B and T memory cells that were induced during the primary immune response. Immune paralysis is the inability to mount a response to a normally immunogenic substance.

48 **The answer is B** *Renal/urinary system / Pharmacology / Diuretics*

Potassium-sparing diuretics act in the distal tubule to inhibit sodium reabsorption, potassium secretion, and hydrogen secretion. Amiloride blocks sodium transport channels, resulting in a decrease in sodium–potassium exchange, and as a result acts as a potassium-sparing diuretic. Furosemide is one of the loop diuretics; their major site of action is the ascending loop of Henle. Acetazolamide is a carbonic anhydrase inhibitor that acts in the proximal tubular epithelial cells. Chlorothiazide and indapamide are thiazide diuretics that act on the distal tubule.

49 **The answer is C** *Respiratory system / Physiology / Lung compliance*

Lung compliance is calculated as the change in volume per unit change in distending pressure. Because alveolar pressure is zero at the beginning and end of inspiration, the transmural (distending) pressure for the lung is zero minus the interpleural pressure. Only the change in interpleural pressure between the beginning and end of inspiration is given. This difference divided into the tidal volume gives the lung compliance during dynamic conditions, or 150 and 60 mL/cm H_2O. Compliance is expressed as volume divided by pressure.

50 **The answer is C** *General principles / Biostatistics / Case-control study*

This is a case-control study design; that is, it begins with the selection of cases of the disease in question (chronic otitis media) and disease-free controls. Both groups are followed backward in time to determine exposure to the putative risk factor (parental history of ear infections).

test 16

Questions

Directions: Single best answer questions consist of numbered items or incomplete statements followed by answers or by completions of the statement. Select the ONE lettered answer or completion that is BEST in each case.

1 The graded dose–response for drug *X* is depicted by *curve B* in the following graph. The curve that best describes the response of the drug in the presence of a noncompetitive antagonist is

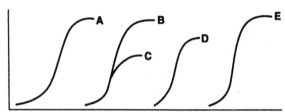

- (A) curve A
- (B) curve C
- (C) curve D
- (D) curve E

2 Which of the following heart sounds is most closely associated with congestive heart failure?

- (A) S_1
- (B) S
- (C) S_3
- (D) S_4
- (E) Fixed splitting of S_2

3 A 6-year-old child is taken to her physician, having had headache, vomiting, fever, and malaise for 2 days. A rash is evident over the child's entire body. A punch biopsy followed by immunostaining confirms *Rickettsia rickettsii* proteins. Which of the following diseases is most closely associated with *R. rickettsii* infections?

- (A) Measles
- (B) Chickenpox
- (C) Lyme disease
- (D) Rocky Mountain spotted fever
- (E) Mumps

4 Which of the following psychosocial stages of cancer is best characterized as a period of short-term focus, when palliation of pain and support of the patient is paramount?

- (A) Diagnosis
- (B) Treatment
- (C) Remission
- (D) Recurrence
- (E) Terminal phase

5 A 23-year-old man has a diffuse palmar and plantar rash accompanied by fever and headache, preceded 4 weeks before by a painless ulcer on his penis. Which of the following organisms is most likely the cause of the patient's symptoms?

- (A) *Treponema pallidum*
- (B) *Neisseria gonorrhoeae*
- (C) *Chlamydia trachomatis*
- (D) Herpesvirus (HSV) 2
- (E) Papillomavirus

6 Which of the following characteristics most correctly describes Turner's syndrome?

- (A) Small, firm testes
- (B) Absence of menses
- (C) 47,XXY karyotype
- (D) Unusually tall build
- (E) Numerous ovarian follicles

7 Which of the following causes or clinical features can be associated with complete renal agenesis?

- (A) Abnormal allantoic regression
- (B) Failure of the inductive interaction between the ureteric bud and the metanephric blastema
- (C) Complete absence of symptoms well into early childhood
- (D) Polyhydramnios
- (E) Increased incidence of Wilms' tumor

8 Which of the following statements correctly characterizes the drug neostigmine?

(A) It irreversibly inhibits acetylcholinesterase
(B) It enters the central nervous system
(C) It is used to stimulate the bladder and gastrointestinal tract, which helps prevent postoperative abdominal distention and urinary retention
(D) It is used to induce the muscle relaxation necessary for surgical procedures
(E) It is useful in the treatment of patients with glaucoma

9 Prostate cancer is the most commonly diagnosed cancer in American men. The pathology of the disease has suggested that androgen ablation is the most effective therapy. If disease is limited to the prostate, prostatectomy is often curative. However, patients with metastatic disease, although not candidates for surgery, still respond to a reduced level of androgen. Using the feedback loop mechanisms regulating androgen synthesis, leuprolide manifests its therapeutic effect by accomplishing which of the following?

(A) It inhibits conversion of testosterone to 5-α-dihydrotestosterone
(B) It inhibits secretion of follicle-stimulating hormone (FSH)
(C) It promotes release of luteinizing hormone-releasing hormone (LHRH)
(D) It promotes estrogen release in males
(E) It competitively inhibits the luteinizing hormone (LH) receptor

10 A 33-year-old woman is diagnosed with marked cardiac insufficiency owing to significant coronary artery occlusion. A blood sample shows the presence of an elevated level of very-low-density lipoproteins (VLDLs) and chylomicrons. Which of the following diseases is the most likely cause of this condition?

(A) Combined hyperlipidemia
(B) Hypertriglyceridemia
(C) Type III hyperlipoproteinemia
(D) Hypercholesterolemia
(E) Lipoprotein lipase deficiency

11 Which of the following is true about blood flow through the liver?

(A) The liver has a triple blood supply from the hepatic artery, the cystic artery, and the portal vein
(B) The caudate and quadrate lobes derive their blood supply in part from the right hepatic artery
(C) Blood supply from the portal vein alone would not provide the liver with sufficient oxygenation
(D) The hepatic sinusoids are lined with a continuous endothelium and substantial basal lamina
(E) Drugs absorbed in the small intestine generally bypass the liver.

12 Oligohydramnios is often caused by

(A) anencephaly
(B) esophageal atresia
(C) renal agenesis
(D) maternal diabetes mellitus
(E) duodenal atresia

13 Sildenafil (Viagra) is effective in the treatment of erectile dysfunction, because it achieves which of the following?

(A) It causes erections by maintaining vasoconstriction
(B) It causes erections by inhibiting nitric oxide release, thus decreasing cyclic guanosine monophosphate (cGMP) levels
(C) It causes erections by inhibiting nitric oxide release, thus decreasing cyclic adenosine monophosphate (cAMP) levels
(D) It causes erections by maintaining cGMP levels
(E) It causes erections by functioning as a prostaglandin analogue

14 A 30-year-old woman has signs and symptoms of hyperthyroidism. She is tachycardic, fidgety, tremulous, and excessively hot, and she complains of a 20-lb weight loss over the past 2 months. Plasma levels of thyroid-stimulating hormone (TSH) are determined, and a diagnosis of Graves' disease is made. The patient is treated with a thioamide, specifically, propylthiouracil (PTU). PTU achieves its effect by which of the following mechanisms?

(A) It blocks thyroid hormone release
(B) It blocks iodide uptake into the thyroid
(C) It antagonizes TSH
(D) It inhibits iodination and peripheral conversion of thyroxine (T_4) to tri-iodothyronine (T_3)
(E) It functions as a nonspecific β-blocking agent

15 An 80-year-old woman is brought to her primary care physician by her son. She complains of stiffness and aches in her shoulders and hips for the last 3 months. She said that she had never had this type of problem in the past and believes that the development of these symptoms have occurred over a short period of time. She has also lost about 15 pounds over the last 3 months. All blood tests are normal except for an elevated erythrocyte sedimentation rate. What is the best diagnosis for this patient?

(A) Osteoarthritis
(B) Rheumatoid arthritis
(C) Septic arthritis
(D) Polymyalgia rheumatica
(E) Dermatomyositis

16 Which of the following statements about the lesion in Figure 63 of the color plate section is correct?

(A) Most patients affected by this lesion are more than 50 years of age
(B) This lesion is associated with chromosome 11; 22 translocation
(C) This lesion is a complication of Paget's disease of bone in some patients
(D) This lesion is the most common bone tumor in adults

17 Oral hyperglycemic drugs offer some patients an effective treatment for type 2 non-insulin-dependent diabetes mellitus (NIDDM). Metformin is a popular biguanide in the United States. Its mechanism of action minimizes the risk of hypoglycemia, as is often noted with the use of another class of hyperglycemic agents, sulfonylureas. Hypoglycemia does not occur as often with patients using metformin because of which of the following properties of this drug?

(A) It promotes glucose release in the liver
(B) It promotes insulin release in the pancreas
(C) It primarily affects the kidney by enhancing glucose secretion into urine
(D) It primarily affects the liver instead of stimulating insulin secretion in the pancreas
(E) It is coupled to glucose that ensures a readily available source of glucose in case of hypoglycemia

18 A 62-year-old woman has dyspnea that has gradually worsened over the past 5 years but recently became more severe after she caught a cold. The physician notices clubbing of the fingers and toes and hears inspiratory crackles. A chest radiograph shows a bilateral basilar reticulonodular infiltrate. A lung biopsy shows a mononuclear cell infiltrate and interstitial scarring with honeycombing. Which one of the following statements is true?

(A) The patient will likely respond well to steroids
(B) This disease is often associated with connective tissue diseases
(C) The patient has bronchiolitis obliterans organizing pneumonia (BOOP)
(D) The abnormalities seen on the biopsy appear temporally homogeneous
(E) The infiltrate seen on the biopsy is diffuse rather than patchy

19 A 46-year-old man with diabetes who is taking an angiotensin-converting enzyme (ACE) inhibitor for hypertension reports having developed vomiting, increasing muscle weakness, and periods in which his heart rate seems uncomfortably fast. An electrocardiogram shows peaked T waves. Which one of the following statements is most likely correct?

(A) The patient is hypokalemic and should be given potassium chloride supplements
(B) The patient is hypokalemic and should be given a β-blocker
(C) The patient is hyperkalemic and should be given a β-blocker
(D) The patient is hyperkalemic and should be given intravenous calcium, followed by insulin and sodium polystyrene sulfonate
(E) The patient is hyperkalemic but does not require treatment other than insulin, if his glucose is uncontrolled, and he should continue the use of the ACE inhibitor

20 An oliguric patient being treated for a gram-negative infection has a sudden increase in his blood urea nitrogen and creatinine ratio. Which one of the following statements would lead to the diagnosis of acute interstitial nephritis rather than acute tubular necrosis?

(A) The patient is taking gentamicin for a gram-negative infection

(B) The patient does not have proteinuria

(C) The patient's urine has dirty brown casts

(D) The patient was taking penicillin for a gram-negative infection and has developed a rash and arthralgia

(E) The patient had a computed tomography scan in which contrast material was used

21 Major histocompatibility complex class I (MHC-I) is an important protein facilitating the immune response. One of its functions is to

(A) present processed antigen to CD4+ T lymphocytes

(B) bind to whole antigens in the antigen-presenting cell's environment for presentation to CD8+ T lymphocytes

(C) regulate the natural killer cell's cytolytic activity

(D) bind to extracellular bacteria to enhance phagocytosis by neutrophils

(E) facilitate cell-to-cell contact between B lymphocytes to enhance antibody production

22 Which of the following statements about non-insulin-dependent diabetus mellitus (NIDDM) is true?

(A) It has no genetic component

(B) Insulin secretion does not change in the late stage of NIDDM

(C) Insulin resistance alone is sufficient for the development of NIDDM

(D) The major environmental component contributing to the development of NIDDM is obesity

(E) NIDDM is rarely controlled by diet and exercise

23 A 50-year-old man dies after an 8-year illness that began with weakness and fasciculations in the left arm. Postmortem analysis of the spinal cord shows disappearance of both corticospinal tract and anterior horn cells. Which of the following is the most likely diagnosis?

(A) Multiple sclerosis

(B) Guillain–Barré syndrome

(C) Amyotrophic lateral sclerosis

(D) Syringomyelia

(E) Tabes dorsalis

24 Poliomyelitis virus causes degeneration of anterior horn cells. Based on this information, which of the following findings would most likely be observed 2 years after the initial infection?

(A) Loss of position and vibration sensation

(B) Muscle hypertrophy

(C) Cogwheel rigidity

(D) Loss of pain and temperature sensation

(E) Flaccid paralysis

25 A 67-year-old woman has spastic paraparesis and sensory ataxia, and she complains of tingling in both of her legs. Physical examination reveals a beefy red tongue, and analysis of her blood indicates decreased hematocrit with an increased mean corpuscular volume (i.e., macrocytic anemia). Given her symptoms, damage to which of the following areas of the spinal cord would be expected?

(A) Ventral spinocerebellar tract

(B) Dorsal horn

(C) Ventral horn

(D) Posterior columns and lateral corticospinal tract

(E) Ventral corticospinal tract

26 A woman with new-onset atrial fibrillation is prescribed warfarin therapy. Ten days later she has a sharply demarcated erythematous lesion on her thigh, which indicates warfarin necrosis. She is most likely to benefit from treatment with which one of the following substances?

(A) Vitamin B_{12}

(B) Tissue-type plasminogen activator

(C) Vitamin K

(D) Erythropoietin

(E) Aspirin

27 A 35-year-old man with chronic hepatitis C viral infection presents with palpable purpura and acute renal failure. A blood sample is collected and maintained at 37°C; the serum is separated from the blood clot, and the serum is cooled to 4°C, resulting in a serum precipitate. A renal biopsy is obtained. Which of the following statements regarding this patient, whose serum precipitate and renal biopsy are depicted in Figure 64 of the color plate section, is true?

(A) The serum precipitate from this patient consists of immunoglobulin (Ig)

(B) The serum precipitate from this patient is composed of fibrin

(C) Serum complement levels are usually normal

(D) Thrombocytopenia is common in patients with this disorder

28 A 30-year-old African American man goes to the emergency department with severe skeletal pain and fever. He has just returned from a skiing vacation in the Rocky Mountains. A diagnosis of sickle cell anemia is made, and hemoglobin S (HbS) is found by electrophoresis. Which of the following statements best describes the abnormality in HbS?

(A) HbS has decreased solubility in the oxygenated state

(B) HbS has increased solubility in the oxygenated state

(C) HbS has decreased solubility in the deoxygenated state

(D) HbS has increased solubility in the deoxygenated state

29 A 20-year-old woman has anemia, splenomegaly, and jaundice. Her mother also was anemic and had a splenectomy as a child. The patient's red blood cells lyse at a higher than normal concentration of saline, and the result of a direct Coombs' test is negative. Which of the following is most likely to be found on the peripheral blood smear?

(A) Target cells

(B) Helmet cells

(C) Burr cells

(D) Spur cells

(E) Spherocytes

30 Propylthiouracil is the prototype of antithyroid drugs of the thiamide type. It is

(A) contraindicated in the therapy of Graves' disease

(B) not used in thyrotoxicosis in pregnancy

(C) inhibits the active transport of iodide in the thyroid gland

(D) interferes with the incorporation of iodine into tyrosyl residues of thyroglobulin

(E) without significant effect on peripheral deiodination of thryoxine to tri-idothyronine

31 A 12-year-old patient who has an insatiable appetite, is short in stature, and is mildly retarded is diagnosed with Prader–Willi syndrome. Knowing that Prader–Willi syndrome involves an imprinted gene on chromosome 15, which one of the following genetic mechanisms could have caused this syndrome?

(A) Trisomy of chromosome 15

(B) Uniparental diploidy

(C) A deletion of a portion of the paternal chromosome 15

(D) Monosomy of chromosome 15

(E) Uniparental disomy of chromosome 2

32 A patient has a partial obstruction of an airway leading to ventilation–perfusion (VQ) mismatch. This scenario leads to an elevated level of the partial pressure of carbon dioxide (P_{CO_2}) and a decreased level of the partial pressure of oxygen (P_{O_2}) in his arterial blood. Which statement concerning the normal physiologic ability to compensate for such a defect is correct?

(A) The patient will be able to compensate for both the elevated P_{CO_2} and decreased P_{O_2}

(B) The patient will be able to compensate for the decreased P_{O_2} but not the elevated P_{CO_2}

(C) The patient will be able to compensate for the elevated P_{CO_2} but not the decreased P_{O_2}

(D) The patient will not be able to compensate for either the elevated P_{CO_2} or the decreased P_{O_2}

(E) Administration of supplemental oxygen would be helpful

33 Which of the following results in metabolic acidosis with an increased anion gap?

(A) Diarrhea

(B) Hyperalimentation

(C) Methanol ingestion

(D) Renal tubular acidosis

(E) Use of carbonic anhydrase inhibitors

34 Which one of the following sets best characterizes respiratory alkalosis?

    (A) pH 7.40, decreased P_{CO_2}, decreased HCO_3^-

    (B) pH 7.51, decreased P_{CO_2}, decreased HCO_3^-

    (C) pH 7.60, increased P_{CO_2}, increased HCO_3^-

    (D) pH 7.49, increased P_{CO_2}, decreased HCO_3^-

    (E) pH 7.55, decreased P_{CO_2}, increased HCO_3^-

35 Concentration of which of the following substances decreases drastically in the proximal tubule under normal conditions?

    (A) Na +

    (B) Urea

    (C) Creatinine

    (D) Glucose

    (E) Cl −

36 A 60-year-old man recently began treatment for essential hypertension. He has a persistent dry cough in the absence of any other pathologic findings. Which of the following drugs is the patient taking to treat his hypertension?

    (A) Verapamil

    (B) Diltiazem

    (C) Nifedipine

    (D) Enalapril

    (E) Furosemide

37 A 50-year-old woman with a history of endoscopic retrograde cholangiopancreatography early in the morning went to the emergency department with acute onset of nausea, vomiting, and severe midepigastric pain radiating to the back. Which of the following findings at admission would adversely affect the survival of this patient?

    (A) Hypertriglyceridemia

    (B) Hyperbilirubinemia

    (C) Serum amylase at 10 times the normal concentration

    (D) Hyperglycemia

    (E) Elevated serum trypsin levels

38 A colleague is designing a clinical trial for a new drug and asks how the study might be affected by patients' adherence to the trial regimen. Which one of the following statements is most accurate?

    (A) Because the researcher is dealing with a serious disease, he does not have to worry about compliance; compliance is a problem only when patients do not believe that they need the therapy to get better

    (B) He should limit his study group to men only, because men are more compliant than women

    (C) The socioeconomic status of his patient group will not affect compliance as long as the patients do not have to pay for the drug

    (D) If there is poor compliance, the trial will overestimate the toxicity of the drug

    (E) If the drug is given in the hospital, he does not have to worry because all of the patients will receive the entire regimen

39 A patient has a transverse fracture of his left humerus. Which one of the following statements is correct?

    (A) The fracture was likely due to compression, because bone is weaker in compression than in torsion or bending

    (B) If a small gap has to be filled in, a hard callus forms instead of cartilage

    (C) Lamellar bone is formed and then is remodeled to cortical bone

    (D) A physis on the radiograph indicates that the patient's skeleton is not fully mature

    (E) If the fracture does not heal by 6 months, it is called a malunion

40 In evaluating a patient who has joint pain, which one of the following statements is characteristic of osteoarthritis but not rheumatoid arthritis (RA)?

    (A) The joint pain is symmetrical

    (B) The patient has morning stiffness that lasts for more than 1 hour

    (C) The patient has swan neck deformities on his second and third fingers

    (D) The patient has pain in the distal interphalangeal joints that is worse after activity and is relieved with rest

    (E) The patient has swelling of the metacarpophalangeal joints

41 Which of the following regarding the abnormality in the cervicovaginal Papanicolaou smear (Figure 65 in the color plate section) obtained from a 20-year-old woman is true?

(A)   The lesion occurs mainly in immunocompromised patients

(B)   The lesion is caused by herpes simplex virus

(C)   The lesion is associated with cervical neoplasia

(D)   Intracellular viral proteins are not demonstrable in the cells depicted

42 A surgeon is considering performing a splenectomy on a 9-year-old girl for staging of Hodgkin's disease. Which one of the following statements is correct concerning the effects of this procedure on the immune system?

(A)   Because the patient has already had all of her immunizations, it is not important that the patient will no longer have a spleen; she will be no more susceptible to disease after the splenectomy

(B)   The patient should have all of her immunizations repeated after the surgery

(C)   *Staphylococcus aureus* is the organism that is of most concern following splenectomy

(D)   The physician should be sure that the patient has had (or receives before surgery) a *Haemophilus influenzae* B vaccination and a Pneumovax vaccination; in addition, prophylactic antibiotics should be prescribed for her after the surgery

(E)   The patient will be highly susceptible to viral infections after the surgery

43 A physician in Guatemala sees a 16-year-old boy who has a slate-blue discoloration on his neck that originally spread from a small, red papule. Lymph nodes in the patient's neck are notably swollen. A diagnosis of pinta is given. Which of the following organisms is the most likely cause of this disease?

(A)   *Borrelia recurrentis*

(B)   *Treponema pertenue*

(C)   *Treponema carateum*

(D)   *Leptospira interrogans*

(E)   *Treponema pallidum*

44 Syphilis is treated with which one of the following antibiotics?

(A)   Amphotericin B

(B)   Ketoconazole

(C)   Trimethoprim

(D)   Rifampin

(E)   Penicillin G

45 At normal pH, which of the following amino acids has a positively charged side chain?

(A)   Glutamic acid

(B)   Proline

(C)   Aspartic acid

(D)   Lysine

(E)   Isoleucine

46 Which of the following statements describes the mechanism of action of lovastatin?

(A)   It lowers serum cholesterol by causing an increase in uptake of low-density lipoprotein

(B)   It strongly inhibits lipolysis in adipose tissue

(C)   It reduces plasma triacylglycerol levels by increasing the activity of lipoprotein lipase

(D)   It binds negatively charged bile acids in the small intestine

(E)   It inhibits 3-hydroxy-3-methylglutaryl (HMG) coenzyme A (CoA) reductase, the enzyme controlling the rate-limiting step in cholesterol synthesis

47 A patient with sweating, narrow pupils, a slow heart rate, and low blood pressure is most likely to have been poisoned with

(A)   *Amanita muscaria*

(B)   methyl alcohol

(C)   chloroform

(D)   heroin

(E)   cocaine

48 Which of the following glycogen storage diseases is caused by deficiency of an enzyme involved in glycogen synthesis?

(A)   Type I—von Gierke's disease

(B)   Type II—Pompe's disease

(C)   Type III—Cori's disease

(D)   Type IV—Andersen's disease

(E)   Type V—McArdle's disease

49 Which of the following statements about pituitary hormones is true?

(A) Luteinizing hormone (LH) and follicle-stimulating hormone (FSH) are both produced in the posterior lobe of the pituitary gland

(B) LH is released continually as a consequence of gonadotropin-releasing hormone (GnRH)

(C) Kallmann's syndrome is characterized by defective GnRH production

(D) LH, thyroid-stimulating hormone, and adrenocorticotropic hormone are typically produced by the same cells in the pituitary gland

(E) Serum LH and FSH are degraded and cleared by the ovaries and testes

50 Which of the following diagnostic tests would be most useful in the diagnosis of autoimmune hemolytic anemia with warm-type antibody?

(A) Coombs' test

(B) Ham's test

(C) Osmotic fragility test

(D) Heinz bodies test

(E) Donath–Landsteiner antibody test

Answer Key

1-B	11-C	21-C	31-C	41-C
2-C	12-C	22-D	32-C	42-D
3-D	13-D	23-C	33-C	43-C
4-E	14-D	24-E	34-B	44-E
5-A	15-D	25-D	35-D	45-D
6-B	16-C	26-C	36-D	46-E
7-B	17-D	27-A	37-D	47-A
8-C	18-B	28-C	38-C	48-D
9-C	19-D	29-E	39-D	49-C
10-A	20-D	30-D	40-D	50-A

Answers and Explanations

1 **The answer is B** *General principles / Pharmacology / Pharmacokinetics*

A noncompetitive antagonist changes the maximal response at high concentration, represented by *curve C*. *Curve A* represents a shift of the dose–response curve to the left, indicating an apparent increase in the potency of drug *X*, which does not occur in the presence of a noncompetitive antagonist. *Curve D* represents the effects of a partial agonist on the drug's dose response. A partial agonist causes less of a response than does a full agonist by itself and acts as a weak competitive antagonist, shifting the dose–response curve to the right. *Curve E* represents a shift of dose response to the right, which occurs in the presence of a competitive antagonist.

2 **The answer is C** *Cardiovascular system / Pathology / Abnormal heart sounds*

Congestive heart failure results in the backup of blood in the venous system, leading to faster than normal ventricular filling. This vigorous filling produces the third heart sound (S_3) in early diastole. S_3 is a dull, low-pitched sound that is best heard with the bell of the diaphragm over the apex of the heart in a patient lying in the left lateral decubitus position. S_1 and S_2 are normal heart sounds. S_4 occurs in late diastole and is produced when an atrial contraction forces the last bolus of blood into a *stiffened* ventricle. Thus, S_4 is commonly associated with pathologic conditions that lead to an increase in ventricular compliance, such as ventricular hypertrophy or myocardial ischemia. S_4 is similar to S_3 in quality. Fixed splitting of S_2 refers to the failure of aortic and pulmonary components of S_2 to fuse during expiration. It occurs when an atrial septal defect is present. It is unlikely to occur in congestive heart failure.

3 **The answer is D** *General principles / Microbiology / Rickettsia rickettsii infection*

Rickettsia rickettsii infection is most closely associated with Rocky Mountain spotted fever. Following entry of the organism into the body, often after a tick bite, a hemorrhagic rash may ensue and cover the entire body, including the palms of the hands and soles of the feet. The appearance of the rash is a result of underlying vascular lesions that lead to the thrombosis of small vessels, fibrin extravasation, and acute necrosis. Despite these features, systemic disseminated intravascular coagulation is rare. Central nervous system involvement, renal failure, upper gastrointestinal bleeding, and hepatic injury may result.

4 **The answer is E** *General principles / Behavioral science / Psychosocial stages of neoplastic disease*

It is important for the physician to recognize the psychosocial stages of patients with neoplastic disease, because the goals and difficulties of the phases differ. The diagnostic phase requires the physician's attention to possible denial of the disease by the patient and to ultimate acceptance of the need for treatment. The actual treatments of neoplastic disease often have serious side effects (malaise, nausea, vomiting) that may promote noncompliance. The period of remission may involve anxious waiting for signs of disease, which can lead to hypochondriacal complaints and lack of return to full functioning. Patients in the terminal phase of cancer need to be in a supportive setting with adequate palliation of pain and discomfort.

5 **The answer is A** *Reproductive system / Microbiology / Etiology of spirochetal diseases*

The etiologic agent of syphilis is *Treponema pallidum*. Humans are the only natural host of the spirochete, and venereal transmission is the most common means of acquiring the infection. In the primary stage, which occurs approximately 3 weeks after contact with an infected individual, a chancre may appear on the penis, cervix, anus, or vaginal wall, marking the site of treponemal entry. The chancre heals spontaneously, even in the absence of therapy. The secondary stage is marked by a diffuse rash on the palms and soles, which may occur in the presence of white lesions of the mouth, fever, arthritis, headache, and lymphadenopathy. These symptoms also resolve spontaneously. The tertiary stage, which can occur years after the initial infection, is marked by inflammatory lesions of the heart, aorta (aortitis), and central nervous system and syphilitic gummas (i.e., lesions in the liver, skin, bone, joints, and subcutaneous tissue). Congenital syphilis occurs when the fetus is infected transplacentally and survives to delivery.

6 **The answer is B** *Reproductive system / Genetics / Turner's syndrome*

Turner's syndrome is an example of gonadal dysgenesis. A patient with Turner's syndrome has a 45,X karyotype. As a result of this genetic anomaly, normal ovaries fail to form. The abnormal ovaries that do form have no follicles in them. Therefore, secondary sexual characteristics, which are normally induced by follicular steroids, are also lacking. Sterility, lack of menses, and a webbed neck are all characteristic of patients with Turner's syndrome. A 47,XXY karyotype and small, firm testes are characteristics usually associated with Klinefelter's syndrome.

7 **The answer is B** *Renal/urinary system / Embryology / Renal agenesis*

Normally, a reciprocal inductive interaction between the ureteric bud and the metanephric blastema leads to the development of the definitive adult kidney. Failure in this inductive system leads to renal agenesis. Failure of allantoid degeneration leads to urinary bladder fistula or to cysts in the umbilical region.
Renal agenesis can be unilateral or bilateral. Unilateral renal agenesis is often asymptomatic and is compatible with a normal life because of compensatory hypertrophy of the single normal kidney. Bilateral renal agenesis is associated with oligohydramnios (decreased volume of amniotic fluid) because of an absence of fetal urine production. A newborn infant with complete renal agenesis can be born and seem normal because of the maternal elimination of fetal nitrogenous wastes by way of the placenta, but the infant will die soon after birth.

8 **The answer is C** *General principles / Pharmacology / Anticholinesterases*

Neostigmine is used for the relief of abdominal distention from a variety of medical and surgical causes. It is used for the treatment of atony of the detrusor muscle of the urinary bladder. Acetylcholinesterase inhibitors, such as neostigmine, are contraindicated in patients with glaucoma because excess acetylcholine at parasympathetic cholinergic synapses in the eye lead to a narrowing of the anterior chamber angle, which reduces drainage through the canal of Schlemm and increases intraocular pressure. Acetylcholinesterase inhibitors do not produce muscle relaxation. Unlike the organophosphorous acetylcholinesterase inhibitor, neostigmine is a reversible inhibitor of the esterase. Neostigmine is a quaternary amine and therefore is only poorly absorbed after oral administration and does not readily cross the blood–brain barrier or enter the central nervous system.

9 **The answer is C** *Reproductive system / Pharmacology; biochemistry / Regulation of gonadotropin function*

Leuprolide is an agonist of LHRH in the hypothalamus. Like LHRH, it stimulates LH release from the pituitary, which initially increases testosterone production by Leydig cells in the testicle. Increased testosterone downregulates LH receptors, leading to a decrease in the release of LH. Decreased LH levels decrease testosterone levels, which is beneficial in treating metastatic carcinoma of the prostate.

10 **The answer is A** *General principles / Genetics; biochemistry / Lipoproteins and genetic disorders*

The defect underlying combined hyperlipidemia is unknown, although research suggests a deficiency in apoprotein CII. In this disorder, serum levels of very-low-density lipoproteins (VLDLs) and chylomicrons are elevated, leading to a combined hyperlipidemia. Alcoholism, diabetes mellitus, and oral contraceptives are also capable of elevating levels of VLDLs and chylomicrons.

11 **The answer is C** *Gastrointestinal system / Anatomy / Hepatic blood supply*

The liver has a double blood supply from the hepatic artery (30%) and the portal vein (70%). The cystic artery supplies the proximal part of the bile duct. The caudate and quadrate lobes derive their blood supply in part from the left hepatic artery and left portal vein, as does the left lobe of the liver. The portal vein carries nutrient-rich blood from the large and small intestine to the liver. Oxygen-rich blood from the hepatic arteries, in addition to portal vein blood, is necessary for proper oxygenation of the liver tissue. The hepatic sinusoids receive blood from the portal vein and hepatic artery and carry it to the central vein. These sinusoids are lined with fenestrated (discontinuous) endothelium. In addition, the basal lamina is discontinuous and even absent in areas.

12 **The answer is C** *Reproductive system / Embryology / Oligohydramnios*

Oligohydramnios, in which the amniotic fluid level is lower than normal, is often caused by renal agenesis. Some digestive tract abnormalities, including esophageal atresia and duodenal atresia, lead to polyhydramnios (i.e., increased levels of amniotic fluid). In addition, maternal diabetes mellitus and anencephaly may cause polyhydramnios.

13 **The answer is D** *General principles / Pharmacology / Mechanism of action of sildenafil*

Sildenafil is a potent inhibitor of cGMP phosphodiesterase type 5. This inhibition maintains elevated levels of cGMP, which promotes smooth muscle relaxation and vasodilation. Increased blood flow to the penis enhances erectile function, and smooth muscle relaxation obstructs venous outflow, further enhancing erectile function. Although prostaglandins also promote vasodilation and increased blood flow to the penis, they do so by a different mechanism. Sildenafil does not function as a prostaglandin agonist.

14 **The answer is D** *Endocrine system / Pharmacology; pathology / Graves' disease*

Graves' disease is caused by the production of antibodies to the TSH receptor in the thyroid. These antibodies actually stimulate the thyroid gland to increase thyroid hormone synthesis. As a result, thyroid hormone levels increase; negative feedback mechanisms then lead to low or undetectable plasma TSH levels. The antibodies act throughout the gland, producing a diffuse enlargement of the thyroid. The presence of a hard nodule or asymmetric enlargement of the gland indicates a malignant process. Thyroglobulin antibodies are characteristic of Hashimoto's thyroiditis, which causes hypothyroidism but does not cause hyperthyroidism. Pharmacologic treatment of Graves' disease relies on inhibitors of thyroid hormone synthesis, such as methimazole and propylthiouracil (PTU). PTU, a thioamide, inhibits the oxidative processes needed for iodination and the coupling of iodotyrosines to form T_3, the metabolically active form of thyroid hormone. Unlike methimazole, it has the advantage of inhibiting T_3 production at the periphery, which brings faster relief of symptoms.

15 **The answer is D** *Musculoskeletal system / Rheumatology / Polymyalgia rheumatica*

The clinical history provided by this patient is highly suggestive of polymyalgia rheumatica. Polymyalgia rheumatica (PR) is disease with a mean onset age of 70 years and is often associated with low-grade fever, weight loss, and depression. Blood tests are usually normal except for an elevated ESR. Physical findings most commonly involve stiffness and weakness in the shoulder and hip girdles that is worst in the morning. The treatment for PR is oral prednisone.

16 **The answer is C** *Musculoskeletal system / Pathology / Osteocarcinoma arising in the metaphysis of the distal femur*

Osteosarcoma is a malignant osteoid-producing bone tumor and is the most common primary bone tumor, excluding myeloma and lymphoma; 1,000 new cases are diagnosed annually in the United States. (Metastatic carcinoma of bone is the most common bone malignancy.) There is a bimodal age distribution: 75% occur in skeletally immature (i.e., growing) bone (in patients younger than 20 years of age), which arises in the metaphysis of long bones. Most other cases arise in the elderly in the setting of Paget's disease, bone infarcts, and prior irradiation. Mutations in the retinoblastoma (Rb) and p53 genes have been described in hereditary forms of osteosarcoma. There is no association with a chromosome 11;22 translocation, which is associated with Ewing's sarcoma and other primitive neuroectodermal tumors. Osteosarcomas arise in mitotically active bone. They account for their origin at the metaphysis in proximity to the epiphyseal plate in growing bone and their association with Paget's disease, bone infarcts, and prior irradiation. Osteosarcomas occur in intramedullary, intracortical, and bone surface locations; they may be solitary or multicentric; and they exhibit several histologic subtypes (e.g., osteoblastic, chondroblastic, fibroblastic, telangiectatic, small cell and giant cell variants). The most common presentation is a young patient with an intramedullary tumor arising in the metaphysis of a large long bone (60% occur in the distal femur or proximal tibia), showing focal osteoblastic differentiation. The tumor replaces the medullary space; it permeates the adjacent cortex and extends into and expands the subperiosteal space, thus inducing reactive subperiosteal bone formation. Radiographically, this periosteal reaction has a sunburst appearance and is associated with a triangular shadow between the cortex and the elevated ends of the periosteum (Codman's triangle). Extension through the periosteum results in the formation of a contiguous soft tissue mass, and penetration through the articular cartilage may result in joint space involvement. Metastasis is characteristically hematogenous, and 20% of patients have pulmonary metastasis at presentation. Long-term survival rates have increased up to 60% with the advent of improved multimodality therapy.

17 **The answer is D** *General principles / Pharmacology / Hyperglycemic agents*

Sulfonylureas stimulate the release of insulin from the pancreas. Although this lowers plasma glucose levels, it carries a risk of hyperinsulinemia and subsequent hypoglycemia. In contrast, metformin decreases circulating plasma glucose levels by inhibiting gluconeogenesis in the liver. Insulin levels are minimally affected because the drug has only a small effect on the pancreas. As a result, hyperinsulinemia does not develop with the use of metformin, and the risk of hypoglycemia is reduced.

18 **The answer is B** *Respiratory system / Pathology / Chronic interstitial lung disease*

These symptoms are typical of usual interstitial pneumonia (UIP), also known as idiopathic pulmonary fibrosis. This disease responds to steroid therapy in only a relatively small percentage of cases. UIP is frequently associated with connective tissue diseases. It can be differentiated from bronchiolitis obliterans organizing pneumonia (BOOP) by the length of time over which the symptoms developed. BOOP generally develops less than a couple of months. Also, BOOP tends to have a ground-glass appearance on chest radiographs, rather than the reticular or reticulonodular appearance seen in UIP. UIP is characterized by a patchy and temporally heterogeneous pattern of injury on examination of the lung biopsy.

19 **The answer is D** *General principles / Physiology / Potassium homeostasis*

Although both cardiac and neuromuscular symptoms can be caused by either hypokalemia or hyperkalemia, the electrocardiogram patterns are distinct for each abnormality. Hyperkalemia is associated with peaked T waves, a wide QRS complex, a prolonged PR interval, absent P waves, and a sine wave pattern. Hypokalemia causes flattened T waves, U waves, and ST segment depression. Treatment of hyperkalemia should include rapid administration of intravenous calcium followed by insulin, albuterol, and sodium bicarbonate and then a potassium-binding agent (e.g., sodium polystyrene sulfonate). Treatment is urgent because cardiac arrest or arrhythmias may occur. ACE inhibitors and β-blockers should be avoided because these drugs, as well as diabetes, are potential causes of hyperkalemia. Treatment of hypokalemia is less urgent but should include potassium replacement along with a search for the underlying cause.

20 **The answer is D** *Renal/urinary system / Physiology / Acute renal failure*

Acute renal failure may be caused by acute tubular necrosis, acute interstitial nephritis, and many other problems. Acute tubular necrosis is frequently incited by aminoglycoside antibiotics, including gentamicin, or by the use of contrast media for radiologic studies. Dirty brown casts are often present in the urine specimen. Urine samples from patients with acute tubular necrosis do not have proteinuria, red blood cells, white blood cells, and white blood cell casts, but these cells are often seen in patients with acute interstitial nephritis. Acute interstitial nephritis is associated with penicillin, dilantin, infections, and radiation. A hypersensitivity response (e.g., fever, rash, and arthralgia) may occur with acute interstitial nephritis but is not seen in patients with acute tubular necrosis.

21 **The answer is C** *General principles / Immunology / Major histocompatability complex class I*

Major histocompatability complex class I (MHC-I) is a protein present on almost all cells of the body. Its function is to sample the intracellular contents and present peptides that come from inside the cell. In the uninfected, noncancerous cell, MHC-I presents normal cell peptides, and there is no immune response. If the cell is infected by a virus or intracellular bacteria or if it is cancerous, the peptides presented by the MHC-I may be recognized as nonself by CD8+ T lymphocytes. Some viruses are able to downregulate the MHC-I expression and avoid detection. Natural killer cells, which are part of the innate immune system and are antigen nonspecific, are inhibited by the presence of MHC-I on the cell surface. Virally infected cells with low expression of MHC-I have an increased risk of being killed by natural killer cells.

22 **The answer is D** *Endocrine system / Pathology / NIDDM*

Pathogenesis of noninsulin-dependent diabetus mellitus (NIDDM) has a very strong genetic component. Concordance rates in monozygotic twins can reach 80%. In fact, the risk to offspring and siblings of parents with NIDDM is higher than in insulin-dependent diabetes mellitus (IDDM). Two major factors are responsible for the development of NIDDM: abnormal insulin secretion and resistance to insulin in target tissues. Although insulin resistance is the predominant finding in early NIDDM, in late stages of the disease, insulin secretion declines sufficiently to cause fasting hyperglycemia and overt diabetes. Insulin resistance alone is not sufficient for the development of NIDDM, because morbidly obese individuals can demonstrate striking insulin resistance and normal glucose tolerance. Obesity, however, is the major environmental factor in the development of NIDDM, and most NIDDM can be controlled with weight loss and diet.

23 **The answer is C** *Central and peripheral nervous system / Neuroanatomy / Spinal cord lesions*

Amyotrophic lateral sclerosis is an idiopathic disease characterized by disappearance of both the corticospinal tract and anterior horn cells. This results in combined signs of upper and lower motor neuron defects, including muscle atrophy, fibrillation, fasciculations, and hyperreflexia; the sensory system remains intact.

24 **The answer is E** *Central and peripheral nervous system / Neuroanatomy / Spinal cord lesions*

Poliomyelitis virus causes degeneration of the anterior horn cells, which results in symptoms of lower motor neuron defects (i.e., flaccid paralysis, fasciculations and fibrillations, muscle atrophy, and hyporeflexia).

25 **The answer is D** *Central and peripheral nervous system / Neuroanatomy / Spinal cord lesions*

Pernicious anemia (i.e., vitamin B_{12} deficiency) causes degeneration of the posterior columns and of the corticospinal tracts, causing proprioceptive loss and upper motor neuron defects, respectively.

26 **The answer is C** *Cardiovascular system / Pharmacology / Warfarin toxicity*

Warfarin functions as an anticoagulant by inhibiting synthesis of vitamin K-dependent clotting factors in the liver. Warfarin necrosis is one of the side effects of warfarin therapy. Warfarin necrosis usually occurs 3 to 10 days after the initiation of therapy. It is more common in women than in men and usually occurs on the breasts, thighs, or buttocks. The lesions are well-demarcated, erythematous, and indurated. Treatment with vitamin K antagonizes both the side effects and therapeutic effects of warfarin, so higher than usual doses of oral anticoagulants are needed when and if such therapy is resumed.

27 The answer is A *Hematopoietic and lymphoreticular system / Pathology / Cryoglobulin precipitate in serum and cryoglobulin thrombi within glomerular capillaries*

Cryoglobulin consists of Ig that precipitates when cooled below 37°C and dissolves when warmed above 37°C. Three types are recognized and are distinguished by immunoelectrophoresis. Type I cryoglobulin typically arises in patients with a plasma cell dyscrasia (e.g., multiple myeloma, Waldenström's macroglobulinemia) and consists of a monoclonal Ig of a single Ig class, usually IgM. Types II and III are mixed cryoglobulins (i.e., they contain two or more immunoglobulin classes, with IgG and IgM the most common combination). Types II and III cryoglobulins are distinguished from each another by the presence (type II) or absence (type III) of a monoclonal Ig component that represents one of the Ig classes. The mixed cryoglobulins are immune complexes with rheumatoid factor activity (i.e., one Ig, usually IgM, binds to the Fc region of the second, usually IgG, forming an immune complex precipitate that is insoluble at low temperatures and is capable of activating complement). Cryoglobulin precipitates may form occlusive microthrombi in the microcirculation, resulting in ischemic injury, or may deposit in blood vessel walls, inciting an inflammatory response that results in small vessel vasculitis. In the kidney, cryoglobulin (usually mixed types) may form occlusive thrombi in the microcirculation and may deposit in glomerular capillary walls and mesangia, most often inducing type I membranoproliferative glomerulonephritis. Ultrastructurally, cryoglobulins often show a tubular–fibrillary substructure. Mixed cryoglobulins often result from an aberrant immunologic response to an antigen, most often chronic hepatitis C virus infection, but they also occur with other infections and autoimmune disorders.

28 The answer is C *Hematopoietic and lymphoreticular system / Pathology / Sickle cell anemia*

Hemoglobin S (HbS) is characterized by substitution of valine for glutamic acid as the sixth amino acid in the β-hemoglobin chain. This substitution decreases HbS solubility in the deoxygenated form. Deoxy-HbS precipitates into a network of fibrous polymers that distort the red blood cells and give them the characteristic sickle cell appearance. Any factor that promotes deoxygenation of HbS, such as unpressurized ascent to high altitudes, increases sickling and sometimes leads to acute infarctive or painful crises. Treatment consists of hydration and pain management.

29 The answer is E *Hematopoietic and lymphoreticular system / Pathology / Hereditary spherocytosis*

Hereditary spherocytosis is characterized on the molecular level by mutations that affect the stability of the red blood cell skeleton. Half of these patients have a defect in ankyrin, a protein that connects spectrin to a membrane-bound protein 3. Loss of the red blood cell membrane leads to the spherical red blood cell shape. The most common mode of inheritance is autosomal-dominant. The most common clinical signs are anemia, splenomegaly, and jaundice. A peripheral blood smear shows spherocytes. Because spherocytes are also present in hemolytic anemias associated with red blood cell antibodies, immunologic causes of spherocytosis must be excluded using a direct Coombs' test. A negative Coombs' test indicates that immune spherocytosis is unlikely in this patient. A family history of anemia or splenectomy is also helpful in the diagnosis.

30 The answer is D *Endocrine system / Pharmacology / Thyroid*

Propylthiouracil, along with methimazole and carbimazole, are a class of antithyroid drugs that interfere with the incorporation of iodine into tyrosyl residues of thryoglobulin. The molecular determinant appears to involve inhibiton of peroxidase enzyme. Propylthiouracil has some of its therapeutic effect by inhibiting peripheral deiodination of thyroxine to tri-iodothyronine and this adds to its utility in treatment of severe hyperthyroidism, such as thyrotoxicosis. In contrast to the other available agents in this class, propylthiouracil does not penetrate the placental barrier very efficiently and thus may be useful in the treatment of thyrotoxicosis in pregnancy. Propylthiouracil is useful for the control of hyperthyroidism in Graves' disease in anticipation of spontaneous remission or in combination with radiotherapy and/or surgery.

31 **The answer is C** *General principles / Genetics / Imprinting*

Genomic imprinting is defined as a difference in the expression of genetic material depending on whether it is maternal or paternal in origin. The mechanisms for this process are not entirely understood. Prader–Willi syndrome is an example of a disease that is caused by lack of a paternal copy of a certain genetic sequence on chromosome 15. Angelman's syndrome is caused by lack of a maternal copy of a nearby sequence. Prader–Willi syndrome may be due to deletion of the specific region of the paternal chromosome 15 or, less commonly, to maternal uniparental disomy of chromosome 15. Although maternal monosomy 15 and maternal uniparental diploidy lead to Prader–Willi syndrome (if only the region of chromosome 15 is considered), these conditions are not compatible with life. Trisomy 15 is also not compatible with life beyond fetal stages, nor does it lead to the absence of a paternal chromosome 15 or Prader–Willi syndrome.

32 **The answer is C** *Respiratory system / Physiology / Ventilation–perfusion mismatch*

In a patient with a ventilation–perfusion (VQ) mismatch, the level of P_{CO_2} increases and the level of P_{O_2} decreases. The decrease in the P_{O_2} raises the rate of ventilation because central chemoreceptors enable the patient to compensate for the elevated P_{CO_2} and keep this value within the normal range. However, the patient cannot compensate for the lowered P_{O_2}. The reason for this failure is that nearly all of the oxygen in the blood is carried by hemoglobin, and under normal conditions the hemoglobin is near saturation of its oxygen-carrying capacity. Thus, even with hyperventilation, an area of high VQ cannot increase the amount of oxygen it is carrying to compensate for an area of low VQ. Increasing the concentration of oxygen of the inspired air would not be beneficial.

33 **The answer is C** *General principles / Physiology / Acid–base disorders*

The anion gap in metabolic acidosis is defined as:

$$\text{Anion gap} = [Na^+] - ([Cl^-] + [HCO_3^-])$$

The normal range for the anion gap is 8 to 12 mmol/L. An anion gap above 12 mmol/L is increased and is caused by the accumulation of acids. Metabolic acidosis with an increased anion gap has either exogenous or endogenous causes. Exogenous causes include ingestion of salicylates, methanol, paraldehyde, or ethylene glycol (antifreeze). Endogenous causes include lactic acidosis, ketoacidosis (i.e., diabetic, starvation-induced, or alcoholic), or renal failure. In contrast, metabolic acidosis with a normal anion gap reflects gastrointestinal problems (e.g., diarrhea, pancreatic fistula) or kidney problems (e.g., renal tubular acidosis). Iatrogenic causes of metabolic acidosis with a normal anion gap include the use of carbonic anhydrase inhibitors, rapid intravenous hydration, and hyperalimentation. Finally, a low anion gap may be a result of decreased concentrations of unmeasured anions (e.g., hypoalbuminemia) or increased concentrations of unmeasured cations (e.g., hypercalcemia, hypermagnesemia).

34 **The answer is B** *General principles / Physiology / Acid–base disorders*

Acid–base disorders are clinically common and are classified as either acidosis or alkalosis. Determination of blood pH, P_{CO_2}, and HCO_3^- is crucial for the investigation of acid–base disorders. In approaching acid–base disorders, it is first necessary to establish whether the disorder is acidosis (i.e., pH < 7.37) or alkalosis (i.e., pH > 7.44), then to determine whether the disturbance is metabolic or respiratory by interpretation of P_{CO_2} and HCO_3^- as follows:

TABLE 16-1

Acid–Base Disorder	Metabolic or Respiratory	P_{CO_2}	HCO_3^-
Acidosis	Metabolic	↓	↓
	Respiratory	↑	↑
Alkalosis	Metabolic	↑	↑
	Respiratory	↓	↓

35 **The answer is D** *Renal/urinary system / Physiology / Urine formation in the nephron*

Some 65% of sodium, chloride, bicarbonate, and potassium in the glomerular filtrate is reabsorbed in the proximal tubule. Sodium concentration, however, remains constant because water readily follows sodium from the lumen into the renal interstitial fluid. Some organic solutes, such as glucose and amino acids, are reabsorbed almost entirely in the proximal tubule. Other organic molecules, such as urea and creatinine, are not as readily reabsorbed, and their concentration actually increases slightly along the length of the proximal tubule.

36 **The answer is D** *Cardiovascular system / Pharmacology / Side effects of angiotensin-converting enzyme inhibitors*

Angiotensin-converting enzyme (ACE) inhibitors, such as enalapril, are commonly used to treat essential hypertension, and 15% of patients treated with ACE inhibitors develop a dry cough. The mechanism for airway irritation is unknown. Verapamil, diltiazem, and nifedipine are calcium channel blockers. Although they are used to treat hypertension, they do not cause dry cough. Furosemide, a loop diuretic, is not generally used in the treatment of hypertension.

37 **The answer is D** *Gastrointestinal system / Pathology / Ransom Imrie criteria for survival in acute pancreatitis*

Pancreatitis owing to endoscopic retrograde cholangiopancreatography is the third-most common cause of acute pancreatitis in the United States. The first two causes are chronic alcohol abuse and gallstones. Acute pancreatitis usually is accompanied by severe midepigastric pain that often radiates to the back, chest, flanks, and lower abdomen. Nausea, vomiting, abdominal distention owing to intestinal hypomotility, and chemical peritonitis are also common. Diagnosis is based on elevated serum amylase or lipase levels. Criteria that adversely affect the survival of patients with acute pancreatitis were developed by Ranson and Imrie and are divided into two groups: findings at admission or diagnosis, and findings in the initial 48 hours. Findings at admission or diagnosis that portend a poor outcome are age above 55 years, leukocytosis above 16,000/μL; hyperglycemia above 200 mg/dL, serum lactate dehydrogenase above 400 IU/L, and serum aspartate aminotransferase above 250 IU/L. Amylase levels are not correlated with the severity of the disease. Although triglycerides, bilirubin, and trypsin are elevated in some cases of acute pancreatitis, these factors do not influence survival.

38 **The answer is C** *General principles / Behavioral science / Patient compliance*

Compliance should be a major concern of physicians, because up to 50% of patients are poorly adherent to some aspect of their treatment regimen. Adherence is a problem even for patients with life-threatening illnesses (e.g., cancer and transplants). Sex, race, and socioeconomic status are unrelated to the level of compliance. However, cost and the complexity of the regimen do affect adherence. Patients are more compliant if they are involved in the planning of the regimen. Even in the hospital, patients do not always receive the prescribed doses at the prescribed times; furthermore, they may refuse to take certain treatments when offered. In terms of research protocols, poor adherence decreases the apparent efficacy of the treatment, but it also underestimates the toxicity of the regimen. Thus, it is an important parameter. It may be assessed by several methods, including pill counting, patient report or daily diary, and biochemical tests.

39 **The answer is D** *Musculoskeletal system / Anatomy / Bone fractures and healing*

Bone is weakest in tension, somewhat stronger in torsion and bending, and strongest in compression. Tension failure also leads to transverse fractures. Once a stable clot forms, cartilage begins to be laid down to stabilize the wound enough for bone to grow (i.e., decrease the strain). However, cartilage formation may not occur if the bone ends are apposed to each other and no motion is allowed. A hard callus forms, and woven bone is laid down; the woven bone is then replaced by lamellar bone. Cortical bone and trabecular bone are subtypes of lamellar bone. A physis on radiograph indicates that the skeleton is not fully mature; the physis disappears once growth is complete. A fracture that does not heal within 6 months is termed a nonunion; a malunion is a fracture that heals in an abnormal position.

40 The answer is D *Musculoskeletal system / Anatomy / Rheumatoid arthritis versus osteoarthritis*

Rheumatoid arthritis (RA) is characterized by symmetrical joint pain; morning stiffness lasting more than 60 minutes; sparing of the distal interphalangeal joints (DIP); involvement of the wrist, metacarpophalangeal joints (MCP), and proximal interphalangeal joints; and systemic symptoms. The pain in patients with RA is relatively constant and not relieved by rest. Swan neck deformities are just one example of the complications that can arise. Osteoarthritis is less commonly symmetrical, involves morning stiffness for 5 to 10 minutes, often involves the DIP joints, typically worsens with activity, and is relieved by rest. It does not cause the vast array of systemic signs that accompany RA. Swelling is uncommon, and the MCP are less frequently involved in patients with osteoarthritis.

41 The answer is C *Reproductive system / Pathology / Human papilloma virus infection with associated koilocytes*

Human papilloma virus (HPV), a sexually transmitted disease, affects the genital tracts of many women worldwide. It occurs in both immunocompetent and immunosuppressed patients. The virus infects squamous cells of the vulva, vagina, and cervix and may also infect endocervical glandular cells. HPV has been associated epidemiologically with approximately 85% of cervical squamous carcinomas and 90% of precancerous lesions. Low-risk HPV serotypes (i.e., 6, 17, 42, 44) are associated with condylomas and low-grade squamous dysplasias; the virus exists in infected cells in an episomal form and is associated with productive viral infection in the mature (i.e., more superficial) squamous cells, resulting in the formation of koilocytes (i.e., squamous cells, often binucleate, with cytoplasmic cavitation, mild nuclear atypia, and intracellular virions). High-risk HPV serotypes (i.e., 16, 18, 31, 33, 35) result in genomically integrated viral DNA and production of E6 and E7 oncoproteins, which bind and inactivate tumor suppressor p53 and Rb proteins. Viral proteins are demonstrable in mature (low-grade) but not immature (high-grade) squamous dysplastic cells. Infection by high-risk serotypes is more closely correlated with high-grade squamous dysplasia and, in some patients, progression to invasive squamous cell carcinoma.

42 The answer is D *Hematopoietic and lymphoreticular system / Immunology / Splenectomy*

Splenectomy does raise susceptibility to infection, but the risks can be reduced if the proper precautions are taken. Encapsulated bacteria, especially *Streptococcus pneumoniae* and *Haemophilus influenzae,* present the greatest threat to patients without a spleen. If possible, vaccinations to both of these organisms should be given to the patient before surgery. Prophylactic antibiotics should be taken following splenectomy, particularly when dental work or other invasive procedures are to be performed. Certain aspects of the immune system remain intact after splenectomy. Thus, it is not necessary to repeat immunizations after surgery. In addition, splenectomy does not significantly increase susceptibility to viral infections or infections by *Staphylococcus aureus*. In fact, adults who have already been exposed to many microorganisms are less affected by removal of the spleen than are children.

43 The answer is C *General principles / Microbiology / Etiology of spirochetal diseases*

Pinta is a tropical disease cause by *Treponema carateum*. It occurs primarily in Central and South America, where it appears to be spread by person-to-person contact. Unlike other treponemal diseases, the lesions of pinta remain local to the skin.

44 The answer is E *General principles / Pharmacology / Syphilis*

Treponema pallidum, which causes syphilis, is susceptible to penicillin G. Amphotericin B and ketoconazole have antifungal activity and do not affect *T. pallidum*. Rifampin inhibits messenger RNA synthesis, and trimethoprim inhibits nucleotide synthesis. Neither of these drugs is needed to treat syphilis.

45 The answer is D *General principles / Biochemistry / Protein structure*

Lysine is a basic amino acid that is positively charged at normal pH. Glutamic acid and aspartic acid are acidic amino acids that are negatively charged at normal pH. Proline and isoleucine are amino acids with nonpolar side chains. They have no net charge at normal pH.

46 The answer is E *General principles / Pharmacology / Antihyperlipidemic drugs*

Lovastatin's mechanism of action is to inhibit HMG CoA reductase, the enzyme that controls the rate-limiting step in cholesterol synthesis. Probucol lowers serum cholesterol by causing an increase in the uptake of low-density lipoprotein. Niacin acts to reduce plasma cholesterol by strongly inhibiting lipolysis in adipose tissue. Clofibrate causes a decrease in plasma triacylglycerol levels by increasing the activity of lipoprotein lipase. Cholestyramine and colestipol reduce serum cholesterol by binding negatively charged bile acids in the small intestine.

47 The answer is A *General principles / Pharmacology /* Amanita muscaria *poisoning*

The mushroom *Amanita muscaria* causes muscarinic effects on the nervous system (i.e., sweating, narrow pupils, a slow heart rate, and low blood pressure); however, in contrast to poisoning with *Amanita phalloides,* patients usually recover without more severe problems. Methyl alcohol may cause blindness, and chloroform causes liver toxicity, which would not produce this patient's symptoms. Nasal bleeding secondary to perforation is a common presentation of cocaine sniffers. In heroin overdose, shortness of breath due to pulmonary edema is often seen.

48 The answer is D *General principles / Biochemistry / Glycogen storage disease*

Type IV glycogen storage disease (Andersen's disease) is caused by a deficiency of glycosyl 4:6 transferase. This enzyme creates branches in glycogen by transferring a chain of five to eight glucosyl residues from the nonreducing end of the glycogen chain (breaking an α-1,4 bond) to another residue on the chain, attaching the two by an α-1,6 linkage. The resulting new nonreducing end and the old reducing end from which the chain came can now be further elongated by glycogen synthase. Pompe's disease is caused by a deficiency of lysosomal α-glucosidase enzyme. McArdle's disease is caused by a deficiency of skeletal muscle glycogen phosphorylase. Cori's disease is caused by amylo-1,6-glucosidase deficiency. Von Gierke's disease is caused by a deficiency of glucose-6-phosphatase. All of these enzymes are involved in glycogen degradation.

49 The answer is C *Endocrine system / Physiology / Gonadotropins*

Luteinizing hormone (LH) and follicle-stimulating hormone (FSH) are synthesized by gonadotrophs in the anterior lobe of the pituitary gland, which are degraded and cleared by the liver and kidney. Immunohistochemical studies have shown that both LH and FSH are present in most gonadotrophs, although a few cells contain one form of the gonadotropins. Pituitary LH is released in pulses as a consequence of intermittent GnRH stimulation. Kallmann's syndrome, a genetic disorder characterized by defective hypothalamic GnRH production, can be treated with GnRH replacement therapy. Although LH, thyroid-stimulating hormone (TSH), and adrenocorticotropic hormone are all made in the anterior pituitary, they are synthesized by distinct cell populations: LH and FSH, gonadotrophs; TSH, basophilic (thyrotropic) cells; and adrenocorticotropic hormone, corticotrophs.

50 The answer is A *Hematopoietic and lymphoreticular system / Hematology / Testing for hematologic disorders*

Although the indirect Coombs' test may give positive results in two thirds of patients with autoimmune hemolytic anemia, the direct Coombs' test demonstrates the presence of autoantibodies, complement, or both on the red blood cell surface. The indirect Coombs' test demonstrates antibodies in the serum, and they are specific to antigens in the donor red blood cells, causing a delayed hemolytic transfusion reaction.

test 17

Questions

Directions: Single best answer questions consist of numbered items or incomplete statements followed by answers or by completions of the statement. Select the ONE lettered answer or completion that is BEST in each case.

1 Which one of the following sets of clinical findings best describes an upper motor neuron lesion?

(A) Negative Babinski sign, hyporeflexia, spasticity
(B) Negative Babinski sign, hyperreflexia, paralysis
(C) Positive Babinski sign, hyporeflexia, spasticity
(D) Positive Babinski sign, hyperreflexia, paralysis
(E) Positive Babinski sign, hyperreflexia, fasciculations, and fibrillations

2 Chronic myeloid leukemia (CML) is characterized by which of the following?

(A) Progressive shrinking and scarring of the spleen
(B) An 8;14 chromosomal translocation
(C) A peak incidence in patients older than 65 years of age
(D) A 9;22 chromosomal translocation
(E) Elevated leukocyte alkaline phosphatase

3 A man shows no detectable signs of Marfan's syndrome (i.e., an autosomal dominant disorder of connective tissue), although his father and two daughters are affected. Which of the following terms most accurately describes this pattern of inheritance?

(A) Allelic heterogeneity
(B) Variable expressivity
(C) Nonpenetrance
(D) Consanguinity
(E) Locus heterogeneity

4 The broad-based budding fungal organism shown in Figure 66 from the color plate section is

(A) Candida
(B) Histoplasma
(C) Cryptococcus
(D) Blastomyces

5 Which of the following reasons correctly explains why penicillin does not readily enter the central nervous system?

(A) It is highly lipid-soluble
(B) Low blood flow to the brain limits its access to this organ
(C) Astrocyte projections serve as a barrier to reduce its penetration
(D) Tight interendothelial cell junctions serve as a site of resistance to its entry to the brain
(E) It is a weak acid (pKa < 3) and thus is primarily unionized in plasma

6 The conversion of glucose to glucose-6-phosphate is a key step in the utilization of glucose. In muscle and fat cells, this step is catalyzed by which of the following enzymes?

(A) Glycogen synthase
(B) Hexokinase
(C) Phosphoglucomutase
(D) Glucokinase
(E) Glucose transporter (GLUT) 4

7 An infant who appeared normal at birth begins to develop hepatomegaly, congestive heart failure, and hypotonia at 9 months of age. Despite intensive medical care, shortly afterward the infant dies of cardiopulmonary failure. A muscle biopsy reveals vacuoles that stain positively for glycogen, and cultured skin fibroblasts show absence or reduced activity of α-1,4-glucosidase. Based on the information provided, which of the following is the most likely diagnosis?

(A) Amylopectinosis
(B) Her's disease
(C) McArdle's disease
(D) Pompe's disease
(E) von Gierke's disease

8 Which of the following embryonic structures gives rise to the ileum and ascending colon?

(A) Vitelline duct
(B) Midgut
(C) Foregut
(D) Hindgut
(E) Cloaca

9 Which of the following brain structures is derived from the mesencephalon?

(A) Pons
(B) Hippocampus
(C) Basal ganglia
(D) Pulvinar
(E) Superior colliculus

10 Which of the following drugs is a popular treatment for chronic asthma, especially when asthmatic symptoms cannot be controlled with adrenergic agents?

(A) Amitriptyline
(B) Phenylephrine
(C) Theophylline
(D) Thalidomide
(E) Tolbutamide

11 Which of the following drugs is a hallucinogen, acting on glutamate receptors, and is an analog of ketamine?

(A) Lysergic acid diethylamide (LSD)
(B) Amphetamine
(C) Mescaline
(D) Phencyclidine
(E) Phenobarbital

12 A 55-year-old woman dies of septicemia after going to the emergency department with severe abdominal pain. She lost 30 lb in the past 2 months and complained of severe pain after meals. Postmortem findings include severe aortic atherosclerosis and a segment of necrotic bowel extending from the splenic flexure to the sigmoid colon. A blockage in which of the following arteries would best support these findings?

(A) Common iliac arteries
(B) Common hepatic artery
(C) Superior mesenteric artery
(D) Inferior mesenteric artery
(E) Splenic artery

13 A patient is taken to the emergency department with pinpoint pupils, a respiratory rate of 8/minute, and a heart rate of 56 bpm. He is largely unresponsive to external stimuli. Which of the following pharmacologic interventions is most appropriate at this time?

(A) Intravenous administration of epinephrine
(B) Intravenous administration of naloxone
(C) Intravenous administration of sodium bicarbonate
(D) Intramuscular administration of insulin
(E) Intravenous administration of lorazepam

14 Alkaptonuria is a rare disorder of tyrosine catabolism characterized by dark urine and arthritis. Which one of the following enzymes is deficient in patients with this disorder?

(A) Homocysteine methyl transferase
(B) Tyrosinase
(C) Homogentisic acid oxidase
(D) Phenylalanine hydroxylase
(E) Dihydropteridine reductase

15 Which of the following treatments of epilepsy is also useful in the treatment of bipolar disorder?

(A) Ethosuximide
(B) Phenobarbital
(C) Phenytoin
(D) Gabapentin
(E) Carbamazepine

16 Which of the following statements about autoregulation of the glomerular filtration rate (GFR) is true?

(A) A decrease in the glomerular filtration rate leads to an increase in NaCl concentration at the macula densa
(B) A decrease in arterial pressure leads to a decrease in renin secretion
(C) Angiotensin II regulates efferent arteriolar resistance
(D) A decrease in NaCl concentration at the macula densa increases afferent arteriolar resistance
(E) An increase in NaCl concentration at the macula densa decreases angiotensin II synthesis

17 Which of the following can lead to prerenal acute renal failure (ARF)?

(A) Hypervolemia
(B) High cardiac output
(C) Systemic vasodilation
(D) Selective renal vasodilation
(E) Ureteric obstruction

18 Which of the following drugs, in addition to being a natural product, is an alkylating agent because it is reduced in the cell and alkylates DNA?

(A) Cyclophosphamide
(B) 5-Fluorouracil
(C) Cytarabine
(D) Vincristine
(E) Mitomycin

19 The parents of the boy indicated with an arrow in this pedigree are seeking genetic counseling because the boy's father and several of his relatives have a genetic disease (shaded in pedigree). This disease causes severe symptoms beginning at about 10 years of age. Their youngest child is now 6 years old, and they would like to know what the chances are that this boy has the disease. The boy and several family members have been tested for a marker of the disease-causing locus that has a θ-value of 0.01. The results are shown below the individuals in the pedigree. What should the family be told about the mode of inheritance and the likelihood that their son is affected?

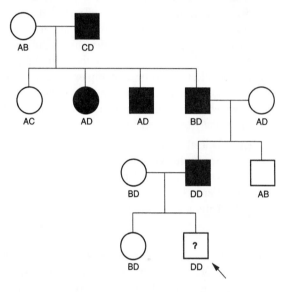

(A) Autosomal dominant, with a probability of 1 that the boy is affected
(B) Autosomal dominant, with a probability of 0.49 that the boy is affected
(C) Autosomal dominant, with a probability of 0.50 that the boy is affected
(D) Autosomal dominant, with a probability of 0.51 that the boy is affected
(E) Autosomal recessive, with a probability of 0.49 that the boy is affected

20 Which of the following is most likely to cause respiratory alkalosis?

(A) Overventilation
(B) Chronic obstructive pulmonary disease
(C) Pulmonary fibrosis
(D) Muscular dystrophy
(E) Myasthenia gravis

21 A 53-year-old woman complains of bilateral loss of sensation in her hands. Neurologic testing shows loss of both pain and temperature sensation in the arms and shoulders. Magnetic resonance imaging indicates a central cavitation in the spinal cord at C5–T5. Which of the following is the most likely diagnosis?

(A) Multiple sclerosis
(B) Guillain–Barré syndrome
(C) Amyotrophic lateral sclerosis
(D) Syringomyelia
(E) Tabes dorsalis

22 A 62-year-old man has lost tactile, position, and joint discrimination and has hyporeflexia in the legs. He also complains of paresthesias and pain in all of these areas. Serologic tests confirm immunoglobulin (Ig) M and IgG antibodies against the cardiolipin–lecithin–cholesterol antigen complex. Based on these findings, he is diagnosed with tabes dorsalis. Lesions to which of the following areas of the spinal cord are most likely to be seen?

(A) Dorsal spinocerebellar tract
(B) Fasciculus gracilis
(C) Lateral spinothalamic tract
(D) Ventral corticospinal tract
(E) Lateral corticospinal tract

23 The tumor depicted in Figure 67 of the color plate section occurred in a 45-year-old woman with hypertension and elevated urinary catecholamines. Which of the following statements is true of the tumor?

(A) This tumor is a frequent cause of hypertension among all hypertensive patients
(B) Half of these tumors occur in association with one of several familial syndromes
(C) Size and cellular pleomorphism are criteria used to distinguish benign and malignant forms of this tumor
(D) About 15% of tumors arise outside of the adrenal gland

24 According to this pedigree, which one of the following statements is true?

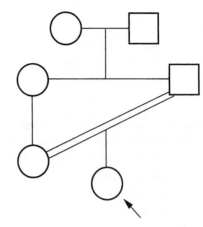

(A) The coefficient of inbreeding for the proband (*arrow*) is 1/8
(B) The coefficient of relatedness for the parents of the proband is 1/2
(C) The coefficient of relatedness for the parents of the proband is 1/8
(D) The coefficient of inbreeding cannot be determined without knowledge of the proband's genotype
(E) If the proband is homozygous at a particular locus, it must be identity by descent
(F) The coefficient of inbreeding of the proband equals the coefficient of relatedness of her parents

25 Ascorbic acid is a six-carbon ketolactone that is

(A) commonly known as vitamin D
(B) required for conversion of proline and lysine residues in procollagen to hydroxyproline and hydroxylysine
(C) synthesized from glucose via conversion of L-gulonolactone in humans
(D) the cause of beriberi
(E) adequately obtained from a diet with liver, meat, fish, or poultry

26 Which one of the following statements concerning smoking cessation is accurate?

(A) A patient who wants help will ask for it; otherwise, it is not useful to ask a patient about smoking

(B) If a patient is going to succeed in quitting, it will likely be in the first attempt with pharmacological treatment only

(C) Most smokers want to quit and have tried to quit at least once

(D) Both withdrawal symptoms and cravings for cigarettes last for several months after smoking cessation

(E) A patient should never quit smoking "cold turkey" but, rather, reduce the number of cigarettes gradually

27 Which one of the following statements about abnormalities that may be present at birth is correct?

(A) A malformation is an abnormality that is caused by intrauterine compression

(B) A cleft lip is a common example of a deformation

(C) Dysplasias are abnormalities of cells and tissues rather than organs; therefore, they rarely are due to a genetic defect

(D) Amniotic bands are an example of a disruption

(E) Associations have only one cause, whereas syndromes are thought to have multiple causes

28 Which one of the following statements about eating disorders is correct?

(A) The difference between anorexia nervosa and bulimia nervosa is that bulimia nervosa involves purging behavior, and anorexia nervosa does not

(B) A patient may be diagnosed with bulimia nervosa even if his or her weight is normal

(C) A patient may be diagnosed with anorexia nervosa even if his or her weight is normal

(D) Although more often diagnosed in women, anorexia nervosa is equally common in men

(E) Eating disorders are acquired conditions that are brought about by societal pressures, not genetic factors

29 Which of the following chemotherapeutic agents is correctly paired with one of its unique toxic effects?

(A) Doxorubicin—cardiac toxicity

(B) Bleomycin—renal toxicity

(C) Cyclophosphamide—pulmonary toxicity

(D) Vincristine—renal toxicity

(E) Methotrexate—neurotoxicity

30 Gingival hyperplasia is a side effect of which of the following antiepileptic drugs?

(A) Valproic acid

(B) Ethosuximide

(C) Phenobarbital

(D) Carbamazepine

(E) Phenytoin

31 Increased circulating levels of insulin trigger a decrease in the level of blood glucose. Which of the following enzymes would most likely be decreased in activity following the release of insulin into the blood?

(A) Protein phosphatase

(B) Glycogen synthase

(C) Glucose-6-phosphatase

(D) Glucokinase

(E) Hexokinase

32 Which of the following tissues cannot use fatty acids as a source of energy?

(A) Liver

(B) Brain

(C) Kidney

(D) Small intestine

(E) Heart

33 Which of the following mutations in a gene or chromosomal translocation is correctly paired with the cancer with which it is most typically associated?

(A) Breast cancer susceptibility (BRCA1) gene—colon cancer

(B) Retinoblastoma gene—pancreatic cancer

(C) t(9;22)(q34;q11) Translocation—acute lymphoblastic leukemia

(D) t(8;14)(q24;q32) Translocation—Burkitt's lymphoma

(E) t(8;21)(q22;q22) Translocation—breast cancer

34 Which of the following is true of the testicular lesion depicted in Figure 68 of the color plate section?

(A) The peak incidence of this lesion is in patients older than 50 years of age

(B) These lesion cells produce testosterone

(C) Tumors arise from a pluripotential cell within the testicular interstitium

(D) Patients with metastatic disease often respond to chemotherapy

35 Syphilis is caused by which one of the following infective agents?

(A) *Trichomonas vaginalis*

(B) *Trichinella spiralis*

(C) *Trypanosoma cruzi*

(D) *Treponema pallidum*

(E) *Trypanosoma gambiense*

36 The region of the brain that is most involved in problem solving is the

(A) parietal lobe

(B) frontal lobe

(C) temporal lobe

(D) cerebellum

(E) occipital lobe

37 Neuroleptic drugs have been shown to block postsynaptic dopamine 2 (D_2) receptors, and these drugs can impair lactation. Blockade of which of the following dopaminergic tracts underlies this impairment?

(A) Tuberoinfundibular tract

(B) Nigrostriatal tract

(C) Mesolimbic tract

(D) Medullary periventricular tract

(E) Incertohypothalamic tract

38 Ablation of the medial forebrain bundle would result in the depletion of which neurotransmitters in the cerebral cortex?

(A) Acetylcholine and dopamine

(B) γ-Aminobutyric acid (GABA) and glycine

(C) Nitric oxide

(D) Serotonin and catecholamines

(E) GABA and dopamine

39 A healthy person eats a meal. In several hours, which of the following tissues will receive lactate, fatty acids, and glycerol while producing and releasing glucose?

(A) Liver

(B) Skeletal muscle

(C) Kidney

(D) Small intestine

(E) Heart

40 A 15-year-old girl has a history of diarrhea, anorexia, and weight loss. She has also been missing her menstrual periods. An intestinal biopsy shows flat mucosa with a significant loss in the microvillus brush border; however, the overall mucosal thickness is maintained. After she starts a diet free of wheat, rye, oats, and barley, her condition greatly improves. Sensitivity to which of the following is most likely responsible for her condition?

(A) Phytol

(B) Monounsaturated fatty acids

(C) Papain

(D) Branched glycogen chains

(E) Gliadin

41 A patient with hypertension, hirsutism, amenorrhea, acne, and an excess of truncal fat with peripheral muscle wasting is referred to an endocrinologist for evaluation. The patient has never taken any form of steroids. The patient has increased levels of cortisol, which are not suppressed by exogenous dexamethasone. The plasma adrenocorticotropic hormone (ACTH) levels are elevated and are not suppressed by dexamethasone. Which of the following disorders is the most likely diagnosis?

(A) Addison's disease

(B) Waterhouse–Friderichsen syndrome

(C) Cushing's syndrome caused by a pituitary tumor

(D) Cushing's syndrome caused by an adrenal tumor

(E) Cushing's syndrome caused by ectopic production of ACTH

42 A pregnant woman has myotonic dystrophy. Her mother also had a mild form of the disease. The patient's symptoms include distal muscle weakness and a hatchet-faced appearance. There is no history of the disorder on her father's side of the family. The patient has two healthy children. Her ultrasound shows that the fetus is a boy. Which one of the following statements is correct?

(A) The fetus is not at risk for having myotonic dystrophy because it affects only females

(B) The fetus has a lower risk of having myotonic dystrophy because the two previous infants did not have the disease

(C) The fetus has a higher risk of having myotonic dystrophy because the two previous infants did not have the disease

(D) If the fetus has myotonic dystrophy, it is likely to be less severe than it is for his mother

(E) If the fetus has myotonic dystrophy, he has a high risk of being more severely affected than his mother

43 A nondiabetic 35-year-old patient has postprandial hypoglycemia. Which one of the following statements is most likely correct?

(A) The patient has insulinoma

(B) The insulin and C-peptide levels are the same; therefore, the patient has factitious hypoglycemia

(C) Alimentary hypoglycemia is consistent with this scenario

(D) An oral glucose tolerance test is required to determine the etiology of hypoglycemia

(E) The patient's history of alcohol abuse is unimportant because alcohol causes hyperglycemia, not hypoglycemia

44 A 38-year-old man complains of pain in his right big toe and ankle. His toe and ankle are erythematous and swollen. The night before he had a large meal, including a steak and "a few" glasses of wine. In the middle of the night he awoke with severe pain. Which one of the following statements is correct?

(A) The patient has pseudogout rather than acute gouty arthritis

(B) That the patient ingested alcohol the previous night makes a diagnosis of acute gouty arthritis less likely because alcohol speeds the excretion of uric acid

(C) This patient will likely develop tophi in the next few weeks

(D) One would expect the synovial fluid to display needle-shaped negatively birefringent crystals under polarized light

(E) Treatment must be administered as soon as possible; otherwise, the patient's symptoms will continue indefinitely

45 Surgical treatment for Parkinson's disease is usually reserved for patients in whom antiparkinsonism drugs are ineffective or poorly tolerated and whose symptoms are particularly severe. Ablation of a subset of inputs into which of the following brain structures accomplishes a relief of the symptoms?

(A) Subthalamic nucleus

(B) Globus pallidus externa

(C) Globus pallidus interna

(D) Substantia nigra pars compacta

(E) Caudate nucleus

46 When the head turns, the eyes shift in the direction opposite to the head motion. Which of the following structures plays an important role in the coordination of compensatory conjugate eye movements during head rotation?

(A) Dorsal medullary raphe

(B) Medial lemniscus

(C) Lateral geniculate

(D) Medial longitudinal fasciculus

(E) Reticular formation

47 Which of the following statements about bile is true?

(A) Bile production by hepatocytes requires the presence of cholecystokinin

(B) Bile salts are hydrophilic

(C) Bile acids are produced by conjugation of taurine or glycine to bile salts

(D) The terminal duodenum actively transports bile acids out of the intestinal lumen, allowing them to be recirculated to the liver

(E) A critical function of the gallbladder is to concentrate the bile

48 Which one of the following statements about energy storage and transfer is true?

(A) Adenosine triphosphate (ATP) can be synthesized from adenosine diphosphate (ADP) by phosphate transfer from 3-phosphoglycerate

(B) Phosphocreatine is an important energy source for muscle tissues

(C) Reactions that have a K_{eq} above 1 have a positive $\Delta G°$

(D) When ATP is hydrolyzed to adenosine monophosphate (AMP) and inorganic pyrophosphate (PP_i), the reaction is endergonic and proceeds spontaneously

(E) The energy of hydrolysis for phosphoenolpyruvate is less than that for pyrophosphate

49 Which of the following statements concerning action potentials recorded simultaneously from the illustrated slow and fast myocardial fibers is correct?

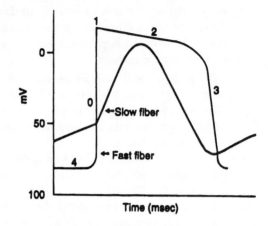

(A) The fast fiber is likely to be present in sinoatrial or atrioventricular nodes

(B) The slow fiber is typical of either atrial or ventricular myocardial cells

(C) In the fast fiber, *phase 0* is caused by opening of K1 channels

(D) In the fast fiber, *phase 2* coincides with an increase in conductance to Ca^21

(E) Application of acetylcholine (ACh) increases the slope of *phase 4* of the slow fiber

50 In a family with myotonic dystrophy, the father has frontal balding, severe weakness, and cardiac arrhythmia; his sister has early-onset cataracts; and his child has electromyographic abnormalities. Which of the following terms most accurately describes this pattern of inheritance?

(A) Consanguinity

(B) Variable expressivity

(C) Locus heterogeneity

(D) Nonpenetrance

(E) Allelic heterogeneity

Answer Key

1-D	11-D	21-D	31-C	41-E
2-D	12-D	22-B	32-B	42-E
3-C	13-B	23-D	33-D	43-C
4-D	14-C	24-A	34-D	44-D
5-D	15-E	25-B	35-D	45-C
6-B	16-C	26-C	36-B	46-D
7-D	17-C	27-D	37-A	47-E
8-B	18-E	28-B	38-D	48-B
9-E	19-C	29-A	39-A	49-D
10-C	20-A	30-E	40-E	50-B

Answers and Explanations

1 **The answer is D** *Central and peripheral nervous system / Neuroanatomy / Motor neuron lesions*

Upper and lower motor neuron lesions each cause paralysis; however, these conditions do not share other clinical findings. Upper motor neuron lesions are associated with spastic paralysis, hyperreflexia, and a positive Babinski reflex (i.e., dorsiflexion of the great toe accompanied by fanning of other toes in response to stroking of the lateral aspects of the sole of the foot). In contrast, the Babinski reflex is absent in lower motor neuron lesions, which are characterized by flaccid paralysis, fasciculations and fibrillations, significant muscle atrophy, and hyporeflexia. Atrophy, fasciculations, and fibrillations are absent in upper motor neuron lesions.

2 **The answer is D** *Hematopoietic and lymphoreticular system / Pathology / Chronic myelogenous leukemia*

Chronic myelogenous leukemia (CML) has a peak incidence in middle-aged people. Patients typically present with a very large spleen and low level of leukocyte alkaline phosphatase. CML is most often characterized by a 9;22 chromosome translocation, which places the c-abl proto-oncogene from chromosome 9 next to the bcr region of chromosome 22. The resulting hybrid bcr-abl gene codes for constitutively active tyrosine kinase.

3 **The answer is C** *General principles / Genetics / Inherited disorders*

A disorder is said to be nonpenetrant when there is no clinical evidence of a mutant allele in a person known to have inherited the gene. The form of gene expression may be highly variable, with some family members being severely affected and others having few signs of the disorder. This common feature of autosomal disorders is called variable expression. Different mutations of either the same gene (i.e., at the same locus) or different genes may give a similar clinical picture. Consanguineous individuals have a proportion of their genes in common by inheritance from a common ancestor. In some villages founded by few settlers, disease alleles may occur in higher frequencies, and a particular recessive disorder may be common in that community.

4 **The answer is D** *General principles / Pathology / Blastomyces*

Blastomycosis is a systemic (deep) mycosis (i.e., it is a noncommunicable fungal infection involving internal organs that occur in immunocompetent patients). Other deep mycoses include histoplasmosis, coccidioidomycosis, and paracoccidioidomycosis. Deep mycoses are contrasted with opportunistic mycoses (i.e., fungal infections predominantly affecting immunocompromised hosts, such as candidiasis, cryptococcosis, aspergillosis, and mucormycosis). The typical portal of entry of deep mycoses is via the respiratory tract through the inhalation of spores.

Blastomycosis is caused by *Blastomyces dermatitidis,* whose natural reservoir is soil or decaying vegetation, mainly in the Mississippi valley. The organism is dimorphic. It exists as fine septate hyphae with round to oval conidia in fungal culture and as large (8 to 15 μm), thick-walled yeasts with an internal substructure and broad-based budding in tissue. In tissue, the organism elicits an intense inflammatory reaction with microabscesses, granulomatous inflammation, tissue destruction, and scarring. Primary infectious presentations include primary pulmonary blastomycosis (mild pulmonary infection with progressive reactivity to skin antigens), advanced pulmonary disease (fever, productive cough, and chest pain associated with pulmonary nodules and hilar adenopathy), and primary cutaneous lesions caused by direct inoculation of the organism into the skin. In some patients, the disease may disseminate hematogenously to the internal organs (e.g., genitourinary tract, bone) and skin. Therapy (e.g., with ketoconazole, amphotericin B) is usually restricted to patients with progressive pulmonary disease and disseminated infection.

Candidiasis is a common opportunistic mycosis and is usually the result of an autoinfection that arises in patients with metabolic (e.g., diabetes) or immunologic disturbances. Clinical presentations include superficial, mucocutaneous, and systemic (i.e., deep) infections. The organism occurs as budding yeasts (4 to 6 μm) and pseudohyphae in patients; the latter form is seen with tissue invasion. Histoplasmosis is a deep mycosis caused by *Histoplasma capsulatum,* a small (3 to 4 μm) yeast in tissue that exists free or as an intracellular pathogen in macrophages. Histoplasmosis, similar to blastomycosis, has both primary pulmonary and disseminated forms.

Cryptococcosis is an opportunistic mycosis caused by *Cryptococcus neoformans,* an encapsulated yeast with narrow-based budding. Primary pulmonary disease and disseminated disease (associated with meningitis) are recognized. The thick polysaccharide capsule exudes India ink (India ink test on cerebrospinal fluid) and stains positively with a mucicarmine stain. The organism exists both free and within macrophages.

5 **The answer is D** *Central and peripheral nervous system / Pharmacology / Blood–brain barrier*

Penicillin is a highly water-soluble weak acid that is primarily ionized in plasma and does not cross plasma membranes very readily. Accordingly, its penetration into the brain is greatly limited by the blood–brain barrier. This barrier exists by virtue of tight interendothelial cell junctions that result in a greatly reduced permeability compared with other organs. Although astrocyte projections are intimately involved with the cerebral endothelium, microscopic tracer studies have clearly indicated that they are not the site of resistance. Blood flow to the brain is high when normalized to brain weight or volume, and thus brain blood flow is never a limiting aspect of transport of small molecules.

6 **The answer is B** *General principles / Biochemistry / Glucose-6-phosphate metabolites*

Hexokinase is found in muscle and fat cells and catalyzes the conversion of glucose to glucose-6-phosphate. This same reaction is also catalyzed by glucokinase, which is the insulin-responsive form of this enzyme found in liver cells. Glycogen synthase facilitates the transfer of glucose from uridine diphosphate–glucose to a nonreducing end of a glycogen fragment. Phosphoglucomutase is involved in the reversible conversion of glucose-6-phosphate into glucose-1-phosphate. In muscle and fat cells, GLUT-4 is the plasma membrane transporter that is responsible for glucose import.

7 **The answer is D** *General principles / Biochemistry / Glycogen storage disorders*

Pompe's disease is characterized by a deficiency of α-1,4-glucosidase (acid maltase), which results in the accumulation of glycogen in vacuoles in the liver, heart, and muscle tissue. In its most severe form, infants have muscle weakness, macroglossia, hepatomegaly, and congestive heart failure, and death often occurs before 2 years of age. In its juvenile-onset form, difficulty in walking, proximal muscle weakness, and respiratory muscle impairment may lead to early death. Amylopectinosis is caused by a deficiency in branching enzyme, whereas McArdle's disease and Her's disease are caused by deficiencies in glycogen phosphorylase isozymes in the muscle and liver, respectively. Von Gierke's disease results from a deficiency of glucose-6-phosphatase.

8 **The answer is B** *Gastrointestinal system / Embryology / Embryonic structures*

The midgut forms the distal small intestine, including most of the duodenum, all of the jejunum, and all of the ileum, as well as the ascending and proximal transverse colon. The cloaca is a hindgut derivative that receives the excurrent ducts of the urinary and reproductive systems. The vitelline duct is a midgut diverticulum that projects into the umbilicus and serves as the axis of rotation of the midgut loop along with the superior mesenteric artery.

9 **The answer is E** *Central and peripheral nervous system / Neuroanatomy / Development of the midbrain*

The mesencephalon, or midbrain, contains the tectum, tegmentum, superior and inferior colliculi, and substantia nigra. The hippocampus and the basal ganglia are telencephalic structures; the pulvinar is a thalamic nucleus and therefore a diencephalic structure. The pons is part of the metencephalon.

10 **The answer is C** *Respiratory system / Pharmacology / Treatment for chronic asthma*

Theophylline is a methylxanthine that acts as a bronchodilator. Although it was once believed that this class of drug worked by inhibiting phosphodiesterase and thus raising levels of cyclic adenosine monophosphate (cAMP), recent evidence suggests that this is not case, and the mechanism of action of these drugs is unknown. Amitriptyline is a tricyclic antidepressant; phenylephrine is an α-agonist that is useful in increasing blood pressure during shock; tolbutamide is an older medication that is useful in diabetes. Thalidomide is a hypnotic that is banned from use during pregnancy because of gross limb-deforming birth defects in the fetus, but it is effective for the treatment of leprosy.

11 **The answer is D** *General principles / Pharmacology / Hallucinogens*

Lysergic acid diethylamide (LSD) acts as a direct agonist at a subset of serotonin receptors. Amphetamine can cause the direct release of catecholamines, especially norepinephrine. Mescaline is a hallucinogenic drug, but it is chemically different from ketamine. Phenobarbital is not a hallucinogen; it acts through activation of GABA receptors. Phencyclidine, an analog of ketamine, is a hallucinogen, acting on glutamate receptors.

12 **The answer is D** *Cardiovascular system / Anatomy / Blockage of the inferior mesenteric artery*

A blockage of the inferior mesenteric artery that supplies the distal third of the transverse colon, descending colon, sigmoid colon, and upper portion of the rectum is most likely responsible for the pattern of necrosis seen in this patient. The common iliac arteries supply the pelvis, perineum, and leg. The celiac trunk gives rise to the left gastric artery, splenic artery, and common hepatic artery, which supply the esophagus, stomach, duodenum, liver, gallbladder, and pancreas. The superior mesenteric artery provides the blood supply to the duodenum, jejunum, ileum, cecum, appendix, ascending colon, and proximal two-thirds of transverse colon.

13 **The answer is B** *General principles / Pharmacology / Opiate overdose*

This patient is showing classic signs of opioid overdose. The pharmacologic treatment of choice is naloxone, an opioid antagonist. Lorazepam would have devastating depressive effects in this patient. Although epinephrine may transiently elevate heart rate and respiratory rate, it does not treat the underlying cause. Sodium bicarbonate and insulin would not be helpful for this patient.

14 **The answer is C** *General principles / Pathology / Alkaptonuria*

Alkaptonuria is caused by a deficiency of homogentisic acid oxidase that leads to excretion of homogentisic acid in the urine, hence dark urine. In addition, high blood levels of homogentisic acid eventually get oxidized and bind collagen fibers, leading to painful arthritis. Homocysteine methyltransferase converts homocysteine to methionine using a methyl moiety from methyltetrahydrofolate, which is converted to tetrahydrofolate. Defects in this enzyme can cause megaloblastic anemia. Defects in tyrosinase lead to albinism and hypopigmentation. Defects in phenylalanine hydroxylase and dihydropteridine reductase cause phenylketonuria.

15 **The answer is E** *Central and peripheral nervous system / Pharmacology / Treatment for epilepsy; treatment for bipolar disorder*

Carbamazepine, like valproic acid, is useful for the treatment of seizure disorders and bipolar disorder.

16 **The answer is C** *Renal/urinary system / Physiology / Autoregulation of GFR*

The glomerular filtration rate (GFR) is kept within a narrow range despite changes in arterial blood pressure by a specialized tubuloglomerular feedback mechanism. This mechanism is implemented by a special anatomic structure called the juxtaglomerular apparatus, which consists of the macula densa cells in the initial portion of the distal tubule and juxtaglomerular cells in the walls of afferent and efferent arterioles. Tubuloglomerular feedback has two components: regulation of afferent arteriolar resistance and regulation of efferent arteriolar resistance. A drop in arterial blood pressure decreases hydrostatic pressure in the glomerulus, thus leading to a decrease in GFR. Macula densa cells move to correct a drop in GFR in two ways. First, they decrease resistance in the afferent arteriole, which increases blood flow to the glomerulus and restores glomerular hydrostatic pressure. Second, they stimulate renin release from the juxtaglomerular cells. Renin, in turn, leads to angiotensin II synthesis. Angiotensin II constricts the efferent arteriole, thus also acting to restore glomerular hydrostatic pressure and GFR.

17 **The answer is C** *Renal/urinary system / Pathology / Etiology of prerenal acute renal failure*

Prerenal acute renal failure (ARF) is the most common form of kidney failure in the United States. It is the generalized response of the kidneys to renal hypoperfusion. Four general processes lead to prerenal ARF: hypovolemia, low cardiac output, systemic vasodilation, and selective renal vasoconstriction. Ureteric obstruction produces postrenal ARF. Thus, any disease entity with any of these properties can result in the decrease and shutdown of blood flow to the kidneys.

18 **The answer is E** *General principles / Pharmacology / Anticancer drug action*

Mitomycin is both a natural product and an alkylating agent. Isolated from a *Streptomyces* species, mitomycin C is reduced by a reduced nicotinamide adenine dinucleotide phosphate-dependent reductase and alkylates DNA. Cytarabine inhibits DNA polymerase and thus kills cells in S phase. Cytarabine nucleotides can be incorporated into DNA and RNA, but the significance of this is not known. Vincristine, a natural product, is an M-phase-specific agent, blocking proliferating cells as the enter metaphase. Cyclophosphamide must be oxidized and activated by cytochrome P450 while the pyrimidine, 5-fluorouracil, must be anabolized to the nucleotide to be active.

19 **The answer is C** *General principles / Genetics / Pedigree analysis*

The mode of inheritance is autosomal dominant. It does not skip generations, and it can be passed from a father to a son or a daughter. The marker that was used is uninformative in this case because it cannot be determined which of the father's alleles was given to the son. The fact that there is a recombination frequency of 1% (θ-value = 0.01) does not affect the probabilities in this case. The son has inherited either the mutant allele of the gene or the normal allele, but it is not known which one. Thus, the probability that he is affected remains the same as before the testing, at 0.50.

20 **The answer is A** *Respiratory system / Physiology / Acid–base disorders*

Respiratory acidosis is characterized by a primary increase in P_{CO_2}, with a compensatory increase in HCO_3^-. The increased P_{CO_2} occurs as a result of decreased alveolar gas exchange. This decreased gas exchange may occur by decreased ventilation (e.g., iatrogenic, narcotic use, cerebrovascular accidents, muscular dystrophy, myasthenia gravis), airway obstruction (e.g., chronic obstructive pulmonary disease, tumor, acute asthma attack), and decreased gas diffusion (e.g., pulmonary fibrosis, massive pulmonary edema, severe pneumonia, pleural effusions).

Respiratory alkalosis is characterized by a primary decrease in P_{CO_2}, with a compensatory decrease in HCO_3^-. The decreased P_{CO_2} results from increased ventilation from either central or peripheral causes or from iatrogenic overventilation. Central causes of hyperventilation include head trauma, cerebrovascular accidents, pain, anxiety, fever (sepsis), and tumors. Peripheral causes include congestive heart failure, pulmonary embolism, mild pulmonary edema, high altitude, and hypoxemia.

21 **The answer is D** *Central and peripheral nervous system / Neuroanatomy / Spinal cord lesions*

Syringomyelia involves progressive cavitation of the central spinal cord or lower brainstem, classically resulting in loss of pain and temperature sensations. This loss of sensation is caused by the destruction of decussating pain fibers in the anterior white commissure.

22 **The answer is B** *Central and peripheral nervous system / Neuroanatomy / Spinal cord lesions*

Tabes dorsalis (locomotor ataxia) is a neurologic manifestation of tertiary syphilis and is associated with degeneration of the posterior columns, which include the fasciculus gracilis and fasciculus cuneatus. Clinical findings in the tabes dorsalis include the progressive loss of peripheral reflexes, loss of joint position (ataxia), and "lightning" pain in the extremities. Other neurologic manifestations of tertiary syphilis include chronic meningitis (meningitic neurosyphilis) and cerebral atrophy, which causes progressive dementia (paretic neurosyphilis).

23 **The answer is D** *Endocrine system / Pathology / Pheochromocytoma arising in the adrenal gland*

The paraganglion system includes neural crest-derived structures (i.e., adrenal medulla and extra-adrenal autonomic nervous system synaptic nodules) producing a variety of catecholamines that are secreted into the blood or that function as neurotransmitters. Neuroendocrine neoplasms originating in the paraganglion system include pheochromocytomas, neuroblastomas, and ganglioneuromas. Pheochromocytomas cause catecholamine-induced hypertension and account for 0.1% to 0.3% of cases of hypertension. Most pheochromocytomas (85%) arise in the adrenal medulla; the remaining 15% occur in the extra-adrenal paraganglia. Approximately 90% are sporadic, and 10% occur in association with one of several sporadic syndromes, such as multiple endocrine neoplasia (MEN) IIA (e.g., medullary thyroid carcinoma, pheochromocytoma, parathyroid hyperplasia), MEN IIB (e.g., MEN IIA plus mucosal neuromas), von Hippel–Lindau syndrome (e.g., renal, hepatic, pancreatic, epididymal cysts; renal cell carcinoma, cerebellar hemangioblastoma, angiomatosis), neurofibromatosis type I (e.g., neurofibromas, café au lait spots, schwannomas, meningiomas, gliomas, pheochromocytomas), and Sturge–Weber syndrome (cavernous hemangiomas of the fifth cranial nerve distribution, pheochromocytoma). Sporadic pheochromocytomas are usually solitary (85%), have a peak incidence between 40 and 60 years of age, and show a slight female predominance. Approximately 70% of familial tumors are bilateral; many arise in a background of adrenal medullary hyperplasia. Tumors range from 1 g to 4 kg, with a mean of 100 g.

Pheochromocytomas are typically gray-pink to brown and lobular; hemorrhage, necrosis, and cyst formation occur in larger tumors. Dichromate fixatives cause a brown-black color reaction owing to oxidation of stored catecholamines (i.e., chromaffin reaction). Microscopically, the tumor consists of basophilic polygonal to spindled paraganglionic cells arranged in nests and trabeculae. These cells are intimately associated with small spindled supportive cells (i.e., sustentacular cells), and individual nests are separated by a rich capillary vascular network. The neoplastic cells stain with neuroendocrine markers (i.e., synaptophysin and chromogranin) owing to the presence of cytoplasmic neurosecretory granules. Malignant behavior occurs in 2% to 10% of adrenal tumors and 20% to 40% of extra-adrenal paragangliomas. The only reliable criterion for malignancy is metastasis; cellular pleomorphism, local invasiveness, and microvascular tumor emboli do not predict malignancy. Patients with pheochromocytoma have intermittent or sustained hypertension with or without paroxysms (i.e., periods of sudden release of catecholamines resulting in headache, diaphoresis, nausea, vomiting, abdominal pain, fatigue, visual alterations). Pheochromocytomas are associated with catecholamine cardiomyopathy (i.e., ischemic myocardial injury secondary to catecholamine-induced vasomotor constriction of the coronary circulation or direct catecholamine toxicity, resulting in myocyte injury or necrosis, inflammation, and fibrosis). Laboratory evaluation for pheochromocytoma includes an assessment of urinary metanephrine and vanillylmandelic acid.

24 **The answer is A** *General principles / Genetics / Inbreeding*

There are several methods to determine the coefficients of inbreeding and relatedness from the pedigree. First, determine the coefficient of relatedness of the proband's parent; this term is used to describe the probability that two people share an allele with identity by descent (IBD). Because a brother and sister have half of their alleles in common, a niece and uncle (as are the parents in this case) would share 1/4 of their alleles IBD because the niece would have half of her mother's alleles IBD. Then the coefficient of inbreeding can be calculated, because it is equal to half of the coefficient of relatedness of the parents. The genotypes are not required for these calculations. If a person is homozygous at a locus, it is not necessarily IBD; it could be identity by state, meaning that the same allele was inherited from separate sources and not a common ancestor.

25 The answer is B *General principles / Biochemistry / Nutrition*

Ascorbic acid or vitamin C cannot be synthesized from precursor glucose in humans (or nonhuman primates and guinea pigs and some bats) and thus must be a critical part of the diet. It is readily obtained from citrus fruits as well as potatoes and other food sources. Ascorbic acid is a cofactor in hydroxylation (and amidation reactions) and is particularly important in collagen synthesis. A deficiency in dietary ascorbic acid leads to scurvy, a disorder typified by defect in collagen synthesis (wound healing defects, rupture of capillaries). The disorder can be treated by ingestion of citrus fruits; orange and lemon juice are particularly good sources, and 60 mg per day is the daily recommended dose for adults. Beriberi is the result of vitamin B_1 (thiamine) deficiency. Deficiencies in nicotinic acid cause pellagra. Nicotinic acid can be maintained by adequate ingestion of animal proteins (in which tryptophan is an important precursor).

26 The answer is C *General principles / Behavioral science / Smoking cessation*

Most smokers wish to quit, and most have tried. Most are unsuccessful in their first attempt; however, many people eventually succeed in quitting long-term. On average, it takes approximately three attempts to quit. It is critical to ask about a patient's smoking habits, because many people who want to quit and who want help will not mention it unless asked. Although cravings may last for a long time, withdrawal symptoms normally abate within 2 weeks. Pharmacologic treatment may be useful, particularly in patients who have withdrawal symptoms, but behavioral counseling is still required to give the person the best chance of succeeding. Quitting "cold turkey" works better than gradual reduction. In fact, a person who is cutting down may be smoking fewer cigarettes but inhaling more deeply and more frequently, thereby providing the same amount of nicotine.

27 The answer is D *General principles / Genetics / Abnormalities of morphogenesis*

Malformations are due to intrinsic processes, and they include abnormalities (e.g., cleft lip). Dysplasias often have genetic causes, but they involve abnormalities of cells or tissues rather than organs (e.g., phacomatoses). Deformations and disruptions are caused by extrinsic factors (e.g., compression and teratogens, respectively). Examples include clubfoot (deformation) and amniotic bands (disruption). A syndrome is a pattern of abnormalities with one cause, whereas an association does not have a single cause.

28 The answer is B *General principles / Behavioral science / Eating disorders*

A diagnosis of bulimia nervosa does not require that the person be below a normal body weight, but it does involve binge eating and compensatory behaviors. The compensatory behaviors may include purging by self-induced vomiting, laxative abuse, and other behavior (e.g., fasting and excessive exercise). A diagnosis of anorexia nervosa is made only when a person's weight is at or below 85% of the ideal and the person has unrealistic concerns about gaining weight. The person may or may not engage in binging and purging. Anorexia nervosa and bulimia nervosa are more common in women than in men, usually with an onset in late adolescence or early adulthood. Although social factors play a role in the development of eating disorders, genetic factors are also important, as concordance rates are higher in monozygotic than dizygotic twins.

29 The answer is A *General principles / Pharmacology / Toxic effects of anticancer drugs*

Doxorubicin administration is limited by cardiac toxicity in high doses. Bleomycin can cause a chronic interstitial pneumonitis in high doses. Cyclophosphamide can cause hemorrhagic cystitis. Vincristine can be neurotoxic, and methotrexate can cause severe gastrointestinal toxicity and bone marrow hypoplasia.

30 The answer is E *General principles / Pharmacology / Side effects of phenytoin*

Gingival hyperplasia is a known side effect of phenytoin and cyclosporine.

31 **The answer is C** *General principles / Biochemistry / Organs and tissues in the postabsorptive state*

Release of insulin by the pancreas helps to decrease the level of blood glucose. Glucose-6-phosphatase converts glucose-6-phosphate into glucose, which can be released into the bloodstream. Its activity is inhibited by insulin. The reverse reaction is catalyzed by glucokinase, whose activity is stimulated by insulin. Hexokinase also converts glucose into glucose-6-phosphate, but its activity is not directly controlled by insulin. Protein phosphatase, which converts glycogen synthase to the active, dephosphorylated state, and glycogen synthase activities are both upregulated by the release of insulin into the bloodstream.

32 **The answer is B** *General principles / Biochemistry / Organs and tissues in the postabsorptive state*

Red blood cells and brain tissue do not use fatty acids as energy sources. Red blood cells lack mitochondria, and fatty acids cannot cross the blood–brain barrier for oxidation, so both of these tissues depend on glucose for their energy needs. All other tissues, including liver, kidney, small intestine, and heart tissue readily use fatty acids as fuel for their homeostatic functions.

33 **The answer is D** *General principles / Pathology / Gene mutations and chromosomal translocations*

t(8;14)(q24;q32) translocations are associated with Burkitt's lymphoma; they involve the production of a fusion protein between c-myc and an Ig heavy chain. Breast cancer susceptibility gene mutations—BRCA1 and BRCA2—have been strongly implicated in both breast and ovarian cancers. Retinoblastoma mutations are the primary etiological event in the development of retinoblastoma and osteosarcoma. t(9;22)(q34;q11) translocations, also known as the Philadelphia chromosome, result in production of a fusion protein, BCR-ABL, which is involved in the development of chronic myelogenous leukemia. The t(8;21)(q22;q22) translocation is associated with acute myelogenous leukemia (M2).

34 **The answer is D** *Reproductive system / Pathology / Mixed malignant germ cell tumor with seminoma and embryonal carcinoma*

Approximately 95% of all primary testicular neoplasms originate in germ cells; the remainder include stromal or sex cord, hematolymphoid, and mesenchymal tumors. Germ cell tumors typically occur in people aged 15 to 34 years and may arise in gonadal or extragonadal locations (i.e., extragonadal tumors arise in midline locations corresponding to the embryologic migratory route of germ cells). The precursor lesion in testicular germ cell tumors is intratubular germ cell neoplasia, an in situ germ cell neoplasm arising from transformed pluripotential germ cells and confined to the seminiferous tubule. Neoplastic progression results in tumor cell invasion into the interstitium, with access to blood vessels and lymphatics leading to metastasis in some patients. Neoplastic germ cells recapitulate all lines of normal germ cell differentiation.

Tumors with spermatocytic differentiation are classified as seminomas; the classic (i.e., most common) type consists of monotonous discohesive cells with clear glycogen-containing cytoplasm and nuclei with single prominent nucleoli. The alternative pathway of differentiation gives rise to the nonseminomatous germ cell tumors (NSGCTs). The least differentiated NSGCT is embryonal carcinoma, which consists of high-grade cohesive tumor cells that grow in glandular, alveolar, and papillary patterns. Somatic differentiation results in teratomas, which are disorganized collections of mature or immature somatic tissues that represent more than one of the three germ layers (i.e., ectoderm, mesoderm, endoderm). Yolk sac differentiation gives rise to a yolk sac tumor (e.g., endodermal sinus tumor), a histologically heterogeneous tumor that recapitulates the embryonic yolk sac. A yolk sac tumor is often associated with an elevation in serum α-fetoprotein. Choriocarcinoma, the most aggressive of the germ cell tumor subtypes, corresponds with placental differentiation; the tumor consists of cytotrophoblasts and syncytiotrophoblasts and is often associated with elevation in the serum β-human chorionic gonadotropin hormone level. Approximately 40% of malignant germ cell tumors have a single histologic pattern, whereas 60% are a mixture of two or more patterns.

Clinically, it is most important to distinguish seminomas from tumors that contain nonseminomatous components. Pure classic seminomas (i.e., 30% of all germ cell tumors) are relatively unaggressive tumors and are radiosensitive; 70% are testicle-confined. Metastasis is typically lymphatic and initially involves retroperitoneal lymph nodes. NSGCTs are metastatic in 60% of patients at presentation. These tumors metastasize via lymphatic and hematogenous routes and are radioresistant, but they usually respond to aggressive chemotherapy (i.e., 80% to 85% achieve complete remission). Isochromosome 12p is a common cytogenetic abnormality that is present in germ cell tumors.

35 **The answer is D** *General principles / Microbiology / Syphilis*

Treponema pallidum causes syphilis. This organism multiplies at the site of inoculation and then spreads widely via the bloodstream. No toxins or virulence factors are known for this organism. *Trichomonas vaginalis* causes trichomoniasis, *Trichinella spiralis* causes trichinosis, *Trypanosoma cruzi* causes Chagas' disease, and *Trypanosoma gambiense* causes sleeping sickness.

36 **The answer is B** *Central and peripheral nervous system / Neuroanatomy / Areas of the brain*

Although the pathology in many parts of the central nervous system (CNS) can impair problem solving, damage to the frontal lobes is the major cause of dysfunctional intellectual processes. The frontal lobe is the area of the brain that is most involved with the ability to solve problems.

37 **The answer is A** *Central and peripheral nervous system / Pharmacology / Effects of neuroleptic drugs*

Lactation (via the tuberoinfundibular tract) and parkinsonism (via the nigrostriatal tract) are both associated with the effects of neuroleptic drugs on postsynaptic D_2 receptors. Some of the antipsychotic effects are also thought to be mediated by dopaminergic blockade, but the brain tracts involved are believed to be the mesolimbic pathway and possibly the mesocortical pathway. There is little evidence that the nigrostriatal and tuberoinfundibular tracts are important in the direct antipsychotic effects of neuroleptics. However, other neurotransmitter systems are probably involved in the neuroleptic effects. Neither the incertohypothalamic tract nor the medullary periventricular tract projects to the pituitary, so they do not affect lactation.

38 **The answer is D** *Central and peripheral nervous system / Anatomy; neuroscience / Neurotransmitters*

Section of the medial forebrain bundle would destroy many of the axons that connect the catecholaminergic and serotoninergic nuclei of the brain stem with the cerebral cortex. Destruction of the medullary raphe would destroy the serotoninergic neurons of the medulla that project to the spinal cord.

39 **The answer is A** *General principles / Biochemistry / Organs and tissues in the postabsorptive state*

The adipose tissue releases fatty acids, which are used by the heart, skeletal muscle, and liver for fuel. Glycerol, which is taken up by the liver and converted to glucose, is also released by adipose tissue. The liver releases glucose into the blood. The glucose, which is derived from glycogenolysis and gluconeogenesis, is taken up and used for fuel by the brain and skeletal muscle. The skeletal muscle releases lactate, formed from glucose via pyruvate, which is taken up by the liver and used as a substrate for gluconeogenesis.

40 **The answer is E** *General principles / Biochemistry / Organs and tissues in the postabsorptive state*

Celiac sprue is caused by sensitivity to gluten, which is present in wheat, rye, oats, and barley. The active ingredient in gluten is gliadin, a protein enriched in glutamine. The presence of gliadin in the small intestine triggers diffuse enteritis that is characterized by a flattened or scalloped mucosa of normal thickness. Some 90% to 95% of patients express the DQw2 histocompatibility antigen, pointing to a genetic basis for the disease. Celiac sprue can cause diarrhea, fatigue, flatulence, anorexia, weight loss, and amenorrhea as long as gluten is present in the diet.

41 **The answer is E** *Endocrine system / Physiology / Cushing's syndrome*

Signs of Cushing's syndrome are hypertension, impaired glucose tolerance, truncal fat, hirsutism, osteoporosis, abdominal striae, and amenorrhea. The causes of Cushing's syndrome include pituitary tumors, adrenal tumors, ectopic ACTH expression, and exogenous glucocorticoid use. Each of these etiologies results in increased levels of glucocorticoids. High levels of dexamethasone, which can act like cortisol through feedback inhibition to block the release of ACTH, can suppress the ACTH and cortisol release in nearly all pituitary tumors that cause Cushing's syndrome. In Cushing's syndrome caused by an adrenal tumor, the ACTH is kept low by the feedback inhibition of high levels of cortisol; however, ectopic production of ACTH, which is most commonly seen in lung cancer, remains elevated. Addison's disease is characterized by low levels of glucocorticoids. Waterhouse–Friderichsen syndrome is also characterized by adrenocortical insufficiency, and it occurs in the setting of sepsis.

42 **The answer is E** *General principles / Genetics / Myotonic dystrophy*

Myotonic dystrophy is an autosomal dominant disorder that may cause myotonia, distal muscle weakness, and mental retardation. It is an expansion disorder. In an affected person, the causative gene contains a repeated sequence that is present in an abnormally high number. The severity of the disease often worsens in successive generations (genetic anticipation). With myotonic dystrophy, genetic anticipation is much more common in passage from the mother than the father. In fact, a child born to a mother with the disease is at risk for neonatal complications including respiratory distress and floppiness. Previous healthy siblings do not change the risk to the fetus. Because the mother has this autosomal dominant disease, each of her children, male or female, will have a 50% chance of getting the disease.

43 **The answer is C** *General principles / Physiology / Hypoglycemia*

Hypoglycemia can be caused by several mechanisms in nondiabetic patients. Because the hypoglycemia occurs postprandially, insulinoma is unlikely, as insulinoma typically causes fasting hypoglycemia. If someone is taking excess insulin that is causing hypoglycemia (factitious hypoglycemia), the level of insulin will be higher than the level of C-peptide because C-peptide is not included in exogenous preparations of insulin. A reactive cause of hypoglycemia (including alimentary and idiopathic) causes postprandial symptoms. In alimentary hypoglycemia, rapid gastric emptying as a result of surgery or other factors causes excessive insulin secretion with meals. Alcohol, pentamidine, and several other drugs may also cause hypoglycemia. Liver damage can be a cause of hypoglycemia; however, more than 80% of the liver mass must be dysfunctional before the rate of hepatic glucose production is reduced. An oral glucose tolerance test is not required for patients with hypoglycemia and may confuse the issue because the results are not consistent for patients in this setting.

44 **The answer is D** *Musculoskeletal system / Anatomy / Acute gouty arthritis*

Painful and swollen big toe and ankle, after consuming alcohol, are common symptoms of acute gouty arthritis. The metatarsophalangeal joint of the first toe is the joint that is most often affected, whereas the ankle is also frequently involved. This differs somewhat from pseudogout, which is a calcium pyrophosphate dihydrate deposition disease. Pseudogout commonly affects the knee; otherwise, pseudogout is symptomatically similar to gout. Acute gouty arthritis is caused by the accumulation of monosodium urate crystals, a byproduct of purine catabolism. These crystals can be seen under polarized light as negatively birefringent crystals that are bright yellow. Alcohol ingestion and dietary excess of purines can precipitate an attack. Alcohol accelerates the degradation of adenosine triphosphate (ATP). Although chronic gout and tophi may develop in this patient, it usually takes about 10 years after the initial symptoms for tophi to develop. In addition, the initial acute attacks are self-limited, and the symptoms resolve in 3 to 10 days without treatment.

45 **The answer is C** *Central and peripheral nervous system / Neuroanatomy / Surgical treatment for Parkinson's disease*

The globus pallidus interna primarily sends inhibitory signals to the thalamus, and hyperactivity of this structure can lead to the bradykinesia and rigidity characteristic of patients with Parkinson's disease. Ablating inputs into the globus pallidus interna (specifically the stimulatory fibers arising from the subthalamic nucleus) can relieve these symptoms in many patients.

46 **The answer is D** *Central and peripheral nervous system / Anatomy / Eye movement*

The medial longitudinal fasciculus plays an important role in the coordination of eye movements, sending reciprocal projections from the abducens nucleus of one side of the brain to the oculomotor nucleus of the other. The dorsal medullary raphe (serotonin projections), medial lemniscus (primary somatosensory input to the thalamus), lateral geniculate (visual pathway), and reticular formation (sleep–wake state) are not involved in this process.

47 The answer is E *Gastrointestinal system / Physiology; anatomy / Bile*

Bile production by the hepatocytes is continuous and does not require initiation by any hormones. Bile salts are amphipathic, rendering them capable of emulsifying lipids. Bile salts are produced when bile acids are conjugated with taurine or glycine. Recirculation of bile acids from the intestine to the liver (enterohepatic circulation) is an important process that mainly begins in the terminal ileum. The terminal ileum actively transports bile acids out of the intestinal lumen. Most of the bile acids are not redirected until they reach this point, giving the majority of the small intestine exposure to the bile acids.

48 The answer is B *General principles / Biochemistry / Energy storage and transfer*

A high-energy bond is defined as a bond that, when hydrolyzed, releases a sufficient amount of energy to drive the synthesis of ATP from adenosine diphosphate (ADP) and inorganic phosphate (P_i). This requires approximately 7.3 kcal/mol. Two intermediates in glycolysis are high-energy compounds: phosphoenolpyruvate and 1,3-bisphosphoglycerate. In the tricarboxylic acid cycle, the conversion of succinyl coenzyme A to succinate releases enough energy to synthesize guanosine triphosphate from guanosine diphosphate and P_i. In muscle tissue, phosphocreatine is a storage form of high energy. The hydrolysis of phosphate from phosphocreatine is coupled with the synthesis of ATP. A reaction that is exergonic is accompanied by a $\Delta G°$ that is less than 0. The relationship between $\Delta G°$ and K_{eq} is $\Delta G° = -RT \ln K_{eq}$. For a reaction to proceed spontaneously, the K_{eq} must be more than 1 and the $\Delta G°$ must be less than 0.

49 The answer is D *Cardiovascular system / Physiology / Myocardial cells*

Fast fibers like those found in nonnodal atrial or ventricular tissue have a rapid depolarization (*phase 0*) caused by the opening of fast $Na+$ channels, followed by a plateau (*phase 2*) secondary to the opening of slow Ca^{2+} channels. Application of ACh or vagal stimulation decreases the slope of *phase 4* of a slow fiber (or pacemaker cell) that is likely to be found in the sinoatrial or atrioventricular nodal tissue. This is owing to increased permeability to $K+$, and it causes a decrease in heart rate in situ.

50 The answer is B *General principles / Genetics / Inherited disorders*

The form of gene expression may be highly variable, with some family members being severely affected and others having few signs of the disorder. This common feature of autosomal disorders is called variable expression. A nonpenetrant disorder is one in which there is no clinical evidence of a mutant allele in a person known to have inherited the gene. Different mutations of either the same gene (i.e., at the same locus) or different genes may give a similar clinical picture. Consanguineous individuals have a proportion of their genes in common by inheritance from a common ancestor. When a population results from only a small number of individuals (founders' effect), disease alleles may be in higher frequencies, and a particular recessive disorder may be common in that community.

Index

X